Determinants of Health

CHILDREN
AND YOUTH

CANADA HEALTH ACTION: BUILDING ON THE LEGACY
PAPERS COMMISSIONED BY THE NATIONAL FORUM ON HEALTH

Determinants of Health

CHILDREN AND YOUTH

ÉDITIONS
MULTIMONDES

FORUM NATIONAL
SUR LA SANTÉ

NATIONAL FORUM
ON HEALTH

Canadian Cataloguing in Publication Data

Main entry under title:

Canada Health Action: Building on the Legacy

Issued also in French under title: La santé au Canada: un héritage à faire fructifier
To be complete in 5 v.
Includes bibliographical references.
Contents: v. 1. Children and Youth.

ISBN 2-921146-62-2 (set)
ISBN 2-921146-45-2 (v. 1)

1. Public health – Canada. 2. Medicine, Preventive – Canada. 3. Children – Health
and hygiene – Canada. 4. Adulthood – Health and hygiene – Canada. 5. Aged –
Health and hygiene – Canada. I. National Forum on Health (Canada).

RA449.C28 1998   362.1'0971   C97-941659-0

Linguistic Revision: Traduction Tandem
Proofreading: Traduction Tandem and Robert Paré
Cover Design: Gérard Beaudry
Graphics: Emmanuel Gagnon

Volume 1: Children and Youth
ISBN 2-921146-45-2   Cat. No.: H21-126/6-1-1997E
Legal Deposit– Bibliothèque nationale du Québec, 1998
Legal Deposit – National Library of Canada, 1998
© Her Majesty the Queen in Right of Canada, 1998

The series The National Forum on Health can be ordered at this address:
Éditions MultiMondes
930, rue Pouliot
Sainte-Foy (Québec)
G1V 3N9 CANADA
Telephone: (418) 651-3885; toll free in North America: 1 800 840-3029
Fax: (418) 651 6822; toll free in North America: 1 888 303-5931
E-mail: multimondes@multim.com
Internet: http://www.multim.com

Published by Éditions MultiMondes in co-operation with the National Forum on Health, Health
Canada, and Canadian Government Publishing, Public Works and Government Services Canada.

In this publication the masculine form is used solely for ease of readability.

FOREWORD

In October 1994, the Prime Minister of Canada, The Right Honourable Jean Chrétien, launched the National Forum on Health to involve and inform Canadians and to advise the federal government on innovative ways to improve the health system and the health of Canada's people. The Forum was set up as an advisory body with the Prime Minister as Chair, the federal Minister of Health as Vice Chair, and 24 volunteer members who contributed a wide range of knowledge founded on involvement in the health system as professionals, consumers and volunteers.

To fulfil their mandate, the Forum focused on long-term and systemic issues. They saw their task as formulating advice appropriate to the development of national policies, and divided the work into four key areas – Values, Striking a Balance, Determinants of Health, and Evidence-Based Decision Making.

The complete report of the National Forum on Health consists of two volumes:
> *Canada Health Action: Building on the Legacy*
> > The Final Report of the National Forum on Health
> and
> *Canada Health Action: Building on the Legacy*
> > Synthesis Reports and Issues Papers

Copies available from: Publications Distribution Centre, Health Canada Communications, PL. 090124C, Brooke Claxton Building, Tunney's Pasture, Ottawa, Ontario K1A 0K9. Telephone: (613) 954-5995. Fax: (613) 941-5366. *(Aussi disponible en français.)*

The Forum based its recommendations on 42 research papers written by the most eminent specialists in the field. The papers are brought together in a five-volume series:

> VOLUME 1 – CHILDREN AND YOUTH
> VOLUME 2 – ADULTS AND SENIORS
> VOLUME 3 – SETTINGS AND ISSUES
> VOLUME 4 – HEALTH CARE SYSTEMS IN CANADA AND ELSEWHERE
> VOLUME 5 – EVIDENCE AND INFORMATION

Individual volumes or the complete series can be ordered from: Editions MultiMondes, 930, rue Pouliot, Sainte-Foy (Québec) G1V 3N9. Telephone: 1 800 840-3029. Fax: 1 888 303-5931. *(Aussi disponible en français.)*

Values

The Values working group sought to understand the values and principles that Canadians hold about health and health care, so that the system continues to reflect and respond to these values. To explore Canadian core values that are connected to the health care system and to understand the implications for decision making, the group conducted some original public opinion research, using scenarios or short stories which addressed many of the issues being investigated by the other working groups of the Forum. The scenarios were tested in focus groups. Quantitative research supplemented the focus groups making the findings more generalizable. The group also contributed to a review of public opinion research on health and social policy. Finally, a review of Canadian and international experience with ethics bodies was commissioned to identify the contribution that such groups can make to continuing the discusssion of values in decision making.

Striking a Balance

The Striking a Balance working group considered how to allocate society's limited resources to best protect, restore and promote the health of Canadians. Attention was given to the balance of resources within the health sector and other sectors of the economy. The group commissioned a series of papers to assist in their deliberations. They conducted a thorough review of international trends in health expenditures, use of resources, and outcomes. They paid considerable attention to public and private financing issues, health system oganization and federal-provicial transfers. The group produced a separate discussion paper on public and private financing, and a position paper on the Canada Health and Social Transfer.

Determinants of Health

The Determinants of Health working group sought to answer the question: In these times of economic and social hardship, what actions must be taken to allow Canadians to continue to enjoy a long life and, if possible, to increase their health status? The group consulted specialists to assist in identifying appropriate actions on the non-medical determinants of health. Specialists were asked to prepare papers on issues of concern to the health of the population related to the macro-economic environment, the contexts in which people live (i.e. families, schools, work and communities), as well as on issues of concern to people's health at different life stages. Each paper presents a review of the literature, examples of success stories or failures, and relevant policy implications.

Evidence-Based Decision Making

The working group on Evidence-Based Decision Making considered how individually practioners and policy makers can have access to, and utilize the best available evidence in making decisions. The group held two workshops with leading authorities to discuss how health information can be used to support and encourage a culture of evicence-based decision making, and to consider what information Canadians need to be better health care consumers and how to get that information to them. The group commissioned papers to: examine the meaning and concepts of evidence and evidence-based decision making as well as cases that illustrate opportunities for improvement; identify the health information infrastructure needed to support evidence-based decision making; examine tools which support more effective health care decision making; and identify strategies for assisting and increasing the role of Canadians in decision making in health and health care.

Members

William R.C. Blundell, B.A.Sc. (Ont.)
Richard Cashin, LL.B. (Nfld.)
André-Pierre Contandriopoulos, Ph.D. (Que.)
Randy Dickinson (N.B.)
Madeleine Dion Stout, M.A. (Ont.)
Robert G. Evans, Ph.D. (B.C.)
Karen Gainer, LL.B. (Alta.)
Debbie L. Good, C.A. (PEI)
Nuala Kenny, M.D. (N.S.)
Richard Lessard, M.D. (Que.)
Steven Lewis (Sask.)
Gerry M. Lougheed Jr. (Ont.)

Margaret McDonald, R.N. (NWT)
Eric M. Maldoff, LL.B. (Que.)
Louise Nadeau, Ph.D. (Que.)
Tom W. Noseworthy, M.D. (Alta.)
Shanthi Radcliffe, M.A. (Ont.)
Marc Renaud, Ph.D. (Que.)
Judith A. Ritchie, Ph.D. (N.S.)
Noralou P. Roos, Ph.D. (Man.)
Duncan Sinclair, Ph.D. (Ont.)
Lynn Smith, LL.B., Q.C. (B.C.)
Mamoru Watanabe, M.D. (Alta.)
Roberta Way-Clark, M.A. (N.S.)

Secretary and Deputy Minister, Health Canada

Michèle S. Jean

Secretariat Staff

Executive Director
Marie E. Fortier

Joyce Adubofuor
Lori Alma
Rachel Bénard
Kathy Bunka
Barbara Campbell
Marlene Campeau
Carmen Connolly
Lise Corbett
John Dossetor
Kayla Estrin
Rhonda Ferderber
Annie Gauvin
Patricia Giesler
Sylvie Guilbault
Janice Hopkins

Lucie Lacombe
Johanne LeBel
Elizabeth Lynam
Krista Locke
John Marriott
Maryse Pesant
Marcel Saulnier
Liliane Sauvé
Linda St-Amour
Judith St-Pierre
Nancy Swainson
Catherine Swift
Josée Villeneuve
Tim Weir
Lynn Westaff

We extend our sincere thanks to all those who participated in the various production stages of this series of publications.

TABLE OF CONTENTS – VOLUME 1

PREVENTING UNINTENTIONAL INJURIES AMONG CHILDREN 175

Barbara A. Morrongiello

YOUTH

STRATEGIES TO PROMOTE THE OPTIMAL DEVELOPMENT OF CANADA'S YOUTH 235

Benjamin H. Gottlieb

MAKING THE TRANSITION FROM SCHOOL TO EMPLOYMENT 275

Paul Anisef

*YOUTH, SUBSTANCE ABUSE AND THE DETERMINANTS
OF HEALTH*

Pamela C. Fralick and Brian Hyndman

STD AND AIDS PREVENTION AMONG YOUNG PEOPLE

Gaston Godin and Francine Michaud

Children

Enriching the Preschool Experiences of Children

JANE BERTRAND
Professor
George Brown College

SUMMARY

The importance of the early experiences of children on later development has been recognized for a long time. Now, overwhelming evidence illustrates both what experiences make a difference and why they do. Children's early years before formal schooling, establish biological, behavioural and psychological systems that will guide them throughout life. The developmental pathways shaped during the early years can be changed, but over time it becomes increasingly difficult to bring about those changes.

Infants are born with biological structures and systems in place to interpret and interact with the world. Experiences shape how these systems develop. Experiences during the early years are particularly powerful in setting the course of development.

This paper considers ways to enrich the preschool experiences of all children, but especially those from disadvantaged backgrounds, to ensure a real head start in life. First, the paper reviews the key conclusions from the literature related to preschool experiences and the impact of those experiences on the broad determinants of health. Next, the paper examines several initiatives designed to enrich preschool experiences and improve children's long-term positive physical, social and mental health. The paper concludes with a discussion of the policy implications.

Key Conclusions

Socioeconomic status affects child development. Socioeconomic status directly relates to outcomes concerning health and longevity. Even before school entry, socially advantaged groups of children tend to outperform less advantaged groups on measures of cognitive and social competence.

A secure attachment with a nurturing adult is critical to the development of young children. The quality of this relationship is connected to a number of outcomes in later childhood and throughout adulthood. Early attachment relationships set down the pattern for later relationships, emotional and social behaviours, and problem solving.

Research both confirms and explains the biological basis for why early experiences determine competence, health, well-being and coping skills in later life. Brain development, including the number of brain cells and how these cells are connected to form neural pathways, is most active during the first few years. Furthermore, patterns of stress reactivity are set early in life and appear to become integrated into a young child's neural organization. Thus coping strategies established during the preschool years can, and usually do, persist throughout life.

During the early years, children develop central conceptual structures that have broad applications and allow children to take advantage of opportunities and challenges for learning skills and acquiring knowledge. Early experiences can support creation and development of the structures related to numeracy and literacy and consequently affect later school learning.

Social, emotional and cognitive readiness to learn in Grade 1 are strong predictors of later competence, coping, health and well-being. Preschool experiences that directly support skills for success in Grade 1 will increase both child and parental expectations of success.

Stories from the Front Lines

Among the initiatives intended to enrich the preschool experiences of children from birth to school entry, numerous examples document the process and outcomes of the intervention or project. This selection of success stories illustrates various approaches and emphasizes longitudinal results where possible.

Staying on Track, a public health program developed by Dr. Sarah Landy and the Public Health Department of the City of Brockville, Ontario, evaluated its cost-effectiveness. The program, which involved a new method of carrying out early identification and intervention, was available for three and a half years to children under four years of age in Brockville. The findings indicated that the level of functioning of participating children improved substantially compared with those not in the program. Furthermore, the program was able to identify three specific problems: maternal depression, early language delays and difficulties in managing feelings. Sociodemographic factors were not as strong a predictor of child outcomes as the quality of parent-child interactions and parental history, suggesting such a program could take a community-wide or universal approach.

The Victoria Day Care Research Project and the Victoria Day Care Research Follow-up Project documented the daily experiences, quality of care and developmental outcomes (immediate and longitudinal) related to participation in three types of child care—licensed family daycare, informal daycare and licensed daycare centres. The original study and the follow-up were designed to explore the interaction of family, caregiving and child variables on child outcomes. The sample included both at-risk and not at-risk children and families. The original study revealed that children from 'low resource' families (those families headed by single mothers with low levels of education, occupation and income) were overrepresented in low-quality care situations and scored significantly lower on language measures. The follow-up study examined the academic, cognitive and social abilities of the children who participated in the original study, who are now adolescents. There are positive developmental outcomes associated with attendance in community-based, licensed daycare centres during the preschool years.

The Children's Television Workshop was established in the early 1960s to produce Sesame Street, *an intervention designed to help disadvantaged children prepare socially and academically for school. A recent study considers the effects of educational television viewing (primarily* Sesame Street*) on academic skills and school readiness of preschool children from lower-income families, and how they adjust to school. The findings indicate a strong positive relationship between viewing educational television such as* Sesame Street *and school readiness.*

One of the best-known preschool intervention programs is the Perry Preschool Project, a preschool enrichment program offered in Michigan in the 1960s to children from low-income families who were assessed as being at significant risk of failing school. The children who participated in the preschool enrichment program were compared with a control group of children. Follow-up studies 27 years later continue to track the two groups, finding that the group that participated in the program has higher incomes, a lower incidence of criminal activity, and higher levels of formal education. The "treatment" group also experienced fewer teenage pregnancies.

A number of Canadian initiatives currently under way are attempting to enrich the preschool experiences of disadvantaged children. Their intention is to improve readiness for learning on school entry and subsequently to improve long-term outcomes. The initiatives build on the knowledge base and experiences to date, understand the interconnections among children, families and communities, and include strong evaluation (usually longitudinal) designs. They include TVO's Get Ready to Learn; 1, 2, 3, GO! in Montreal; Better Beginnings, Better Futures in Ontario; and the federal government's Community Action Plan for Children projects.

Policy Implications

A variety of preschool experiences within a child's social context can make a long-term difference in the development of health, well-being, competence and coping skills. Many of the factors that affect healthy child development are related to other determinants of health. There is increasing evidence that intervening before the critical transition to school has great potential to positively influence later health and well-being. The question for policymakers is how policies and programs can be organized to best support preschool initiatives.

There is a need to consider interrelationships between the child care needs of families and early childhood education programs while recognizing the political and financial barriers to a comprehensive, public child care system. Attention should be directed at reorganizing the current resources, building community capacity and focusing on parents and caregivers.

Supports to children and their families should be available to all children community-wide. At the same time, programs should be in place that focus on children at increased risk. These focused programs can be delivered within the same operating framework.

The effect of various experiences on children's development can be measured and should be tracked over longer periods. Measuring results and using the information in policy decisions will help to maximize scarce resources.

Socioeconomic status is a persistent factor related to how children do during the preschool years. It is a determinant of health and well-being throughout life. Mechanisms to address the distribution of adequate economic resources to families with preschool children must be addressed as part of any proposal to ensure a real head-start in life for all children.

TABLE OF CONTENTS

KEY CONCLUSIONS FROM THE LITERATURE

Much research examines preschool experiences and the effect of these experiences on child development and other broad determinants of health. The relationship between the experiences of children during their early years and their later developmental outcomes has long been recognized in many different cultural contexts. Recent studies provide strong evidence verifying the relationship. Drawing on findings from a number of disciplines including psychology, biology, education, early intervention, family studies, economics, public health and sociology, we can identify how development progresses during the early years and what kinds of experiences make a difference. We can also identify how much early development may influence later health, competence and coping abilities. This section briefly summarizes the findings and identifies key conclusions that emerge from this body of research. In particular, the discussion of the key research findings emphasizes the establishment of biological, behavioural and psychological systems during the preschool years.

Socioeconomic Status and Child Development Outcomes

A child's socioeconomic status, determined by family income, parental occupations and parental education levels, strongly influences development outcomes from conception on.

Child poverty has serious consequences. Children from poor families are more likely to

- have difficulties at birth (Hanvey et al. 1994),
- die during the first year (Hanvey et al. 1994),
- get sick more often (Hanvey et al. 1994),
- have emotional and behavioural problems (Offord, Boyle, and Racine 1989; Duncan, Brooks-Gunn, and Klebanov 1994), and
- do less well intellectually during their years before school than children from more well-to-do families (Burchinal, Lee, and Ramey 1989; Burchinal et al. 1995; Wright 1983).

Nevertheless, there is debate about how poverty affects child development and what kinds of poverty are more damaging to children (Bolger, Patterson, and Thompson 1995; Dodge, Petit, and Bates 1994; Steinhauer 1995). One American study (Dodge, Petit, and Bates 1994) identified eight factors that seem to mediate the negative effect of low income on behaviour. The factors included harsh discipline, lack of warmth, interactions with aggressive adults, maternal aggressive values, family life stressors, mother's lack of social support, peer group instability and lack of cognitive stimulation. Poverty increases the likelihood that these factors will be present in the child's home (Bolger, Patterson, and Thompson 1995; Dodge et al. 1994). Preschool children in low-income families are more likely to lack stimulating play materials and to have limited opportunities for exploration (Wright 1983; Ross, Shillington, and Lochhead 1994). Children from low-income families are more likely to receive poor-quality nonparental child care (Goelman and Pence 1988). Simply put, poor children seem to get less nurturing and stimulation, the very things that would help to counter the negative effects of poverty.

Researchers have also considered the impact of short-term versus persistent or long-term poverty. A study recently conducted in the United States (Bolger, Patterson, and Thompson 1995) found that children living in chronic poverty experienced more behaviour difficulties than children living in families that had experienced short-term periods of poverty. (As expected, children who did not live in poverty experienced the fewest difficulties.) Duncan, Brooks-Gunn and Klebanov (1994) found behavioural and emotional problems more pronounced for children at age five in chronically poor families.

But the relationship between socioeconomic status and consequences for child development is not just about the negative effect of poverty. Nor would eliminating poverty reduce all difficulties related to emotional and physical health, intellectual functioning, and behaviour.

In a number of areas, where information about child outcomes can be analyzed by income quintile, there is a relationship between higher incomes and healthy child development or how well children do (Ross, Scott, and Kelly 1996). Both infant mortality and low-birthweight rates improve with each income level (Statistics Canada reported in Hanvey et al. 1994). In a study examining children's understanding of numbers, kindergarten children demonstrated different levels of attainment and these differences were related to family socioeconomic status (Griffin, Case, and Siegler 1994). When asked whether 5 or 4 was more, more than 90 percent of the children in the highest income group were able to answer correctly. The percentage of correct answers dropped as the socioeconomic status dropped, with only 15 percent of the lowest income group answering correctly.

In other areas, the data do not exist to examine the differences in child development outcomes beyond poor and nonpoor. Offord (personal communication 1995) suggests "there is a threshold above which additional income confers no advantage on children in terms of emotional and behavioural adjustment, and school performance. This threshold should be somewhere between $25,000 and $35,000 annual family income."

Children who are poor have higher rates of intellectual, emotional and behaviour difficulties but the majority of preschool children who are having difficulty are not poor. While the elimination of poverty could be expected to reduce the incidence of these problems, it is unlikely it would reduce the rate for the nonpoor children. As the Ontario Health Study (Offord, Boyle, and Racine 1989) points out, the chances of a reported behaviour problem are greater for poor children; however, there are, in total, more nonpoor children with difficulties.

Attachment and Relationships with Others

Caring relationships with others are known contributors to health and well-being for all age groups. Attachment refers to a strong, primary connection between two people who care about each other and who act in ways that keep the relationship going. Infant attachment is a close emotional bond between an infant and one or more nurturing adults.

There are many theories and numerous studies about infant attachment. Most often, infants form an attachment relationship with their mother, although many infants will have a close emotional bond with their fathers, other family members and nonfamily members. Studies with monkeys (Harlow and Zimmerman 1959) and with high-risk children (Werner and Smith 1982) show the potential value of an attachment relationship with a nurturing "surrogate" adult who is not a biological parent.

Both temperament and experience affect attachment. Infants with a predisposition toward low stress tolerance who are raised by caregivers (parents and others) who are responsive are likely to be securely attached. But the same infants raised with rigid, less responsive caregivers are more likely to have difficulties developing secure attachment relationships (Kagan, in press). Research studies of child-rearing practices in rhesus monkeys have reached the same conclusions (Suomi 1993). Monkeys with a low stress tolerance that were placed with highly nurturant foster mothers developed secure attachments and had positive later developmental outcomes. However, other monkeys with the same temperament that were raised by punitive foster mother monkeys showed extreme reactions to new situations and stress throughout their lives.

In a longitudinal study following infants into adulthood (Werner and Smith 1982), the most important factor in surviving traumatic and difficult events, including absent, abusive or unresponsive parents, was at least one consistent, trusting relationship with an adult.

Considerable research evidence links secure attachment to social and academic competence and other positive developmental outcomes. Early attachment relationships seem to lay down a pattern for later relationships (Beckwith 1990; Bretherton and Waters 1985; Main 1990). Patterns of communicating and relating to others, interpreting information, problem solving, and emotional expression and behaviour are all influenced by the quality of early attachment relationships (Beckwith 1990; Keating 1993). Other longitudinal studies report that children securely attached as infants had better grades and fewer conflicts with others in primary school (Egeland 1989).

Human infants usually form attachment relationships during the first year of life. Children who do not form attachment relationships during the first year of life may do so in later years, but it is much more difficult to establish this relationship.

The Neural System

Cellular and molecular biologists are learning more about how the nervous system works. Technological innovation has led to more powerful brain-scanning equipment enabling researchers to measure the brain's growth and development and understand how the environment affects what the brain does.

Babies and young children cared for by nurturing adults in a stimulating environment usually do better than children in less optimal situations. Not only do they do better as children, but they are also more competent, better able to cope and healthier as adults. The importance to later life of the experiences in the first few years are well documented and generally accepted. A recent report from the Carnegie Corporation of New York (1994), *Starting Points*, provides an excellent summary of the research findings.

First, brain development during prenatal stages and the first year of life is dramatic (Carnegie Corporation of New York 1994). At conception, life begins as one cell. A full-term newborn baby has a brain and nervous system with more than 100 billion nerve cells or neurons. But they are not yet fully connected with each other. During the first year of life, the brain matures as connections or synapses are formed between the neurons. The part of the neuron that receives information actually branches out to connect with other neurons. The numbers are incredible: each neuron forms up to 15,000 synapses. These connections create pathways or the brain's map for learning.

The brain is very vulnerable to early experience, however (Carnegie Corporation of New York 1994). There are critical periods for the brain development necessary to support some sensory systems. A critical period is the limited and fixed time for a specific developmental process to take place. If the environment is unable to provide the stimulation or input needed during that sensory system's critical period, there can be a permanent disruption in how that sensory system works. For example, studies of reduced visual stimulation during the critical period (a brief period during the first year of life) indicate that full development of the visual cortex in the brain is impeded (Cyander 1994). There is growing evidence that critical or sensitive periods may exist for other brain functions outside of those involved with sensory systems (Cyander 1994; Carnegie Corporation of New York 1994). This strongly suggests that periods of deprivation during the first years of life could impair brain development and reduce cognitive and language capacities.

The environment affects not only the number of brain cells and connections, but also the way they are wired (Carnegie Corporation of New York 1994). A newborn has an oversupply of neurons and synapses. The wiring process establishes pathways between neurons and synapses that are used frequently and eliminates those that are inactive. It shapes competence, coping, health and well-being, and is a complicated interactive process about which scientists still have much to learn. This process is most active during the first years of life but does continue through adolescence. Although genetic programming plays a part in determining neural pathways of the brain, experience through sensory stimulation also seems to be important.

Stress experienced early in life can have negative effects on how the brain develops and functions (Carnegie Corporation of New York 1994). Stress is an event or circumstance that strains or stretches an individual's ability to cope. Stress produces both psychological and physiological reactions. Reactions to stress activate the immune system and the nervous system. The adrenal glands release corticosteroids or stress hormones. Corticosteroids over a prolonged period can weaken the immune system and interfere with memory and learning functions of the brain (Cyander 1994).

For example, it is well established that abuse and neglect experienced in early childhood affect a child's ability to establish relationships. Many studies (reported in Keating 1993) suggest negative interpersonal relationships that involve abuse and neglect may also reduce cognitive flexibility and interfere with immune system functioning. The stress induced by abuse and neglect results in neural changes that affect biological and cognitive functioning.

Early experiences in learning to cope with stress affect the basic biological reactions and establish relatively stable patterns in later years (Keating 1993). Effective coping abilities reduce strain on the immune system and related endocrine system, promoting better health and cognitive functioning.

Research is moving toward the conclusion that experience shapes the brain. Genetics may provide the foundation of potential capacities but it is really the quality and quantity of experiences that determine actual capacities.

Cognitive and Language Competencies

During the preschool years, children acquire basic cognitive and language competencies that influence later abilities and expertise (Keating 1993). Recent investigations suggest that central conceptual structures that facilitate cognitive and language competencies emerge during this period (Case 1992; Volpe et al. 1994). The intellectual functioning of children is reorganized into conceptual structures that are not specific to particular skills such as reading or counting.

The emergence of central conceptual structures are dependent on previous experiences and seem to occur at certain key periods during the preschool years. This is consistent with evidence described earlier in this paper that suggests actual critical or sensitive periods for cortical brain development related to cognitive functions.

The way children acquire language skills supports the idea of a central conceptual structure that develops in response to environmental influences. The ability of children to master the complexity of human verbal communication emerges within the first few years. There is general agreement that a biological predisposition exists. Yet, without environmental experiences and stimulation, language is not acquired or is seriously inhibited.

Numeracy, or a basic understanding of numbers and how to manipulate them, lays down the foundation for later mathematical knowledge and understanding. Recent evidence suggests a general structure termed "a mental counting line" (Case 1992) emerges between 4 to 7 years. This conceptual structure is needed to understand and manipulate numbers. It also seems to be dependent on related experiences. The research is suggesting that if it does not emerge in the early years, it, like later language acquisition, will be more difficult to develop.

Social Context

Attachment, neural development, and acquisition of cognitive and language competencies are important developmental tasks during the preschool period (Keating 1993). There appears to be a period of inherent readiness, sometimes termed a "sensitive period," for experiences to stimulate social, emotional, physical, neurological and cognitive development. "There is consistent evidence, relating to a variety of areas of function, that if appropriate stimulation is missed at a specific time in early childhood, the function can be developed through other forms of stimulation later in life. It may just be harder to do" (Hertzman 1995, 11). The child's social context or environment shapes the experiences he has, directly influencing attachment, neural development and emerging competencies.

The immediate social context of children includes their families and child care settings. Secondary environments that influence the child directly and indirectly include neighbourhoods, workplaces, specialized health and social services, faith organizations, and recreational facilities. Government policies on income redistribution, public services, and equity and social justice may be more removed from children's immediate environments but they too influence other levels of the environment.

Children who experience nurturing and stimulating environments tend to do better in accomplishing the developmental tasks (attachment, neural development, and acquisition of cognitive and language competencies) of the preschool years. Unmet developmental needs predict serious difficulties both during the preschool years and in later development across social, emotional, cognitive and physical domains (Keating 1993; Tremblay and Craig 1994; Offord et al. 1992; Doherty 1995).

Many prevention and intervention initiatives are directed at children identified as "at risk" according to socioeconomic status, family status and parent difficulties. Both family support and early childhood education programs have demonstrated success in reducing the impact of these risks on developmental outcomes (Doherty 1992; Keating 1993; Tremblay and Craig 1994; Volpe et al. 1994). Many of these studies involve relatively small samples, have inherent methodological difficulties and have access to unsustainable demonstration funding. It may be problematic to generalize from the individual findings, but collectively they point in the same direction. Almost unanimously, they report improved short-term outcomes; those that have included a follow-up component report a number of long-term benefits. None of the initiatives report negative outcomes (Tremblay and Craig 1994; Doherty 1992).

But it is not just the at-risk population that needs support. Changes in demographic factors and parental, particularly maternal, labour participation rates, mean that the majority of Canadian families with preschool children require regular nonparental child care arrangements while parents work or attend school (Lero et al. 1992). There is strong evidence that quality child care settings support healthy development outcomes for all children (Doherty 1995; Whitebook, Howes, and Phillips 1990; Clarke-Stewart 1989). On the other hand, poor-quality child care has negative effects that can have a long-term impact on development (Vandell et al. 1988). A review of Canadian, U.S., British and European studies reported consistent findings that poor-quality child care negatively affects social, emotional and cognitive development during the preschool years and in later life (Doherty 1995). The majority of preschool children are not in high- or even adequate-quality child care settings (Lero et al. 1992; Whitebook, Howes, and Philips 1991; Galinsky et al. 1994). Sole-support parents, dual-income parents and parents who are working full time in the home all can benefit from a range of family support programs, regardless of income level.

The quality of nurturing and stimulation available to preschool children is the key determinant of healthy child outcomes (Ontario. Premier's Council on Health, Well-Being and Social Justice 1994; Keating 1993). Both family support and good-quality early child care and education programs contribute to the social context of preschool children. At the same time, these programs cannot remove the effect of neighbourhoods, social services and health care, public policies, income distribution, economic circumstances and social justice.

Transition to School: An Outcome and a Determinant

Successful entry to formal schooling (Grade 1) is both a measurable outcome of development from birth and an important predictor of later academic success and positive social-emotional development (Offord et al. 1992; Tremblay et al. 1992; Alexander and Entwisle 1988; Rutledge 1993).

Children who are successful in Grade 1 are ready, socially and cognitively, to learn. They are able to concentrate, have the necessary social skills to work in a group and solve problems, and see themselves as learners (Ontario. Royal Commission on Learning 1994). They have acquired basic literacy and numeracy during their preschool years (Keating 1993) and have developed the central conceptual structures needed for further learning.

Children who have positive experiences during the first two grades build both their competencies and confidence for continued academic and social success in schools. Of course, the dynamics of the school experience itself can negatively or positively contribute to the child's outcomes in later years, but the initial transition is important (Ontario. Premier's Council on Health, Well-Being and Social Justice 1994). In one U.S. study, the first year of formal schooling (Grade 1) was a significant contributor to school achievement, particularly for ethnic minority children (Alexander and Entwisle 1988).

STORIES FROM THE FRONT LINES

The following four initiatives illustrate a variety of approaches to enriching children's preschool experiences.

Staying on Track

The Staying on Track project was designed, implemented and evaluated to promote the healthy development of all children and their families in the Brockville, Ontario, area (Landy et al. 1993).

Actions on Nonmedical Determinants of Health

The project established and evaluated an early identification, tracking, intervention and referral system for young children in Brockville, and in the Leeds-Grenville counties. Components of the project included setting up and running a community-wide identification and tracking system from birth to 5 1/2 years of age; establishing a database to examine the impact of a number of variables on developmental outcomes at 5 1/2 years; providing counselling and information related to parenting; identifying problems and appropriate interventions; and increasing cooperation among various service providers from health, social services and education sectors. In addition, the project was set up to evaluate the effectiveness of the intervention components and to conduct a cost-benefit analysis of the effectiveness of a tracking and intervention system.

Staying on Track was available for three and a half years (from 1990– 1992) to children under four years of age and their families. Eligible families were those with children born between April 1990 and June 1991, with children 18 months of age (toddler) in 1990, with children 3 1/2 years old (preschooler) in 1990 and with children 5 1/2 years old (control) in 1991.

Public health nurses were trained to use screening and assessment tools to measure self-regulatory behaviour, developmental level, social relationships, and physical characteristics and health. Home visits were arranged for the newborn group; the toddler group's initial contact was at the Public Health Unit. Prekindergarten registration in the school provided the opportunity for the initial visit with the preschool group. Initial visits included the administration of assessment tools and completion of questionnaires, discussion of growth, development and health information, and counselling on issues identified by the parents. Follow-up visits were determined by assessment results with a group or cluster of variables suggesting potential developmental risk, a concern about a child, parent or family identified by the public health nurse, or a concern identified by a parent at any time during the program. If a problem persisted after follow-up by the public health nurse, the family was referred to an appropriate agency or service.

A total of 723 eligible families were contacted to participate in the Staying on Track project. The average participation rate across the different groups was 70 percent. The families who agreed to participate in the program had similar employment status and income levels as other families living in the area. The participants did have a higher educational levels than the local population as a whole.

The interventions significantly improved the outcomes for children in the infant group compared with those not in the program. There was less improvement for the toddler group and no significant effects measured for the preschool group. More than 90 percent of the parents who participated in the program stated that the program should be a regular part of the health care system and 83 percent wanted to continue with the program. The program was able to identify specific problems such as maternal depression, early difficulties in language development and early difficulties in managing feelings, in addition to providing appropriate services or supports.

Staying on Track provided important information about how risk factors, protective factors and pathways mediate developmental outcomes. The findings from the project indicated different variables were more likely to predict outcomes at each of the ages in the study. Parent-child interactions, as well as the mother's own perceptions of her parenting abilities, and the mother's own childhood experiences and her attitude toward her baby were the most predictive variables for the youngest group studied. At 5 1/2 years of age, adjustment to school and to peers were identified as more important variables with a direct impact on the child's development. Overall, socio-economic factors were not as predictive of child outcomes as was the quality of parent-child interactions and parental history, suggesting a community-wide approach for this type of program would be appropriate.

Reasons for the Initiative

Staying on Track was initiated to explore further a cost-efficient model of identifying at-risk populations of very young children and providing early intervention as needed using public health nurses. Although governments and communities recognize the need for health promotion, prevention and early intervention initiatives to improve overall health outcomes, public health units are being reduced and are concentrating on home visits to new mothers. Involvement of public health nurses with infants, young children and their families is becoming more focused on at-risk families. The physical problems of infants are the most common indicators of "at risk" status. Standardized measures are not generally used. Nonphysical determinants of child development outcomes, such as emotional health, behaviour and intellectual functioning, are usually not included.

Players

Staying on Track was a collaboration of front-line service providers (public health nurses, related health and social service providers, and educators), clinical experts and researchers. A community advisory board included representatives of the health, social service and education sectors and consumers of these services. Approximately 600 children and their parents were involved in the project. The project was implemented in 1990 by the Leeds, Grenville and Lanark District Health Unit and Beechgrove Children's Centre.

Dr. Sarah Landy of the C. M. Hincks Treatment Centre and Dr. Ray DeV. Peters of Queen's University were responsible for the research design of the project. Landy selected the initial assessment tools after completing a review of the literature and after consulting with Peters and other experts. Landy and Peters, together with Dr. Brian Allen and Faye Brookes, were the project managers. The public health nurses, including the part-time coordinator, were hired from the Leeds, Grenville and Lanark District Health Unit and were responsible for implementing the program.

The project established a community advisory committee before the program actually began. The responsibilities of the advisory committee included facilitating interagency collaboration, developing strategies for

greater interagency cooperation, monitoring agency and consumer satisfaction, and identifying gaps in service delivery for infants, young children
and their families. The advisory committee included 22 members
representing the health care sector, local school boards and social service
organizations, as well as parents and small business. The final report indicates
that the make-up of the advisory committee contributed to cooperation
and support for this project. However, parents and business were each
represented by one person, and two people are not likely to make a substantial
consumer contribution.

The final report indicates the advisory committee was satisfied that the
program was successful and 90 percent indicated that it should be integrated
into the health care system. Slightly more than 50 percent of the advisory
committee members indicated that interagency collaboration increased.
Although the advisory committee had 22 members, only nine members
appear to have completed the survey questionnaire on satisfaction with the
project.

Analysis of the Results

Overall, the project suggests an innovative approach to improving developmental outcomes for children. By introducing a broader, more systematic
assessment method into the traditional, but disappearing, public health
nurse visits to newborns, the project demonstrated an effective, simple system
for identifying and tracking infants and young children. Data and analysis
suggest several variables that are predictive of later development outcomes,
although they have not been emphasized in the literature on risk and
protective factors. The immediate costs of the program are documented,
but the long-term cost-benefit analysis is difficult to assess without more
longitudinal data.

There is no clear evidence in the report that the project has fostered
collaboration among local early intervention services. This may be explained
simply by the fact that coordination and collaboration among specialized
social service and health agencies was already reasonably effective. Brockville
is a small community with only a few agencies and organizations, which
probably makes coordination easier. There was also a well-established
Children's Services Advisory Group that had effectively coordinated related
services in the area for several years.

The final report does note limitations on the research. First, the 3 1/2
year timespan does not permit full assessment of the interventions over the
5 1/2 year period before school entry. Some of the measures used were
designed specifically for this project and do not have known validity. Service
providers were limited to assessment tools they could use easily in a
community setting. Perhaps most importantly, it is unknown whether
positive outcomes connected to this intervention will, in fact, continue

into the school years and beyond. It is possible to suggest that early interventions into basic parent-child interactions and parenting attitudes will have a lasting effect on parenting abilities and expectations, and, therefore, will positively influence parent-child relationships and child outcomes. Follow-up study would be useful in exploring these issues. Given the small size and relatively stable population of Brockville, it might be feasible to track these children throughout their school years.

The final report suggests that further research could compare this model of intervention with a similar design using paraprofessionals. This raises the question of the level of professional and expert direction in the design and implementation of the project as a whole. The project was directed and implemented by professional service providers and research experts. There is very little indication that the residents who participated in the study or the two community advisory board committee members who represented community interests (parents and business) had input into actual design or implementation of the project.

Replicability of the Initiative

The project recommends tracking, identification and early intervention systems for infants, young children and families in all communities, beginning at birth and continuing until school entry. The recommended system is based on a three-tiered approach including a basic level of support to all children and families, more specialized information for those who have specific problems, and referral to appropriate service agencies for those who are identified as at risk. The recommendations also suggest specific tools for tracking and identifying families that need additional resources.

At present, the Hincks Centre is replicating the work of Staying on Track under the leadership of Dr. Sarah Landy in Jamestown, an inner city area in Toronto. The Hincks Centre is collaborating with the City of Toronto Public Health Department, the Cabbagetown Youth Centre and the Toronto Board of Education.

Funding

In total, the Staying on Track project cost $675,000 over the course of 3 1/2 years. The Premier's Council on Health, Well-Being and Social Justice funded the cost of project design, research and full implementation. The annual cost per child in the program is calculated at $454.

Evaluation

The final report (Landy et al. 1993) describes the evaluation of the early identification, tracking, intervention and referral system established in this project. The variables studied are grouped into four categories: child-related, sociocultural, parent-related and parent-child interactional. Numerous measures were used for each category of variables.

Victoria Day Care Research Project

The Victoria Day Care Research Project was conducted in Victoria, British Columbia, in the early 1980s to examine the effects of three different daycare settings. The focus was on the interaction of family, caregiving and child variables on child language development outcomes (Goelman and Pence 1988). In 1992–1993, the Victoria Day Care Follow-up Research Project contacted families from the original study and collected data on the children's current cognitive, language and academic performance. This is a unique Canadian longitudinal study that follows a nontargeted group of children who attended community-based child care from their preschool years into their school years (Pence 1995).

The results from the two studies are important to considerations of public policy directions because more than 70 percent of Canadian preschool children are regularly placed in nonparental care (Lero et al. 1992).

Actions on Nonmedical Determinants of Health

This particular initiative did not undertake a specific action or intervention but studied the impact of three types of child care, comparing the effects of high and low levels of quality on children and accounting for variation in family characteristics.

The original research study in the early 1980s was one of the first to examine the effects of interaction between parents, children and caregivers. Using an ecological framework, the study revealed interesting relationships.

The follow-up study was designed to explore the longitudinal impact of the initial findings. Ten years later, the original families were contacted and, where possible, the children and their families were interviewed and assessed (Pence 1995). The purpose of the follow-up study was to collect data on child outcomes and trace patterns from the original study. The findings of the follow-up study are not ready for publication but should provide a uniquely Canadian report of the long-term impact of child care of varying quality.

Reasons for the Initiative

Studies on the impact of early childhood education and child care experiences on children's development, particularly those outcomes related to academic performance, have focused primarily on children identified as at risk. At the time of the Victoria Day Care Research Project, most research had focused on either compensatory part-time early childhood education programs or highly resourced child care settings that often operated as laboratory facilities connected to an academic or research institution. The impact of such settings are generally positive (Doherty 1995; Lazer and Darlington 1982), but the costs are high. While arguments justifying the investment based on future cost savings are compelling (Barnett and Escobar 1990; Schweinhart et al. 1993), it is necessary to consider what is possible within current fiscal realities. It is also necessary to recognize part-time, compensatory, early childhood education programs do not provide the child care arrangements needed by parents who are working, attending school or training opportunities.

Most preschool children in the early 1980s, like children today, were not at risk and were participating in child care regularly. Many children at risk, as defined by low income and other family characteristics, are also in regular child care. The focus of this study is on the kinds of "regular" child care arrangements many Canadian children experience. The National Child Care Study (1992) found that unregulated home daycare is the most common (27 percent) form of nonparental care. Licensed home daycare is used by very few (2 percent) families in Canada. Care given by relatives is the second most common arrangement (23 percent) for children under the age of six, and licensed child care is the third most common arrangement (14 percent). Therefore, it is valuable to examine the impact of the child care that is typically available to families.

Another important aspect of this initiative is that it considers the impact of various child care arrangements within an ecological framework that permits examination of the interactions between quality of care and quality of family life. The follow-up study provides valuable information about the subsequent school performance of these children and provides further analysis of the data that suggests relationships between quality of care and later outcomes. Finally, the study was conducted in Canada. U.S. and European longitudinal studies on the impact of child care experiences are useful when considering policy for Canada, but it is better to ensure applicability to the Canadian context.

Actors

In total, 125 children and their families, caregivers and child care establishments participated in the study. The study included 61 boys and 64 girls, and 64 children from lone-parent families and 61 children from two-parent families. All children in the study had been attending their current child care for at least the previous 6 months, they were either the eldest child in their family or only children, and their parents worked or attended school for at least 30 hours each week. Child variables, including age of entry into nonparental child care, and parent variables, including education, income and occupation, were similarly represented in each of the three care arrangement groups.

Fifty-four children were enrolled in licensed community child care programs, 38 in licensed home daycares and 33 in unlicensed home daycares. The licensed daycares were found through local licensing authorities, and unlicensed daycares were found through newspaper advertisements and neighbourhood bulletin boards. Caregivers who wanted to participate approached their clients and, when their parents agreed to participate, children were selected according to the criteria described earlier.

It seems reasonable to assume that caregivers who had volunteered to participate in the program, particularly in unlicensed home daycares, saw themselves as providers of good-quality care.

Analysis of the Results

The Victoria Day Care Research Project set out to examine and compare three different types of child care. The establishments are set up specifically to provide nonparental care for preschool children and, therefore, their overall goals probably include nurturing and stimulating children. The caregivers were the point of initial contact for the study and volunteered to participate.

The results and analysis of the research study produced several interesting findings. First, it did not concur with studies that link higher-quality child care settings with better child language outcomes (Doherty 1995; McCartney 1984). Second, the original findings found greater variation in the quality of family home daycares, both regulated and informal. Children in higher-quality home daycares scored significantly higher than those in the lower-quality home daycares. This finding has been corroborated by more recent studies (Galinsky et al. 1994, Clifford et al. 1993). The activity patterns of children varied with the quality of the home daycare. Children in high-quality home daycares participated in all types of activities (fine motor, gross motor, information and reading) more frequently. Children in low-quality home daycares watched more television, both educational and non-educational, than children in higher-quality home daycares. The quality of regulated home daycares was higher than the quality of unregulated home daycares. Third, family characteristics, such as maternal education, were significant predictors of children's language development in all types of child care.

However, the most compelling finding from this research is the clustering of children from "low resource" families in lower-quality daycare, in contrast to the clustering of children from "high resource" families in higher-quality daycare.

Replicability of the Initiative

The child care establishments used in the study were not developed or implemented for the study. The study used a sample of child care arrangements already in place. It would, therefore, be possible to replicate the study and examine a sample of children, parents and caregivers and their child care arrangements in a specific geographical area. A larger-scale replication of this project would provide further information about the effects of interrelationships between various types of child care in a child's life. Such a study would also help policymakers decide how to promote optimal child care alternatives for all children. Further study would probably continue to confirm the positive impact of high-quality settings and the negative impact of low-quality settings on immediate and longer-term child development outcomes.

Funding

The Social Sciences and Humanities Research Council of Canada provided funding for the original research study. The child care establishments were funded through regular fees for service paid by parents. The child care establishments participating in the study received no additional funding to do so. Parents of children in licensed daycares were eligible for government funding in the form of fee subsidies, subject to criteria in place at the time. Information about fees or the expenses of the child care establishments is not included in the project documentation.

Evaluation

The original research project used a variety of methods to gather information about the child care arrangements, the kinds of daily experiences children had in these arrangements, the attitudes and perceptions of parents and caregivers about each arrangement, and relationships between the children's experiences, family characteristics and child language development outcomes.

The overall quality of the physical setting and program activities of the daycare environments were measured with the Early Childhood Rating Scale (Harms and Clifford 1980) for the centres and the Day Care Home Environment Rating Scale (Harms, Clifford, and Padan Belkin 1983). Both scales are accepted as valid assessment tools in the literature (Doherty 1995). The Child Observation Form (Goelman 1983) was developed for direct observation and recording of children's activities in both home daycares and daycare centres during this research project. Parents and caregivers completed a one-hour structured interview that gathered information about their perceptions of the child care setting. The Peabody Picture Vocabulary

(Dunn 1979) and the Expressive One-Word Picture Vocabulary Test (Gardner 1979) assessed each child's language skills three times during the two-year study. Both tests are widely accepted as valid measures of preschool children's language development.

Sesame Street

The best-known children's educational television show in North America is *Sesame Street*. It would be difficult to find children who are not familiar with its cast and characters. The approaches and style of this television series are probably not only copied in other educational productions and entertainment for children but also influence North American perceptions and expectations of television programming for preschoolers (Bertrand 1994). In the 1960s, *Sesame Street* got its start in the environment that fostered the Head Start Program in the United States and the Canada Assistance Plan in Canada. Based on both ideology and research, efforts such as *Sesame Street* were designed to fight poverty and improve life chances and opportunities for all children. *Sesame Street* runs in Canada today, adapted to Canadian education needs and culture.

The potential of television as both an educational tool and a contributor to aggression, violence and passive, inattentive habits is well documented in the literature (Liebert and Sprafkin 1988; Garbarino 1995). While recognizing the well-documented, negative impact of television on the lives of children, most of this discussion will focus on the impact of *Sesame Street*.

Actions on Nonmedical Determinants of Health

In 1968, the Children's Television Workshop began to produce a television program for disadvantaged preschool children (Liebert and Sprafkin 1988). The daily program was designed to foster intellectual and social development. The curriculum was designed to teach children specific skills, such as letter and numeral recognition, counting and vocabulary expansion, as well as to promote prosocial skills, such as cooperation and willingness to accept ethnic diversity (Liebert and Sprafkin 1988).

A recent review prepared for TVOntario of public television and its effect on children (Volpe et al. 1994) reports that 98 percent of Canadian households have at least one television set and 70 percent of Canadian households have videocassette recorders. It also states that preschool children (between two and six years of age) watch 19 to 22 hours of television a week. Given the prevalence of television in Canadian homes, the rapid expansion of cable systems that offer numerous channels, the availability of VCRs and the amount of time preschool children spend watching television, it is likely that most Canadian preschool children watch *Sesame Street*. The success of *Sesame Street* as popular entertainment is clear. There is also evidence that it helps prepare children to learn.

Reasons for the Initiative

As mentioned earlier, the Children's Television Workshop produced *Sesame Street* as an early intervention for improving the social and academic skills of disadvantaged children and, therefore, helping them succeed at school. The initial program proposal stated that *Sesame Street* would respond to "the national demand that we give the disadvantaged a fair chance in the beginning" (Liebert and Sprafkin 1988, 219).

The producers of *Sesame Street* intended to bring stimulation and opportunities for learning into disadvantaged children's homes through the television to compensate for resources presumed to be available to affluent families. The characters and scenes presented were designed to depict racially, linguistically and culturally diverse role models in constructive, cooperative situations. Conflict resolution, acceptance of differences and a celebration of diversity were and are the common themes of *Sesame Street* episodes, vignettes and songs.

The design of *Sesame Street* was based on the premise that learning is a process that takes place from the outside in and moves from simple to complex. Learning readiness is related to mastering simple patterns, concepts and skills in preparation for more complex concepts. Motivation is perceived as directing attention. Children who are disadvantaged were seen as needing exemplars to teach the skills and attitudes necessary for successful entry to school. Television was a good way to reach all children, regardless of social circumstances (Volpe et al. 1994).

Actors

The Children's Television Workshop, which created *Sesame Street*, was established in 1968, with both private and public funds, to produce a daily program for children. The founding groups financing the initiative included the Carnegie Foundation, the Ford Foundation and various U.S. federal government departments. Like the Head Start initiative, begun in 1966, the Children's Television Workshop was responding to both a growing interest in the potential of early interventions to improve development of children, and popular and political support to end (or at least reduce) poverty. It was supported by some of the same funders, educators and researchers as the Head Start program.

The early design and production of *Sesame Street* brought a high-calibre creative team into contact with child development and preschool education experts (Liebert and Sprafkin 1988). Their task was to produce an entertaining television program that would capture the attention of preschool children and motivate children to watch the program. Lessons to build pre-academic or readiness skills and to model prosocial behaviours were embedded in the show. The series developed around an ensemble of regular characters, including Big Bird, and several Muppets™, including Kermit the Frog, Cookie Monster, Ernie and Bert. An impressive range of entertainment and sports celebrities have appeared as special guests.

More recent views on using television to support learning opportunities for children recognize the importance of children's immediate and broader social context (Volpe et al. 1994; Singer et al. 1993). The inclusion of parents and caregivers in outreach strategies and the recognition of diverse social networks are now incorporated into the development of educational television for preschoolers, but were not part of the original strategy of *Sesame Street*.

Analysis of the Results

In the late 1960s, the creators of *Sesame Street* set out to intervene in the lives of disadvantaged preschool children and provide the stimulation they would need to be ready to learn on entry to school. The goal was to narrow the gap between advantaged and disadvantaged children at school entry.

Initial studies found that disadvantaged children who viewed *Sesame Street* did better, based on academic and social measures, than children who did not (Liebert and Sprafkin 1988). A few years later, studies questioned the extent of that impact (Cook et al. 1975). Twenty years later, studies have again concluded that viewing *Sesame Street* is positively related to school readiness.

The impact of *Sesame Street* on outcomes in later school years or beyond school has not been assessed. It is quite possible that the initial advantage gained from higher skill levels at school entry disappears over time. This would be consistent with research that assessed the impact of Head Start programs on academic performance (McKey et al. 1985). However, the impact of *Sesame Street*, like the impact of early childhood education intervention programs (Lazer and Darlington 1982), may be related to higher expectations of school performance of both children and parents, and consequent behaviour outcomes.

Since its first appearance, *Sesame Street* has been hugely popular with audiences worldwide. It is still going strong after 25 years in continuous production and broadcast. It would be a rare preschooler who has access to television and has not watched *Sesame Street*. The toy market is well supplied with *Sesame Street*–related materials, including dolls, figurines, books, games, audio and video recordings, and interactive CDs, using series characters to motivate attention and the show's methods of instruction to teach skills and concepts. *Sesame Street* is now an integral part of North American mass culture.

The target audience, disadvantaged children, is not the show's only audience. In fact, children in more affluent families probably watch more *Sesame Street* than the target audience (Liebert and Sprafkin 1988; Wright and Huston 1995). Researchers have not yet examined the impact of *Sesame Street* on advantaged preschool children's learning outcomes, but *Sesame Street* may have helped broaden the skill gap for disadvantaged children entering school. At the same time, the virtually universal appeal of *Sesame Street* has earned it a reputation as entertaining, educational television for preschoolers, not as an early intervention program. This may make it attractive in disadvantaged households where viewers would not welcome programming that implied that their poverty made them less likely to succeed in life.

Assessing the impact of *Sesame Street* is inherently complex. It is difficult to control for confounding variables known to affect child outcomes. The most recent study assessing the impact of *Sesame Street* viewing on school performance (Wright and Huston 1995) controls for several family variables but does not control for attendance at a preschool or child care program. It is probably impossible to find a North American control group that is not familiar with *Sesame Street*.

The success of *Sesame Street* may have had other unintended results. *Sesame Street* is produced to meet high technical and aesthetic standards. The style, format and accomplished performances engage young viewers and claim their full attention. The animated vignettes that highlight concepts to be learned punctuate the storyline dialogue among the series characters. This format appeals to young children, perhaps partly because it resembles commercial programming in which the storyline is framed by commercials that target particular products. On the other hand, *Sesame Street* may be merely teaching children to watch television with regular commercials. Are children who grow up watching *Sesame Street* more attentive viewers of commercial television than children who do not grow up watching *Sesame Street*?

Replicability of the Initiative

It is difficult to envision how or why another *Sesame Street* would be created in North America. Other educational programs for children have become popular, and these are frequently seen as complements to *Sesame Street* (Wright and Huston 1995), but none have achieved such extensive popularity or exposure.

In 1996, TVOntario launched Get Ready to Learn, an educational series for preschool children, caregivers and parents that builds on current programming for children. The program design of Get Ready to Learn is influenced by the experiences, evaluations and success of *Sesame Street*. Get Ready to Learn is discussed further in the section New Community Directions.

The Children's Television Workshop has developed other children's programs, including *Electric Company*, directed at reading skills; *3-2-1 Contact*, designed to stimulate interest in science and technology in children 8 to 12 years old; and *Square One TV*, designed to stimulate interest in mathematics in children 8 to 12 years old, (Liebert and Sprafkin 1988). As with *Sesame Street*, the later programs were developed through collaborative effort, involving creative teams, marketing experts, child development experts and educators, to bring about an entertaining presentation of well-designed instruction and sound information.

Perhaps the most valuable lesson from *Sesame Street* lies in its enormous popularity. The size of its regular audience indicates that television is the most effective method for gaining access to preschool children and their parents and caregivers.

Funding

The Children's Television Workshop is a nonprofit organization; it received its initial funding from both private and public organizations. *Sesame Street* received $8 million in development funding (Liebert and Sprafkin 1988), and generates its own operational, research and development funding.

Evaluation

Because *Sesame Street* was designed to be educational, independent evaluation of its effectiveness was built into the initial project (Liebert and Sprafkin 1988). During the first year of production (1969), the Educational Testing Services measured the impact of viewing the show across the United States. This initial evaluation study (Ball and Bogatz 1970; Bogatz and Ball 1971) demonstrated that children who watched *Sesame Street* improved more than nonviewers on the language and numeracy skills targeted by the series. Also, skills and abilities not directly included in the programming, such as reading and printing one's name, improved more among children who viewed *Sesame Street* than among nonviewers. Children who watched *Sesame Street* also had more positive perceptions of and attitudes toward visible minorities, especially African Americans and Hispanics.

A later analysis of the initial evaluations questioned the positive findings (Cook et al. 1975). The effect identified among *Sesame Street* viewers was largely attributed to encouragement from their mothers, rather than the program. The variations in skill acquisition were largely due to rote learning, not improvement in overall ability to think and comprehend.

After the initial summative evaluation of the impact of *Sesame Street* on child outcomes, several short-term studies of curriculum content were made. These largely supported the effectiveness of *Sesame Street* (Wright and Huston 1995).

A recent four-year longitudinal study examined television viewing by low-income children (with a particular focus on *Sesame Street*) and its relationship to later academic skills, school readiness and school adjustment (Wright and Huston 1995). The research findings indicate that, until 5 years of age, there is a strong positive relationship between watching *Sesame Street* and time spent being read to, reading and in other educational activities. For children 2 and 3 years old, *Sesame Street* viewing predicted language skills (letter recognition, vocabulary size), math skills and school readiness as measured by age-appropriate standardized achievement tests. For children in the first two grades of school, preschool regular viewing of *Sesame Street* was a positive predictor of reading comprehension and overall school adjustment, according to teachers' assessment. The research design controlled for other variables, such as parents' education, quality of the home environment and family income.

Perry Preschool Project

The Perry Preschool Project is the most frequently referenced early childhood intervention. It is a longitudinal study on the effects of a preschool education program for children 3 and 4 years old in the early 1960s. The findings, which dramatically endorse the social and financial benefits of early childhood education, find their way into most discussions of the nonmedical determinants of health.

Actions on Nonmedical Determinants of Health

The Perry Preschool program ran from October to June, and included a 2 1/2 hour activity program five mornings a week, and 1 1/2 hour weekly home visits by the children's preschool teachers. Most children attended the program for two years, at 3 and 4 years of age. The trained teachers worked closely with child development and educational experts to develop a cognitive-developmental program based on Piagetian theory of cognitive development (Weikart et al. 1967).

The curriculum that grew out of the preschool program became the foundation for the High/Scope Foundation, which now includes demonstration programs for infant-toddlers, preschoolers and children of school age; preservice and in-service training programs for teachers; the High/Scope Press; and a large educational research facility. It is a multi-million dollar operation producing curricula and multimedia research materials for worldwide distribution.

The Perry Preschool Project was a longitudinal study that tracked the progress of the participants in the original preschool program through the school years and into early adulthood (Schweinhart, Barnes, and Weikart 1993). It found that individuals who attended the Perry Preschool program during the 1960s fared better in high school (academically and socially) and continue to report more positive outcomes as adults (higher earnings, fewer arrests, etc.).

It is important to clarify that Perry Preschool was neither a Head Start project nor a child care program. It was a part-time, early childhood, compensatory-education program with a home visit component.

Reasons for the Initiative

The Perry Preschool program was developed to enrich the lives of disadvantaged preschool children by providing a stimulating educational program and by educating and supporting parents, particularly mothers. It also provided an excellent opportunity to use an experimental design to study the long-term effects of such an initiative.

As stated earlier in this paper, the 1960s in the United States and Canada were marked by attention to poverty and its effects on young children. In the United States, civil rights struggles highlighted the inequities faced by African American children. There was a strong belief that, with "catch-up" support during their preschool years, children would enter school with equal opportunities to succeed (Zigler 1990). The Perry Preschool program, like Head Start and *Sesame Street*, was attempting to provide that catch-up support.

The Perry Preschool Project, on the other hand, was a much smaller, more focused initiative. It began as part of a strong research design and curriculum development project. Measuring the results and developing a practical curriculum that applied Piagetian principles were also important reasons for this initiative.

Actors

The Perry Preschool Project studied 123 children from African American families who lived in the neighbourhood around the Perry Elementary School in Ypsilanti, Michigan (near Detroit), in the 1960s. The children were all assessed as having low IQs and their families as low income (Barnett and Escobar 1990). Approximately 50 percent of the children (58) attended the program; the rest (65) did not attend the program and were the control group.

Every classroom had 8 to 13 children, and two teachers qualified as public school teachers with specific early childhood education and special education training (Barnett and Escobar 1990). The child-centred curriculum, based on Piagetian cognitive development theories, was largely designed by David Weikart, who worked with the classroom teachers in ongoing design, implementation and evaluation.

Analysis of the Results

All interpretations of the results indicate that the Perry Preschool program made a positive impact on outcomes for this group of children, in both the short and the long term. Consistent with findings from other research done on early education intervention programs (Doherty 1992), the children were better prepared for school (academically and socially) and achieved greater school success.

The later findings, which report greater success in adolescence and early adulthood, have not been repeated in other studies (Doherty 1992). First, very few longitudinal studies have included such long-term follow-up. Those studies that have followed participants into adolescence do not find the same level of dramatic difference between those who attended a preschool program and those who did not. This probably reflects the complicated interaction between home, school and neighbourhood, as children move into and through adolescence. The Perry Preschool Project sample was small and very specific, so it is difficult to generalize the findings relating later adolescent and adult positive experiences to the preschool program without corroboration from other research findings.

Perhaps the most compelling aspect of the Perry Preschool Project is its elaborate cost-benefit analysis. The projected savings from reduced expenditures in social services, education and justice were factored into the costing. Although the program itself was well resourced and quite expensive compared with regular community-based preschool programs, the overall estimated savings were enormous. The researchers reported that the bottom line was a $1 expenditure in preschool programming could save $7 in later special education, social services, justice and remediation costs (Schweinhart, Barnes, and Weikart 1993).

The Perry Preschool Project results can be interpreted to emphasize the positive impact of two years' preschool programming, including: higher high school graduation rates, lower teenage pregnancy rates, higher incomes, fewer arrests and less dependence on social assistance. However, it is also evident that the children who attended the preschool grew up to achieve far less than comparable children in more affluent families (Hertzman 1995).

Another consideration is the involvement of the program designers and managers in the evaluation process. As with *Staying on Track*, although appropriate research protocols are reported, the potential for conflict of interest or bias in the research methodology must be acknowledged.

Replicability of the Initiative

In Canada, Wright (1983) implemented a preschool compensatory program at the University of Western Ontario at London, Ontario. The curriculum resembled the cognitive-oriented program developed for the Perry Preschool.

The program was half-day in duration and included children from both low-income and higher-income families. The children who attended for two years were compared with children who attended the program for only one year, and the low-income children were followed into kindergarten and compared with children who did not attend the preschool program.

Several problems arose with the methodology of the program. Comparatively few low-income children attended the program, which was located on a university campus rather than in a low-income community. Also, the follow-up data were weakened by substantial attrition in the sample. Nevertheless, although they are less dramatic than the Perry Preschool Project findings, the findings of the London study suggest that the compensatory preschool education program had positive effects on the intellectual abilities and language skills of children in low-income families. However, Canadian reviews of compensatory preschool education have raised concerns about the applicability of the Perry Preschool experience, based on 123 low-income, African American children in the early 1960s living near Detroit, to Canada in the 1990s (Wright 1983; Ontario. Ministry of Community and Social Services 1989).

Funding

The Perry Preschool Project originally received funding for the operation and research components of the project from charitable foundations. The cost of the half-day preschool program would have exceeded the average cost of a nursery school program at the time.

Research follow-up continues with the support of the High/Scope Research Foundation, which supports itself through publishing and offering extensive training services.

Evaluation

The Perry Preschool was a small, half-day program that operated for only five years. Almost 30 years since it closed, policymakers, advocates and researchers still frequently cite data from it as evidence of the benefits of preschool programs.

The experimental research design of the Perry Preschool Project contributed significantly to its overall credibility. Unlike most educational and psychological research involving children, the Perry Preschool Project assigned children randomly to the experimental group, which attended the preschool program, and a control group, which did not. Attrition over almost 30 years has been remarkably low—99 of the original 123 children participated in the follow-up.

The Perry Preschool Project also indicates the power of longitudinal data (Zigler and Styfco 1994). The evaluation has followed graduates for more than 25 years and continues to monitor outcomes. There is a lack of longitudinal evaluation monitoring long-term impact of early childhood experiences.

Canadian Community-Based Initiatives

In Canada, many practitioners and researchers are developing and implementing approaches to support healthy development outcomes for preschool children, adopting an ecological model that recognizes the interactions between the immediate and more distant environments of preschool children. A few of these initiatives are summarized here; results are not yet available but the outlook is promising.

Get Ready to Learn

TVOntario (TVO) is a public broadcaster licensed as the Ontario Educational Communications Authority. TVO has spearheaded Get Ready to Learn to enrich the learning environment of preschool children. Get Ready to Learn is a project bringing together educational programming for children with strategies to support parents and caregivers in their ability to care for and educate young children. Most preschool children have access to television and are in informal daycare or at home with a parent on a regular basis. Many do not have optimal stimulation in these environments (Volpe et al. 1994).

Educational programming for preschoolers, such as *Sesame Street,* is designed to foster cognitive and linguistic skills for later use at school. Get Ready To Learn is designed to promote health in the environment of preschool children by enhancing resources, supporting parents and caregivers, and building on the community's capacity to create opportunities. To accomplish this goal, TVO intends to bring together the potential of both broadcast and nonbroadcast technology for parents, other caregivers and the community.

TVO contracted with child development and educational experts to review the literature on early childhood education, intervention and the role of public television (Volpe et al. 1994). The Get Ready to Learn project has built partnerships with various stakeholder groups involved with Ontario families, children and caregivers. The extensive advisory committee includes representation from service providers (from early childhood services including child care centres, family home child care and family resource centres), educators and trainers, professional organizations representing early childhood educators and teachers, and government agencies representing children, families, communities, health, social services and education. Community outreach strategies include sessions to permit parents and caregivers to express their views and needs in getting children ready to learn.

Information gathered in such sessions will be used in developing on-air programming and interactive, nonbroadcast, programming strategies for reaching adult caregivers. Parents, caregivers and local agencies will develop ways to reach parents and caregivers who do not respond to initial efforts. The project also includes monitoring its effects on children.

Better Beginnings, Better Futures Project

The Better Beginnings, Better Futures Project is a demonstration and longitudinal research project in Ontario (Peters and Russell 1994). It is funded by the Ontario ministries of Health, Education and Social Services and the federal departments of Indian and Northern Affairs and Canadian Heritage. The project funds 12 communities to provide services designed to meet local needs and preferences. After an initial program planning and development year, four years of operations will be funded. The research will track the progress of children, their families and their communities for 20 years.

The Better Beginnings model is based on research on prevention programs and a key informant survey of Canadian prevention programs. The model combines what is known about effective home visits to mothers with newborns, child care, and ecological primary school programs with community development and integration of services.

The extensive, multisite comparative research is led by a multidisciplinary consortium of researchers. The focus is on children up to eight years of age who live in 12 disadvantaged communities in Ontario. The communities selected all agreed to provide for meaningful, significant involvement of residents in decision making, and to create, integrate and enhance local services.

The project is now in its third year of full program implementation. Outcome data will not be available for several years but, in the interim, changes are occurring. At least 50 percent of all committee and subcommittee members are parents and community leaders working with service providers and educators. Committee members wrote the job descriptions, hired staff and made funding decisions. Increased control over services and education led to stronger self-evaluation and community evaluation. Parents and community leaders are now more confident and optimistic about their capacity to foster child development.

1, 2, 3, GO!

The community mobilization project 1, 2, 3, GO! is located in six low-income Montreal neighbourhoods. It is designed to improve developmental outcomes for children up to the age of 3. The project brings together the community's financial, human and material resources to support activities for the children and their families.

The evaluation component will include measures of child outcomes (cognitive and social) and documentation of successful strategies in mobilizing community support (Bouchard 1995).

POLICY IMPLICATIONS

Methods for enriching the lives of disadvantaged preschool children in Canada must appreciate that children are part of immediate and extended families, and that families are part of neighbourhoods and cultural communities. Children and their families are influenced by work environments, health care services, social services, information and entertainment media, schools and recreation facilities. Children, families and their environment, in turn, are affected by governments, business, legislation and broader issues of social justice.

In time, these environments and systems are influenced by what happens to children during their preschool years. A good start in the preschool years does not guarantee success or immunize children against later difficulties, but it does seem to set children on the path to improved chances for health, happiness, competence and coping abilities in later childhood, adolescence and adulthood. The Canadian workforce and Canadian society need skilled people who can adapt to change and continue to learn. Such citizens begin with investment in children, their families and their communities.

An approach that recognizes the interconnections between the immediate and more distant environments of children is useful, and much is already known or strongly suspected about enriching preschool experiences.

Family Support, Child Care and Early Childhood Education

High-quality early childhood education fosters language development, social skills and cognitive abilities. At the same time, working parents need high-quality child care to help them meet their child-rearing responsibilities. It does not make sense to separate child care and early childhood education needs and experiences for children. Good child care and good early childhood education happen together. Good child care and early childhood education programs are, implicitly, family support programs, and many include specific, explicit efforts directed at parents and other family members. Other services that are viewed primarily as family support include interventions and information that provides or contributes to child care and early childhood education.

Nevertheless, Canadian policies and programs related to child care and early childhood education often separate family support, child care and early childhood education. For example, national child care policy, research and funding for child care programs are responsibilities of Human Resources Development Canada. At the same time, Health Canada is responsible for several programs and initiatives related to early childhood education and family support.

Currently, significant financial and political issues are hindering the establishment of a comprehensive child care and early childhood education program, including family support initiatives, in Canada. However, there is still no justification for maintaining the status quo; the evidence of immediate and long-term benefits is too convincing. We propose three guidelines for action in this area.

Begin with what exists – Parents may receive child-rearing support from family members, informal neighbourhood networks, home-visiting programs, health care professionals, participation in early childhood programs with their children, parenting courses or groups, family resource centres, television, electronic communication or print materials. Child-rearing skills are not instinctive—the capacity to nurture may be inherent, but the skill required to care for and guide an infant through to adulthood must be learned, and is influenced by social context.

The vast majority of Canadian children experience a combination of parental and nonparental care during their preschool years. The combined quality of that care makes a big difference to their immediate and long-term development. Nonparental arrangements range from in-home care to regulated or unregulated home daycare, to licensed child care to kindergarten. Arrangements may be occasional, part time or full time. From the child's point of view, all nonparental care arrangements contribute to learning and development, although the contribution may not always be positive.

The range of family supports and early childhood services currently available is neither adequate nor equitable. Some families have real options because of their socioeconomic circumstances, resourcefulness or geographic location. Others are left to piece together mediocre or inferior care arrangements for their preschool children. Many have almost no family supports.

Nevertheless, the range of family supports and early childhood services currently available is the starting point. Recognition and acceptance of the true range of options is essential to expanding and extending both the quality and quantity of Canada's early childhood services and family supports.

Remove legislative, bureaucratic and funding barriers to early childhood services – Many ways and means for enriching preschool experiences are not mutually exclusive and can work together to improve children's life chances. For example, preschool initiatives and the school system must collaborate. Schools are the community's focal points for children. However, collaboration must respect family and community values, preferences and needs. It must involve cooperative problem solving, intersectoral partnerships, and sharing of resources and decision making, rather than appropriation of available programs and services.

Canadian policies and programs related to early childhood services often separate family support, child care and early childhood education. As mentioned above, national child care policy, research and funding programs for child care are responsibilities of Human Resources Development Canada. However, the Child Care Expense Deduction, a taxation measure, is administered by Revenue Canada—Taxation, and Health Canada is responsible for several programs and initiatives related to early intervention programs and family support. When the federal government separated child care funding from funding for family support and early intervention, it created a new barrier.

Communities can come together to support families and young children – Communities have the human and financial capacities to find innovative, flexible, effective ways to care for and educate preschool children and to support families in their child-rearing responsibilities (Garbarino 1995; Healthy Child Development Project 1995). No solution is universal, and community-level players are most likely to respond appropriately to local needs.

Employers can promote family-friendly work policies that allow parents to participate in their children's early education or take time to care for their children when they are sick. Schools can work with other community partners and with parents to develop after-school care and activities, and preschool programs. In some communities, adjusting school hours could help parents juggle their work schedules and help community agencies provide out-of-school programming.

Effective community solutions need the support of financial, legislative and bureaucratic practices at all levels of government. They will be damaged, if not destroyed, by governments that off-load social responsibilities.

Focus on parents and caregivers – Policy efforts related to early childhood care and education programs, including family support initiatives, must focus on parents and caregivers. Quality of parental and nonparental care is a determinant of healthy child development during the preschool years (Ontario. Premier's Council on Health, Well-Being and Social Justice 1994). The skills and abilities of parents and caregivers are the most important factors in determining the quality of care (Doherty 1995; Keating 1993; Volpe et al. 1994) The results of specific preschool programs are related to complex *interactions* between skills, interests, information, opportunities, challenges, expectations and relationships. The social experiences of preschool children are directly linked to their families. Neighbourhoods, communities, workplaces, social services, health care and public policies influence the development of preschool children through their families. Culture, gender, social class and diverse individual characteristics present both challenges and opportunities for preschool and later school experiences. Initiatives for enriching the preschool experiences of disadvantaged children must adapt to and respect diversity.

Early childhood education practices and parenting practices should reflect the growing understanding of conceptual structures that emerge during the preschool years. They should focus on changing relationships and expectations, and developing social and academic skills required for success in primary school.

Universal and Specific Programs

Programs intended for specific economic or cultural groups are problematic. Because they identify a group as needing special support, they can stigmatize that group. The negative effects of stigmatization tend to interfere with outcomes. Furthermore, strict set criteria are just as likely to exclude children who can benefit from the program as they are to exclude children who do not need the program. As discussed earlier in this paper, many children are in trouble and at risk although their families are not disadvantaged (Keating 1993; Offord et al. 1992; Vandell et al. 1988).

At the same time, universal programs designed to provide equal opportunity, such as the public school system, have failed for many (Keating 1993). Equal opportunity to participate gets everyone in the door, but some need more support to attain equitable outcomes (Offord, personal communication 1995). Both research and front-line experience suggest that a community-wide access approach, with additional support for families that need it, is the best way to ensure equitable benefits. Universality means all children and their families have equal access to family supports and early childhood services, and those who are disadvantaged or at risk receive the additional resources they need to ensure equitable outcomes.

Cost is the main argument against universal approaches. However, equal access and equitable outcomes do not exclude user fees. High-quality early childhood services require broad public support, but it is quite reasonable to assume that much of the costs will be assumed by individual families. Also, public expenditure on preschool children is a long-term investment, not a consumption expense (Mustard 1996). In less than 20 years, the Canadian workforce will begin to shrink as the baby boom generation begins to retire. Canadian productivity depends on skilled, competent workers who can sustain a growing elderly population. Even increased immigration will not make this possible if large numbers of young adults are not prepared socially and cognitively to participate in a knowledge-based economy and live in culturally diverse communities (Keating 1993; Mustard 1996). Finally, ample evidence demonstrates that failure to invest in preschool children increases remediation costs through the educational, health, social service and justice systems in later years (Mustard and Keating 1993; Offord et al. 1992; Schweinhart et al. 1993; Tremblay and Craig 1994). These represent consumption spending to repair available damage. In the absence of strong investment in preschool years, these expensive services are overwhelmed and unable to help those in greatest need.

A commitment to invest in children's early years carries cost implications. Careful accounting of all current spending on related programs, benefits and services is needed. The next section of this paper discusses the importance of measuring results and allocating resources accordingly.

Canada's financial situation should improve over the next decade. There will still be competition for resources, including calls for tax cuts and for better benefits and tax considerations for Canada's aging population. Investment in early childhood services and family supports will be possible only with heightened awareness of the importance of such investments, both now and in the future.

Measuring the Results

Decisions are made about public policies and government spending on programs related to preschool children and their families with surprisingly little information on the results that can be expected. Also, little data on impacts is collected.

As governments and communities must examine their spending carefully, how children are doing and what makes a real difference to outcomes is critical information. Information is needed at national, provincial and local levels, and should include both measures of child outcomes and of the primary environments in which children live. Three current initiatives are producing data on how children are doing: the *National Longitudinal Study of Children* (Human Resources Development Canada, Statistics Canada), the *Progress of Canada's Children* (Centre for International Statistics) and *Achievements and Well-Being of Children and Youth* (Ontario. Premier's Council on Health, Well-Being and Social Justice).

The *National Longitudinal Survey of Children* demonstrates how children's development is influenced by life experiences, individual characteristics, and family, household and community environments over time. The survey will produce national data to indicate how children are doing and where to proceed with policies and programs. The future of the survey is currently under review (SPR Associates 1996).

The *Progress of Canada's Children* is an annual report that pulls together various aspects of child and family well-being, including environmental indicators and progress indicators. Data for the report is collected by the *National Longitudinal Survey of Children* and other sources. Its format resembles that of the UNICEF publication, *The Progress of Nations*.

Achievement and Well-Being of Children and Youth is a reporting tool for communities to use for collecting precise data about their children and youth. Data collection questionnaires are in the final stages of development (Offord, personal communication 1995).

These three initiatives are important contributions to social reporting and decision making. They will complement each other and help decision makers at all levels understand how best to organize resources for children and youth, including preschool children, and how to promote better outcomes for all. Public financial support will be needed to continue current work.

Large Canadian longitudinal studies are needed to determine whether small-scale prevention and intervention strategies studied elsewhere can work for the general Canadian population. Such research will show governments and communities what combinations of family supports and early childhood services are most effective (Offord, personal communication 1995; Tremblay and Craig 1994). The initiatives discussed earlier (now under way across Canada) are an excellent start in this direction.

Social and Economic Public Policies

The literature reporting interventions to enrich the lives of disadvantaged preschool children and the results of the projects reported here concur with Edward Zigler's statement that:

> The ecological model has clear implications that we not oversell what we can realistically accomplish with current early intervention programs. In many instances these programs simply cannot change enough of the ecology or the larger environment to make a real difference in the lives of families. The problems of many families will not be solved by early intervention efforts, but only by changes in the basic features of the infrastructure of our society. No amount of counselling, early childhood curricula, or home visits will take the place of jobs that provide decent incomes, affordable housing, appropriate health care, optimal family configurations, or integrated neighbourhoods where children encounter positive role models (Zigler 1990, xiii).

Reducing child poverty in Canada would not give all children the head start they need, but it would make a big difference. Societies in which the gap between the wealthiest and poorest citizens is narrow have fewer gradient effects on several outcomes, including those related to child development (Mustard and Keating 1993).

Changing the economic circumstances of low-income families with preschool children is one important step in reducing the gap between higher-income and lower-income Canadian families and in reducing child poverty. Low family incomes can be raised in two ways: higher income transfers or higher wages. A combination of these strategies would best serve the needs of disadvantaged preschool children.

Lone mothers with preschool children are less likely to work outside the home than mothers in two-parent families. The Canadian National Child Care Study found only 35.6 percent of lone mothers with preschool children work outside the home, compared with 47.3 percent of mothers in two-parent families (Lero et al. 1992). Lone mothers are more likely to work outside the home if they can get adequate child care. Their child care decisions are particularly sensitive to cost (Cleveland and Hyatt 1996). An expansion of family support and early childhood services, building on currently available services, will require increases, not reductions, in public spending. However, some of these investment costs will be offset by increased employment rates and income levels of lone mothers with preschool children. As well, public assistance payments should decrease.

The Child Benefit Tax Credit geared to family income effectively transfers income to families with children. An increase in this benefit could reduce the gap between higher-income and lower-income families, and address the problem of falling incomes among young families with preschool children. It reaches both families that receive social assistance and families with low-wage breadwinners. An expanded Child Benefit Tax Credit could also provide a more substantial bridge for parents who want to work outside the home but need assistance until their earnings rise.

SUMMARY OF POLICY IMPLICATIONS

Research findings and front-line experience discussed in this paper indicate several policy directions:

Early childhood services – Recognize all currently available forms of early childhood education, child care, early intervention and family support initiatives. Remove legislative, funding and bureaucratic barriers to service. Build on and support community-based efforts. Focus on improving the skills and abilities of parents and caregivers.

Community-wide access – Ensure that all children have access to early childhood services. Some children and their families will need additional support or services to be able to participate fully.

Monitor the health and well-being of children – Support complementary initiatives such as the *National Longitudinal Survey of Children*, the *Progress of Canada's Children* annual report and the *Achievement and Well-Being of Children and Youth* community survey.

Ensure that public and economic policies address child poverty – Ensure that child care is an early childhood service accessible to job seekers, particularly lone mothers. Expand the Child Benefit Tax Credit program to provide a bridge between social assistance and employment income.

> Investment in early childhood is an investment in our productivity. The relationship between the quality of nurturing and adequacy of nutrition in early childhood and health risks in later life has implications not only for health policies, but for policies concerning the competence and coping skills of the population—for the human capital. Fraser Mustard 1996

Jane Bertrand *is a faculty member in the Early Childhood Education Program at George Brown College and has studied child development and early education methodology at the Ontario Institute of Studies in Education. She has participated in a number of policy development initiatives related to early childhood services to young children and their families. She is a strong advocate of expanded child care and family support programs.*

BIBLIOGRAPHY

ALEXANDER, K. L., and ENTWISLE, D. R. 1988. Achievement in the first two years of school: Patterns and processes. *Monographs of the Society for Research on Child Development* 53 (2, serial no. 218).

BALL, S., and BOGATZ, G. A. 1970. *The First Year of Sesame Street: An Evaluation*. Princeton (NJ): Educational Testing Service.

BARNETT, W., and ESCOBAR, C. 1990. Economic costs and benefits of early intervention. *Handbook of Early Childhood Interventions*, eds. S. MEISELS, and J. SHONKOFF. New York: Cambridge University Press.

BECKWITH, L. 1990. Adaptive and maladaptive parenting—Implications for intervention. In *Handbook of Early Childhood Intervention*, eds. S. MEISELS, and J. SHONKOFF. New York: Cambridge University Press.

BERTRAND, J. 1994. Caring for the children. *Putting the Pieces Together: A Childcare Agenda for the '90s*. Toronto: Ontario Coalition for Better Child Care.

BOLGER, K., PATTERSON, C., and THOMPSON, W. 1995. Psychosocial adjustment among children experiencing persistent and intermittent family economic hardship. *Child Development* 66: 1107–1129.

BOGATZ, G. A., and BALL, S. 1971. *The Second Year of Sesame Street: A Continuing Evaluation*. Princeton (NJ): Educational Testing Service.

BOUCHARD, C. 1995. *The Case for 1, 2, 3, GO!* Montreal: 1, 2, 3, GO!

BRETHERTON, I., and WATERS, E. Eds. 1985. *Growing Points of Attachment Theory and Research*. Chicago: University of Chicago.

BURCHINAL, M., LEE, M., and RAMEY, C. 1989. Type of day-care and preschool intellectual development in disadvantaged children. *Child Development* 60: 128–137.

BURCHINAL, M., RAMEY, S., REID, M., and JACCARD, J. 1995. Early child care experiences and their association with family and child characteristics during middle childhood. *Early Childhood Research Quarterly* 10: 33–61.

CARNEGIE CORPORATION OF NEW YORK. 1994. *Starting Points: Meeting the Needs of Our Youngest Children*. New York: Carnegie Corporation of New York.

CASE, R. 1992. *The Mind's Staircase: Exploring the Conceptual Underpinnings of Children's Thought and Knowledge*. Hillsdale (NJ): L. E. Erlbaum.

CENTRE FOR INTERNATIONAL STATISTICS. 1995. *The Progress of Canada's Children*. Ottawa: Centre for International Statistics.

CLARKE-STEWART, K. A. 1987. Predicting child development from child care forms and features: The Chicago study. In *Quality Child Care: What Does the Research Tell Us?*, ed. D. PHILLIPS. Washington (DC): National Association for the Education of Young Children, pp. 21–41.

CLEVELAND, G., and HYATT, D. 1996. On the edge: Single mothers' employment and child care arrangements for young children. *Canadian Journal of Research in Early Childhood Education* 5(1):13–25.

CLIFFORD, R., HARMS, T., PEPPER, S., and STUART, B. 1993. Assessing quality in family day care. In *Family Day Care: Current Research for Informed Family Policy*, eds. D. PETERS and A. PENCE. New York: Teachers College Press.

COOK, T. D., APPLETON, H., CONNER, R. F., SHAFFER, A., TAMKIN, G., and WEBER, S. J. 1975. *Sesame Street Revisited*. New York: Russell Sage.

CYANDER, M. 1994. Mechanisms of brain development. *Daedalus, Journal of the American Academy of Arts and Sciences*, fall 1994.

DODGE, K., PETIT, G., and BATES, J. 1994. Socialization mediators of the relation between socioeconomic status and child conduct problems. *Child Development* 65(2): 649–665.

DOHERTY, G. 1992. *Addressing the Issue of the Lack of School Readiness in Preschoolers.* A paper prepared for the Prosperity Steering Group. Ottawa: Prosperity Initiative, Government of Canada.

DOHERTY, G. 1995. *Quality Matters: Excellence in Early Childhood Programs.* Toronto: Addison-Wesley Publishers.

DOHERTY, G. 1996. *The Great Child Care Debate: The Long-Term Effects of Non-Parental Childcare.* Occasional Paper no. 7. Toronto: Childcare Resource and Research Unit, University of Toronto.

DUNCAN, G. J., BROOKS-GUNN, J., and KLEBANOV, P. K. 1994. Economic deprivation and early childhood development. *Child Development* 65: 296–318.

DUNN, L. M. 1979. *Peabody Picture Vocabulary Test* (revised). Circle Pines (MN): American Guidance Service.

EGELAND, B. 1989. *Secure Attachment in Infancy and Competence in the Third Grade.* Paper presented at the American Association for the Advancement of Science, San Francisco. January 1989.

GALINSKY, E., HOWES, C., KONTOS, S., and SHINN, M. 1994. *The Study of Children in Family Child Care and Relative Care.* New York: Families and Work Institute.

GARBARINO, J. 1995. *Raising Children in a Socially Toxic Environment.* San Francisco: Jossey-Bass, Inc. Publishers.

GARDNER, M. F. 1979. *Expressive One-Word Picture Vocabulary Test.* Novato (CA): Academy Therapy Publications.

GOELMAN, H. 1983. *Manual for Child Observations in the Victoria Day Care Project.* Unpublished manuscript. Vancouver: University of British Columbia.

GOELMAN, H., and PENCE, A. 1988. Children in three types of child care: Daily experiences, quality of care and developmental outcomes. *Early Childhood Development and Care* 33: 67–76.

GRIFFIN, S., CASE, R., and SIEGLER, R. S. 1994. Rightstart: Providing the central conceptual prerequisites for first formal learning of arithmetic to students at risk for school failure. In *Classroom Lessons: Integrating Cognitive Theory and Classroom Practice*, ed. K. MCGILLY. Cambridge (MA): MIT Press/Bradford Books.

HANVEY, L., AVARD, D., GRAHAM, I., UNDERWOOD, K., CAMPBELL, J., KELLY, C., and GALLANT, L. 1994. *The Health of Canada's Children: A CICH Profile.* Ottawa: CICH.

HARLOW, H., and ZIMMERMAN, R. 1959. Affectional responses in the infant monkey. *Science* 103: 421–432.

HARMS, T., and CLIFFORD, R. 1980. *The Early Childhood Environment Rating Scale.* New York: Teachers College Press.

HARMS, T., CLIFFORD, R., and PADAN BELKIN, E. 1983. *The Day Care Home Environment Rating Scale.* Chapel Hill (NC): Homebased Day Care Training Project.

HEALTHY CHILD DEVELOPMENT PROJECT. 1995. *Healthy Children: Healthy Communities: A Compendium of Approaches from across Canada.* Ottawa: Healthy Child Development Project.

HERTZMAN, C. 1995. *Child Development and Long-Term Outcomes: A Population Health Perspective and Summary of Successful Interventions.* CIAR Programs in Human Development and Population Health. Working Paper no. 4.

KAGAN, J. In press. Biology and the child. *Handbook of Child Psychology.* Cambridge (MA): Harvard University Press.

KEATING, D. 1993. *Developmental Determinants of Health and Well-Being in Children and Youth.* Working paper. Toronto: Premier's Council on Health, Well-Being and Social Justice.

LANDY, S., PETERS, R. DeV., ALLEN A. B., BROOKS, F., and JEWELL, S. 1993. *Staying on Track: An Early Identification, Tracking, Intervention and Referral System for Infants, Young Children and Their Families.* Toronto: Premier's Council on Health, Well-Being and Social Justice.

LAZER, I., and DARLINGTON, R. 1982. *Lasting Effects of Education: A Report from the Consortium for Longitudinal Studies.* Monographs of the Society for Research in Child Development, 47 (serial no. 195): pp. 2–5.

LERO, D., GOELMAN, H., PENCE, A., BROCKMAN, L., and NUTALL, S. 1992. *The Canadian National Child Care Study: Parental Work Patterns and Child Care Needs.* Ottawa: Statistics Canada—Catalogue 89–529E.

LIEBERT, R., and SPRAFKIN, J. 1988. *The Early Window: Effects of Television on Children and Youth.* 3rd ed. New York: Pergamon Press.

MAIN, M. 1990. Cross-cultural studies of attachment organization: Recent studies, changing methodologies, and the concept of conditional strategies. *Human Development* 33: 48–61.

MCCARTNEY, K. 1984. Effects of quality of day care environment on children's language development. *Developmental Psychology* 20(2): 244–260.

MCKEY, R. H., CONDELLI, L., GANSON, H, BARNETT, B. J., MCCONKEY, C. and PLANTZ, M. C. 1985. *The Impact of Head Start on Children, Families and Communities.* Washington (DC): Department of Health and Human Services.

MUSTARD, F. 1996. *Why National Projects?* Presentation at the Symposium on National Projects for a New Canada. March 2, 1996. Toronto: Glendon Campus, York University.

MUSTARD, F., and KEATING, D. 1993. Social and economic factors and human development. *Family Security in Insecure Times.* Ottawa: Canadian Council on Social Development.

OFFORD, D. 1995. Personal communication.

OFFORD, D., BOYLE, M., and RACINE, Y. 1989. *Ontario Child Health Study: Children at Risk.* Toronto: Queen's Printer for Ontario.

OFFORD, D., BOYLE, M., RACINE, Y. A., FLEMING, J. E., CADMAN, D. T., et al. 1992. Outcome, prognosis, and risk in a longitudinal follow-up study. *Journal of American Academy of Child and Adolescent Psychiatry* 31: 60–67.

ONTARIO. MINISTRY OF COMMUNITY AND SOCIAL SERVICES. 1989. *Better Beginnings, Better Futures.* Toronto: Queen's Printer for Ontario.

ONTARIO. PREMIER'S COUNCIL ON HEALTH, WELL-BEING AND SOCIAL JUSTICE. 1994. *Yours, Mine and Ours.* Toronto: Queen's Printer for Ontario.

ONTARIO. ROYAL COMMISSION ON LEARNING. 1994. *For the Love of Learning.* Toronto: Queen's Printer for Ontario.

PENCE, A. 1995. Personal communication.

PETERS, R. DEV., and RUSSELL, C. 1994. *Better Beginnings, Better Futures Project: Model, Program and Research Overview.* Toronto: Queen's Printer for Ontario.

ROSS, D., SCOTT, K., and KELLY, M. 1996. *Child Poverty: What Are the Consequences?* Ottawa: Centre for International Statistics, Canadian Council on Social Development.

ROSS, D., SHILLINGTON, E., and LOCHHEAD, C. 1994. *The Canadian Fact Book on Poverty.* Ottawa: Canadian Council on Social Development.

RUTLEDGE, D. 1993. *Education, Justice and Well-Being.* Working paper. Toronto: Premier's Council on Health, Well-Being and Social Justice.

SCHWEINHART, L. J., BARNES, H. V., and WEIKART, D. P. 1993. *Significant Benefits: The High/Scope Perry Preschool Study through Age 27.* Monographs of the High/Scope Educational Research Foundation, 10. Ypsilanti (MI): High/Scope Press.

SINGER, J. L., SINGER, D. G., EVANS, K. K., LEVIN, C., TARPLEY, T., and WORRAL, S. F. 1993. *A Role for Television in the Enhancement of Children's Readiness to Learn.* Report presented to the Corporation for Public Broadcasting.

SPR ASSOCIATES. 1996. *Background: A Short Overview of the Survey Designs and Instruments Used in the 1994–1995 Cycle of the NLSC.* Toronto: SPR Associates.

STEINHAUER, P. D. 1995. The effects of growing up in poverty on developmental outcomes in children: Some implications of the revision of the social security system. *The Canadian Child Psychiatric Bulletin* 4(2): 32–39.

SUOMI, S. 1993. Social and biological pathways that contribute to variations in health status: Evidence from primate studies. *Prosperity, Health and Well-Being.* Proceedings of the 11th Honda Foundation Discoveries Symposium, October 16–18, 1993, Toronto. pp. 105–112.

TREMBLAY, R., and CRAIG, W. 1994. *Developmental Prevention of Crime from Pre-Birth to Adolescence.* CIAR Program in Human Development Working Paper no. 6.

TREMBLAY, R. E., MASSE, B., PERRON, D., LeBLANC, M., SCHWARTZMAN, A. E., and LEDINGHAM, J. E. 1992. Early disruptive behaviour, poor school achievement, delinquent behaviour and delinquent personality: Longitudinal analyses. *Journal of Consulting and Clinical Psychology* 60: 64–72.

VANDELL, D., HENDERSON, V. K. and WILSON, K. S. 1988. A longitudinal study of children with day care experiences of varying quality. *Child Development* 59: 1286–1292.

VOLPE, R., PETERSON-BADALI, M., CORTER, C., CASE, R., and BIEMILLER, A. 1994. *Possible Roles for Public Television in Getting Ontario's Children Ready to Learn.* Toronto: TVOntario.

WEIKART, D.P. 1967. *Preschool Intervention: A Preliminary Report of the Perry Preschool Project.* Ann Arbor (MI): Campus Publishers.

WERNER, E., and SMITH, R. S., 1982. *Vulnerable but Invincible: A Longitudinal Study of Resilient Children and Youth.* New York: McGraw-Hill.

WHITEBOOK, M., HOWES, C., and PHILLIPS, D. 1990. *Who Cares? Child Care Teachers and the Quality of Care in America. The National Child Care Staffing Study.* Oakland (CA): The Child Care Employee Project.

WRIGHT, J., and HUSTON, A. 1995. *Effects of Educational TV Viewing of Lower Income Preschoolers on Academic Skills, School Readiness, and School Adjustment One to Three Years Later. A Report to the Children's Television Workshop.* Lawrence (KS): Department of Human Development, University of Kansas.

WRIGHT, M. 1983. *Compensatory Education in the Preschool: A Canadian Approach.* Ypsilanti (MI): High/Scope Press.

ZIGLER, E. 1990. Foreword. In *Handbook of Early Childhood Interventions,* eds. S. MEISELS and J. SHONKOFF. New York: Cambridge University Press.

ZIGLER, E., and STYFCO, S. Eds. 1994. *Head Start and Beyond: A National Plan for Extended Childhood Intervention.* New Haven and London: Yale University Press.

Developing Resiliency in Children from Disadvantaged Populations

PAUL D. STEINHAUER, M.D., FRCP(C)

Professor of Psychiatry, University of Toronto
Chair, Sparrow Lake Alliance
Chair, Voices for Children

SUMMARY

This paper reviews the different ways that resiliency has been defined in the professional literature, and defines resiliency as "unusually good adaptation in the face of severe stress, and/or an ability of the stressed person to rebound to the prestress level of adaptation." Based on this definition, the paper reviews biological, psychological, familial and social factors related to disadvantage that undermine the development of the precursors of resiliency, and lists factors that protect the potential for resiliency in each of these areas.

The paper then proceeds chronologically through a number of stages— conception through birth, infancy, the preschool years, the school years— examining for each stage the risk and protective factors within the child, the family and the community relevant to the achievement of resiliency. For each of these, it lists crucial developmental tasks and then examines how risk and protective factors influence the achievement of these tasks and preparation for resiliency. Next, the paper defines the goals and models of interventions specific to each stage that have been shown to foster the development of the precursors of resiliency by counteracting the major risks experienced during that stage. These are illustrated by 12 "success stories": established programs that have either proven their ability to help significant numbers of disadvantaged children achieve resiliency, or are well-designed and promising ongoing projects worthy of continued scrutiny while their effectiveness and efficiency are being established.

The paper concludes with 10 recommendations for policy that, if instituted, would allow significantly greater numbers of disadvantaged children to transcend adversity and achieve their developmental potential.

TABLE OF CONTENTS

LIST OF FIGURES

LIST OF TABLES

DEFINITION AND SOURCES OF RESILIENCY

The professional literature makes it clear that there is no single accepted definition of resiliency. Rather, the kind of positive outcomes used to define the resilient child vary depending on the outcome definitions used in each individual study (Kaufman et al. 1994).

This paper defines resiliency as unusually good adaptation in the face of severe stress (Beardslee 1989) and/or the ability of the stressed person to rebound to the prestress level of adaptation (Garmezy 1991a). This implies that the resilient child has gradually, over time, developed the resources needed to cope—and even to become stronger—while rising to the challenge of difficult conditions (Garmezy 1993; Prevention and Children Committee 1995; Egeland, Carlson, and Sroufe 1993).

Many sources of resiliency allow some children to transcend adversity and are often mutually reinforcing. They include:
- the child's genetic makeup and health;
- the "goodness of fit" between child and parents;
- the capacities of the parents—as individuals and as a couple—to support optimal development;
- the level of chronic stress—environmental, interpersonal or psychological—experienced by the family and the child;
- the perspectives of the parents and the child when confronted with stress.

It is these protective factors—within the child, the family, and their social environments—with which this paper is primarily concerned.

Many children experience high levels of chronic stress and adversity in regard to their health or their environment as they develop. But risks experienced within one aspect of their life, for example chronic illness, maltreatment or growing up in poverty, may be counteracted by protections provided by other aspects in what is called the protective triad (i.e., individual opportunities, close family ties and external support systems, including the school and the community: Garmezy 1991b). Given such supports, some children become resilient despite chronic exposure to disadvantage, and some are even strengthened by their struggle against adversity (Sinnema 1991; Cicchetti et al. 1993).

Resiliency is multidimensional: highly stressed adolescents with superior social skills are able to overcome major difficulties in both emotional adjustment and other areas of school competence (Luthar, Doernberger, and Zigler 1993).

Protective personal characteristics that help some children transcend environmental disadvantage include social competence (Ibid.), problem-solving skills and autonomy (Steinhauer, Santa-Barbara, and Skinner 1984), and a resilient perspective (Benard 1991; Sheppard and Kashani 1991). Children with a resilient perspective are basically optimistic. They have a sense of meaning and purpose, the will to overcome, confidence, self-esteem, and the inclination and ability to recruit social support. They are creative problem solvers, able to rebound and persevere in the face of hardships, frustration and even initial defeat (Fine 1991; Garmezy 1991a; Wolin and Wolin 1993; Williams, Wiebe, and Smith 1992), and they have a spiritual dimension that overlaps with hope (Danieli 1994).

One experience common to the development of many of these protective personal qualities is that of having had a secure attachment within a cohesive and supportive family (see figure 1).

Protective factors in families and schools that foster resiliency include:
- caring and support (Gribble et al. 1993);
- high but achievable expectations;
- opportunities for children to participate and contribute (Baumrind 1989); and
- in families, the strength to endure and cope despite chronic stress and repeated crises (McCubbin, McCubbin, and Thompson 1992).

As Bronfenbrenner (1985) has shown, *living in a civic society*—according to an African proverb, it takes a whole village to raise a child—supports the family and favours the development of competence and of the precursors of resiliency. In communities with less social capital and little societal cohesion, more parental involvement and better child management are needed to raise resilient children. Even these may not be enough to counteract the overwhelming effects of extreme disadvantage and an uncivic community (Garbarino et al. 1992; Richters and Martinez 1993; Capaldi and Patterson, in press).

THE ACHIEVEMENT OF RESILIENCY
IN THE FACE OF DISADVANTAGE

How can we best help children achieve resiliency despite disadvantage? The term "disadvantage" is often used as a synonym for poverty. The undermining effect of poverty is cumulative (Garmezy 1991b). Children growing up in poverty show almost three and one-half times the conduct disorders, almost twice the chronic illness, and more than twice the rate of school problems, hyperactivity and emotional disorders (Ross, Shillington, and Lochhead 1994) than those who are not poor. In one large study, the deeper the level of poverty, the higher the incidence of violence in children (three times greater in girls; five times greater in boys: Tremblay et al. 1994).

However, it is more the degree of inequity—that is, the extent of the gap between rich and poor in a society—and the degree of powerlessness and lack of control over one's life rather than the economic deprivation itself that most strongly undermines physical and mental health (Marmot, Kogevinas, and Evans 1987; Davey Smith, Bartley, and Blane 1990; Hertzman, Frank, and Evans 1990; Canadian Institute of Advanced

Figure 1

Secure attachment as a precursor of resiliency

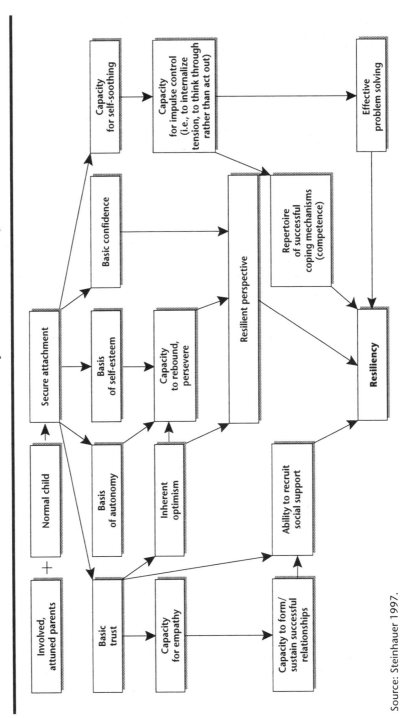

Source: Steinhauer 1997.

Research 1991). Any situation that increases inequity, including attempts by governments to cut their economic deficits in ways that aggravate their social deficits, can be expected to increase health and mental health problems (including suicides) and crime rates. New Zealand is often used as a shining example of what trickle-down economics can do for a country's economic woes. But what *has* happened in New Zealand since 1984, when it decided to tackle the economic deficit while ignoring the social deficit? While its cash flow problem has indeed been solved, the total national debt is double what it was in 1984. And, over the dozen years that New Zealand has been correcting its economic situation:

- its youth suicide rate—the highest in the world—has doubled since 1985;
- its crime rate (1993) is the highest of the industrialized countries;
- its poverty rate rose 40 percent from cuts to welfare and unemployment—nearly 25 percent of New Zealand children are being raised in poverty;
- its unemployment (using 1984 definitions) tripled in four years to 12.7 percent;
- its middle class has decreased;
- the gap between rich and poor, in both income and education, has increased substantially; and for the first time in its history, New Zealand has a large impoverished underclass (Canadian Broadcasting Corporation 1995).

In such circumstances, children are probably affected through increases in parental stress, family conflict, violence and abuse, through decreased supports and services in school and the community, and by identifying with their parents' alienation and sense of marginalization and betrayal.

There are different kinds and degrees of disadvantage. Poverty aggravates parental stress and family tension in many ways. It serves as a source of stress in its own right. It erodes parents' limited psychosocial resources and magnifies interpersonal and psychological problems. It aggravates parenting problems (Avison 1994) and lessens opportunities for temporary escape from sources of stress. But evidence is mounting that, even for poor children, it is the combined effects of multiple environmental stresses (Rutter 1979a; Rae-Grant 1991) and the clustered effects of the psychosocial deprivations that often coexist with poverty—particularly maternal depression, parental substance abuse, parental violence and paternal criminality—rather than just low income that undermine competence and resiliency (Dembo et al. 1992; Ontario Mental Health Foundation 1994; Byrne et al. 1996; Steinhauer 1995a). Also, the transient poverty and life experience of immigrant children in supportive families differ from the type of disadvantage experienced by children raised in families trapped in a permanent underclass (Steinhauer 1995a).

Children do not have to be poor to be disadvantaged. Children of chronically neglectful, conflicted, violent and abusive families are also disadvantaged, whether or not they are poor. Changing economic patterns, the increased need for two parents to work (Hanvey et al. 1994, 119; Avard and Chance 1994), higher levels (by more than 10 times) of marriage breakdown since the Second World War (Barr 1993), and the mobility that has, for many families, made extended family less available to share child care, have left many parents with less time and energy to devote to parenting (Hewlett 1991a; Scrivener 1994). In the 60 years that records have been kept, never have children and parents spent as little time together (Watkins, Menken, and Bongaarts 1987), a situation that Mattox (1990) termed the "Family Time Famine." These days, about 65 percent of families with young children need two incomes to escape poverty (Vanier 1994). This has greatly increased the need for affordable high-quality extrafamilial child care. Without it, many families face a Hobson's choice: one parent can stay home to care for the children (thereby dragging the family into poverty), or they can settle for the only child care available, the quality of which may be far from adequate.

This paper now examines how biological, familial and environmental risks inherent in disadvantage undermine the potential for achieving competence and resiliency. Next it considers protective factors and processes that have helped many disadvantaged children rise above adversity, thereby fostering their development of resiliency. It concludes with models of selected interventions that nurture resiliency at personal, familial and community levels from conception through adolescence.

HOW DO THE RISKS INHERENT IN DISADVANTAGE UNDERMINE THE POTENTIAL FOR RESILIENCY?

How do the risks inherent in disadvantage tend to undermine, at different ages, the potential genetic, familial, environmental and psychological sources of resiliency?

From conception to birth, the major risks faced are primarily *biological*, though some are environmental. What is commonly termed low birthweight really refers to two overlapping conditions: some babies are born too small (growth impaired), while others are born too soon (preterm delivery: Paneth 1995). While most low-birthweight babies now survive because of improved neonatal care—including many weighing as little as 750 grams at birth—the lower the birthweight, the greater the risk of preserving the infant's life at the cost of significant lifelong health and developmental problems. These may prevent the child from ever leading a full and productive life, while greatly increasing the cost to the community for expensive and often insufficiently available health care and remedial education (Allen, Donohue, and Dusman 1993; Hack et al. 1994). Low-, and especially very low, birthweight babies are almost twice as likely to die at birth or during their first year. They have almost twice the risk of lifelong disease and disabilities, including cerebral palsy, visual problems, attention deficit hyperactivity disorder, learning disabilities and respiratory problems (Canada 1992; McCormick, Gortmaker, and Sobol 1990).

Families from the poorest neighbourhoods are 1.4 times as likely as those from the richest neighbourhoods to have low-birthweight babies (Hanvey et al. 1994, 123), but it is not yet clear how much of such babies' less severe but more common developmental delays are a result of the disadvantaged environments in which low-birthweight children are more likely to live and grow. Certainly a disadvantaged environment aggravates the cognitive and behavioural disabilities that originate in biological deficiencies (Watkins, Menken, and Bongaarts 1987; Shiono and Behrman 1995).

Biological factors that increase the risk of low or very low birthweight include extremes of maternal age (less than 20; over 45 years), multiple births, black race (independent of level of disadvantage: Paneth 1995, 26; Shiono et al. 1986), maternal smoking and poor maternal diet. At least some of the social class gradient follows from the fact that the poorest mothers are the heaviest smokers (Institute of Medicine 1985; Rush and Cassano 1983). Smoking, which retards fetal growth, is the single largest modifiable risk factor contributing to low birthweight and infant mortality. Smoking during pregnancy, low maternal weight gain and low pregnancy weight account for nearly two-thirds of all growth-retarded infants (Kramer 1987). Up to 20 percent of all cases of low birthweight could be prevented by eliminating smoking in pregnancy (Chomitz, Cheung, and Lieberman 1995). The abuse of alcohol and other drugs during pregnancy is also associated with low birthweight and preterm birth (Schneider, Griffith, and Chasnoff 1989; Rodgers 1989; Canada 1992).

Other biological risks during this period include fetal brain damage (e.g., Fetal Alcohol Syndrome), which often results in hyperactivity, difficulties in impulse control, dysphoric mood and inability to be soothed. These symptoms frequently result from maternal drinking or drug (especially cocaine) abuse during pregnancy. Fetal brain damage increases the rates of attachment failure, academic failure, oppositional/defiant and antisocial behaviour, and psychiatric problems in adult life (Mannuzza et al. 1993).

Social factors increasing the risk of low or very low birthweight include isolation, lack of psychosocial supports, and chronic high stress and abuse of the mother during pregnancy (Goodyer 1990; Garmezy 1991b; Carnegie Corporation of New York 1994). Anything that combats isolation and counteracts the psychosocial stresses often associated with poverty also helps prepare for attachment, bonding and other precursors of resiliency in the neonatal period (see Jacobson and Frye 1991, diagram 1). Preterm delivery, which causes most low birthweight in the United States is, like fetal growth impairment, very much related to social class, and is a greater cause of infant mortality in developed nations than fetal growth impairment. Maternal smoking and poor nutrition—which are linked to fetal growth retardation—affect preterm delivery less than they do growth impairment.

In summary, decreasing maternal isolation, improving nutrition, and lowering smoking and alcohol and drug use during pregnancy can cause a significant though modest increase in the number of healthy and potentially resilient babies born to relaxed, prepared mothers.

From birth through the toddler years, the main threats remain biological and environmental, but the quality of the family environment becomes increasingly important as either a threat to or a potential source of resiliency. Increasing evidence suggests that consistently neglectful or abusive parenting (i.e., chronic stress) during the first one to two years of life may be associated with permanent brain damage. The ongoing development of the still immature—and highly vulnerable—infant brain is significantly influenced by the quality and quantity of stimuli received from the child's environment during periods of heightened sensitivity during the first three years. Thus, environment during this period has a major influence on brain development and thereby on cognitive potential and the capacity for control over intense feelings, including anxiety and aggression (Carnegie Corporation of New York 1994; Keating 1992; Perry, in press).

Another biological factor that can undermine potential resiliency is a physiologically (and at least at times genetically) low threshold of response by the brain's limbic system to unfamiliarity and change, which leads to a high and persistent level of arousal of the sympathetic nervous system (Garcia-Coll, Kagan, and Reznick 1984; Kagan, Reznick, and Snidman 1987). Such infants are more vulnerable both to insecure attachment and to behavioural inhibition (Manassis et al. 1994) and, with age, are prone to avoid new or stressful situations whenever they can. Avoidance decreases anxiety, but it does so in ways that keep the infant from developing more effective coping strategies. The lack of effective coping strategies denies the child a sense of mastery, favours habitual avoidance and predisposes the child to the development of anxiety disorders (Biederman et al. 1990; Hirshfeld et al. 1992). Secure, involved, sensitively attuned parenting may help children develop more effective means of coping, thus protecting their potential for mastery, competence and resilience.

Probably the strongest single familial factor protecting the potential for resiliency during this period is anything that supports the establishment of a secure attachment to a primary caregiver. A secure attachment is favoured by a relaxed, secure, supported mother who is involved with and sensitively attuned to her child. It can be undermined by the mother's own unresolved attachment difficulties. Such residual difficulties often stem from the neglect and abuse the mother experienced—or believes she experienced—in her own childhood (Main and Goldwyn 1984). The risk of attachment failure can also be decreased by: freedom from isolation; adequate social supports during the neonatal and toddler periods; effective treatment of maternal depression, psychosis or drug abuse; and support for the mother in the face of chronic friction, abuse or abandonment by her partner (Garmezy 1991b). The child's secure attachment to the father can also help compensate for the effect of an insecure attachment to the mother (Fox, Kimmerly, and Schafer 1991).

But not all attachment failures stem from parental deficiencies. Such infant-related factors as prematurity, deformities or chronic illnesses, especially if they limit contact between infant and parents and bar the parents from ministering to the infant during long hospital stays or interfere with the infant's capacity to participate in the bonding process, can undermine the processes of attachment and bonding (Minde 1980). Hospital procedures that encourage parents to be actively and physically involved in the care of their child will foster attachment and protect the capacity for resiliency. Child characteristics, including difficult temperament, may interfere with "goodness of fit," that is, the child's basic temperament and other inherited characteristics may fail to meet the needs of the parents. When a poor fit occurs, it can undermine the bonding process central to the achievement of competence and resiliency. On the other hand, an easy (i.e., "laid back") temperament can buffer the child's reactions to stress and increase the child's adaptability, favouring goodness of fit and successful attachment (Werner 1984; Raine, Venables, and Williams 1990). However, too low a level of arousal (too little anxiety) has its own risks for the development of delinquency and adult criminality (Magnusson, Klinteberg, and Statton 1991; Raine, Venables, and Williams 1990; Tremblay et al. 1991).

The vulnerability of an infant with a low threshold of response and high sympathetic arousal to insecure attachment may be increased if the primary caregiver is herself[1] insecure or has an anxiety disorder (Manassis et al. 1994). The response of an anxious, depressed or insecure parent to an inhibited (anxious and shy) child may, if the response is critical and lacking in encouragement, undermine the child's development of the coping mechanisms that could otherwise guard against internalizing disorders and protect his capacity for resiliency (Weissman et al. 1987; Kochanska 1991; Baldwin, Baldwin, and Cole 1990). In the preschool and school-age years, the opportunity for free play with peers, if successful, may enhance social skills, reduce avoidance behaviours and decrease the child's anxiety and inhibition, thus favouring the achievement of resiliency (Rubin 1982).

---

1. I refer to the primary caregiver as "she" because, in the vast majority of Canadian families, the mother assumes most responsibility for infant care, thus becoming the primary attachment figure. In families where the father does most of the child care, he would be the primary attachment figure.

Throughout the *toddler, preschool and school-age years,* the major factor protecting the potential for resiliency will be the ability of the disadvantaged child's parents, as individuals and as a couple, to meet that child's developmental needs. Illness or disability, which often undermine the achievement of competence, can, in some children, actually spur the achievement of resilience (National Center for Youth Disabilities 1991; Sinnema 1991). How a child responds to stress may be influenced by that child's sex. Girls are more likely to respond by developing internalizing disorders (especially separation anxiety disorders and depression), while boys are more prone to externalizing disorders (Attention Deficit Hyperactivity Disorder, Oppositional Defiant Disorder, Conduct Disorder: Offord et al. 1989; Last et al. 1987) (see table 1).

Table 1
Six-month prevalence of individual psychiatric disorders by age and sex

Age and sex groupings	Conduct disorder (%)	Hyperactivity (%)	Emotional disorder (%)	Somatization (%)
4–11				
Boys	6.5	10.1	10.2	—
Girls	1.8	3.3	10.7	—
12–16				
Boys	10.4	7.3	4.9	4.5
Girls	4.1	3.4	13.6	10.7

Source: Derived from data in D. R. Offord et al. 1989.

Factors in individual parents that commonly undermine successful parenting cannot always be controlled. Individual parent characteristics that affect the achievement of resiliency in children can be genetic and/or psychodynamic.

At a genetic level, factors transmitted to the child that favour resiliency include freedom from congenital diseases or such psychiatric disorders as affective disorder, schizophrenia, anxiety disorders, substance abuse and developmental disabilities. An important protective genetic factor would be the presence of at least adequate intelligence (Luthar and Zigler 1992). Children who have one parent who has had a major depression are between two and four times as likely to have a psychiatric disorder themselves. Although this is often depression, the child's vulnerability to both anxiety disorders and behavioural problems is also increased (Beardslee et al. 1993; Rutter and Quinton 1984; Pape et al. 1996).

Children of parents with an anxiety disorder are more likely to have anxiety disorders but, although the familial transmission of anxiety disorders has been established, it is not clear whether the familial influence is hereditary, environmental or a combination of the two (Reeves et al. 1987; Turner, Beidel, and Costello 1987; Messer and Beidel 1994; Thapar and McGuffin 1995).

A boy born to a family with an older criminal member is two and a half times as likely to become delinquent himself, although here again the relative role of genetic and environmental factors in the transmission is not clear (Fisher 1985; Gabel and Schindledecker 1993).

At a psychodynamic level, mental health in a parent may—but will not necessarily—favour the achievement of resiliency. How much parental mental illness will undermine the achievement of resiliency will vary depending on how the illness undermines the child's development. This in turn will depend on the age and developmental status of the child, the nature, severity and periodicity of the parent's disorder, side effects of the parent's treatment, the presence in the home of another caregiver able to meet the needs of the children and to buffer them from the effects of the other parent's illness, and indirect effects of the illness on the marital relationship.

Particularly likely to undermine the potential for resiliency are parental disorders that interfere with attachment, including anything that will block a primary caregiver's capacity for full involvement with and sensitive attunement to the developing infant. These include the direct influence on the parent's pattern of relating or parenting caused by the major mental illnesses such as affective disorder, schizophrenia or any other conditions or personality traits that, either themselves or from the effects of the medications used to treat them, contribute to parental preoccupation and withdrawal or to episodes of unpredictable, erratic or hostile parental behaviour that frighten the infant (Resnick, Harris, and Blum 1993; Beardslee et al. 1993).

The residual effects on parents who were themselves neglected or abused during their own upbringing—and it is the parent's current perception rather than what actually occurred that counts—may undermine attachment or any other aspects of parenting, while proving extremely difficult, though not impossible, to overcome (Main and Goldwyn 1984). Parental substance abuse also undermines the child's capacity for resiliency while often resisting attempts at remediation (Reich et al. 1993). After successful attachment has been achieved, parental psychopathology affects child development primarily indirectly through its corrosive effects on the marriage and on parent-child relationships.

Parental psychopathology does not invariably undermine the capacity for resiliency. Some people, despite considerable psychopathology, parent surprisingly effectively. Also, adversity can spur the development of the personal resources needed to achieve resiliency, especially in temperamentally favoured individuals who have been securely attached[2] (Beardslee 1989;

---

2. Paul Zindel's play *The Effect of Gamma Rays on Man-in-the-Moon Marigolds* bears eloquent testimony to this pattern of familial adversity serving as a spur to the achievement of resiliency.

Garmezy 1991a; Cicchetti et al. 1993). When this occurs, however, the availability and supportiveness of the other parent or some mentor outside the immediate family—a relative, teacher, youth leader, neighbour or therapist who genuinely cares about the child and is sufficiently involved to serve as a parent surrogate, usually for an extended period of time—is often crucial (Rutter 1979b).

Marital harmony fosters the capacity for resiliency (see figure 2). Marital conflict, however, makes consistent expectations and regular follow-through by both parents less likely, thereby predisposing children to poor impulse control and socialization (Fergusson, Horfwood, and Lynskey 1992; Pedersen 1994). As well as raising the level of family tension, marital conflict affects children in a number of ways. It polarizes parents, which invariably undermines consistency. It also "triangulates" one or more children who are trapped between the conflicting expectations of the battling parents. If the conflict is sufficiently intense or chronic, it may precipitate family violence, and that will increase the risk that the child will become aggressive, lower his capacity for empathy, and increase his vulnerability to psychiatric disorders and antisocial behaviour, even if the child is not the one being abused (Hinchey and Gavelek 1982; Lewis et al. 1983; Jaffe et al. 1986; Moore et al. 1989; Widom 1989).

Finally, severe and chronic marital conflict frequently ends in marriage breakdown. This in turn results in one or more of the following consequences: the child being raised by a single parent (doing the work of two); the single-parent family being mother-led (as 84 percent of Canadian single-parent families are: Hanvey et al. 1994, 6); abandonment by the father (loss of emotional and possibly economic support: Hewlett 1991b); the mother-led single-parent family falling below the poverty line (as more than 60 percent of such families do: Hanvey et al. 1994, 117); and the child being raised in a reconstituted family (which also increases the risk of poor developmental outcomes: Philp 1995). Thus, often the hazards of family breakdown are potentiated by the sequelae of the separation, all of which—but especially poverty—involve significant risks of their own.

The *parenting style* of an intact family that combines a high level of caring and involvement with high but reasonable expectations is most likely to help children develop the confidence, the competence (and the associated feeling of well-being), the coping skills needed to maintain competence, and the sense of perspective that shapes how they react to stress. The interaction of these factors contributes to the achievement of resiliency (Garmezy and Masten 1991; Barnes and Farrell 1992; Resnick, Harris, and Blum 1993; Dodge, Pettit, and Bates 1994; Campbell 1995) (see figure 3).

Authoritative parents, as defined by Baumrind (1989), combine high but reasonable demands, high involvement and sensitive attunement to the needs of their children, and a high level of cognitive involvement. In infancy and through the preschool years, cognitive involvement consists primarily

62

Figure 2

Marital conflict and its effect on the development of resilience

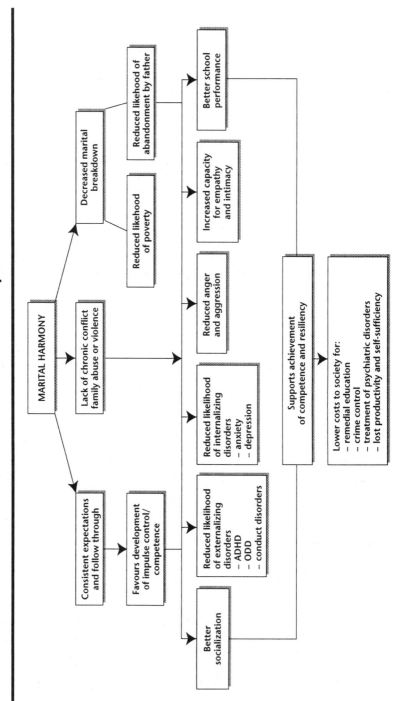

of cognitive and language stimulation. With age, however, cognitive involvement increasingly takes the form of encouraging children to speak up for themselves and negotiate successfully with others, a skill that is a forerunner of effective problem solving. Authoritative families show consistently high levels of reciprocity, in that members are sensitive and responsive to each others' needs. Without reciprocity, children tend to resent and oppose even reasonable parental limits and expectations. Authoritative families typically have clear and consistent expectations of their children, backed up by a predictable, noncoercive and nonrestrictive form of discipline that serves as a model of problem solving and effective conflict resolution.

Authoritative families do not avoid confrontation when it is needed but, since their confrontations are not coercive, they confront in a way that encourages socialization and models effective problem solving. Since these families are nonintrusive, they encourage their children to assume responsibility for and to learn from the consequences of their own behaviour. They avoid the extremes of excessive parental passivity (habitual non-confrontation) and parental coercion, both of which undermine effective socialization. Children typically respond to parental coercion with anger and rebellion. Their preoccupation with the unfairness of the parental assault keeps them from learning to reflect on and take responsibility for the inappropriateness of their behaviour. Authoritative families consistently produce highly competent children, and are least likely to raise incompetent children. Competence achieved in the face of adversity, as was discussed above, is a prerequisite for resiliency.

Parenting style affects boys and girls somewhat differently. Parental warmth, for example, increases social responsibility in both boys and girls, but improves intellectual competence in boys only. Similarly, while cognitive responsiveness increases general competence and social assertiveness, it fosters social responsibility in boys only. Firm but not coercive parental controls increase social competence in both girls and boys, but in girls they do so by increasing social assertiveness, while in boys they do so by enhancing social responsibility (Baumrind 1989).

During the school-age years, disadvantaged children are generally less likely to develop the cognitive, emotional and social skills needed for success in school. They are also more likely than children from affluent areas to have attention difficulties, to be hyperactive and to have poor impulse control. Boys are more likely to show these forms of behaviour than girls (Tremblay et al. 1995). Such children are generally at greater risk for school failure and delinquency. Already denied initial success, they begin school at risk. Their experiences there can further undermine both their confidence and their competence. However, good child care—in their families or in high-quality alternative care or early child care and education (ECCE)—can help disadvantaged children attain the control required to sit still, to focus their attention and to work independently. Readiness to learn in

Figure 3
Parenting style and its effect on the development of resilience

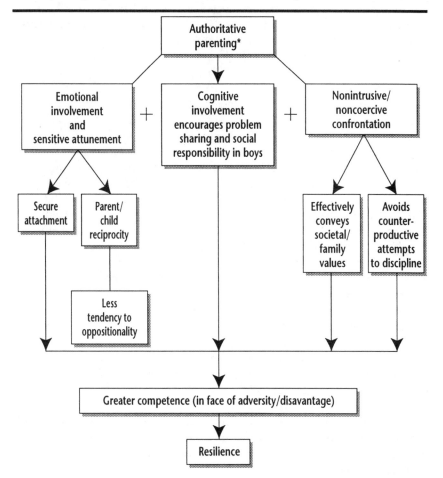

• As defined by Baumrind (1989), authoritative parenting combines high but reasonable demands, with high parental involvement and responsiveness.

kindergarten is the strongest predictor of success in mathematics in eighth grade and is a protective factor against the development of delinquency (Fuchs and Reklis 1994). Those who have mastered, before starting school, the social skills and the control over aggression that they will need to succeed with peers and to accept a teacher's authority are, like their non-disadvantaged peers, primed for academic, social and emotional success. Children who, because of secure attachments, possess the basic trust that enables them to use their teacher as a learning partner, along with the associated self-esteem and confidence they will need to take the chances required for successful learning, are candidates for early academic success. This will, in turn, reinforce their confidence, self-esteem and resilient perspective.

Boys are more likely than girls to have trouble in Grade 1, because of their greater cognitive immaturity and because boys have a higher incidence of genetically based learning disabilities. Again, effective parenting can help overcome disadvantage by providing the will, skills, motivation and ongoing supervision of homework required for school success. The less time senior public school students spend unsupervised, the less likely they are to abuse drugs and the more likely they are to be good students (Richardson et al. 1989). In fact, by age 14, success in school—especially in English and history—is related more to what is going on in a child's family than to what is happening in the child's school (Coleman and Hoffer 1987). With 20 percent of Canadian public school children spending time unsupervised while parents work or attend school, parents and schools can help maximize academic and social competence by giving children sufficient, intersectoral, after-school services integrated with the educational system in a seamless day (Hanvey et al. 1994, 7).

School failure and inadequate control over aggression frequently coexist and potentiate each other. Boys who are impulsive and hyperactive, low in anxiety and lowest in reward dependency in kindergarten (age five) are at risk for becoming violent and antisocial in adolescence (Tremblay et al. 1994; Magnusson, Klinteberg, and Statton 1991). Boys who are violent in kindergarten are more likely to remain violent if they do poorly in school (Tremblay et al. 1991). By Grade 2, the learning problems that often accompany delinquency are well established: in one study, 45 percent of conduct-disordered children were already behind in reading and 36 percent were behind in writing (Meltzer et al. 1984). Poor school performance and a weak bond to school are often complicated by poor school behaviour. This elicits disciplinary action by the school, initiating a struggle that, escalating through primary and secondary school, often leads to both delinquency and dropping out by adolescence (Loeber and Keenan 1995). Involved and effective parenting, supplemented when required by high-quality child care or ECCE before school entry, can significantly improve children's cognitive and language development, their social competence, their control over their aggression, their compliance with adult instructions and their readiness to learn, while decreasing the number of behaviour problems reported by Grade 1 teachers (Bertrand 1993).

A school that provides a stimulating and supportive alternative environment able to buffer for many children the effects of disadvantage can help even poorly prepared children transcend adversity by preparing them to succeed in school. Such schools create a safe environment in which children feel secure, respected, challenged and cared for, despite the occasionally undermining effects of family and community. These schools present high academic and behavioural expectations along with the structure, support and enrichment needed to help students achieve their potential. They have teachers who genuinely care about their students and who are prepared to become involved with them and to serve as mentors for students willing to use them in that way. In such schools, the ethos supports respectful and reciprocal relationships, and actively defines bullying as unacceptable. Such schools work at building bridges between the school and the community, and welcome the community as a true partner in the shared task of helping children achieve their potential in school and in life (Rutter et al. 1979b; Sylva 1994; Comer 1985, 1988).

A child's peer relationships can do much to shape his attitudes and behaviour during the school years and, increasingly, through adolescence. Peer relationships provide another chance for children to learn the interpersonal skills so important to social competence. They provide a community in microcosm that can either support or undermine the child's mastery of problem solving, self-esteem and control over emotions (including aggression), while helping the child move toward increasing independence. Informal or supervised group recreational activities may be a significant source not only of fun, but of skills that in themselves can help children succeed in spite of disadvantage (Kellam 1990; Jones and Offord 1989). Successful experiences with peers help children learn to follow rules and take turns. For socialized children, group activities can offer an antidote to boredom and important opportunities for the successful sublimation of aggression. Well-supervised group activities offer not only all of the above, but also provide another opportunity for an ongoing association with a mentor, an experience frequently found in the history of children who achieve resiliency in the face of disadvantage (Kellam 1990). For some highly anxious children, particularly those with anxious parents, successful relationships with peers can provide the models and experience that stimulate the formation of the coping mechanisms that help counteract excessive anxiety and the drift toward increasing avoidance (Manassis and Bradley 1994).

Children and youth whose family and school experiences have for any reason been alienating may turn to their peers for the sense of belonging and status they are not finding at home or in school. The choice of peers can be a strong influence supporting either prosocial or antisocial attitudes and behaviour. Often an oppositional child or teenager finds acceptance and support in a peer group based on shared resentment and rejection of family, school, adults, authority, other ethnic or racial groups, or the mores of the society from which he feels alienated. If that group feeling is then cemented by partying (based on the communal consumption of alcohol or street drugs) or by shared antisocial behaviour, the youth is assured a readily available source of support that serves as an antidote to loneliness and a model for identification. During adolescence, such a peer group may be the predominant social influence, reinforcing increasingly antisocial attitudes and behaviour (Henggeler and Borduin 1990). Until recently, such unofficial or official gangs consisted largely of males, but criminologists and police report that gangs of teenage girls are a new, rapidly spreading and worrying phenomenon (Matthews 1993).

But how does *life in a disadvantaged community* undermine poor children's opportunities to achieve their developmental potential? Both the hyperactivity and conduct disorders so frequently associated with academic failure and inadequate socialization are more than twice as common in poor children as in those who are not poor (Ross, Shillington, and Lochhead 1994; Tremblay et al. 1994). A Quebec study of 4000 children has shown that the deeper the level of poverty, the higher the level of violence, especially for girls (Tremblay et al. 1991). We suspect that this stems from the sense of hopelessness that comes from feeling powerless and marginalized. We know that in uncivic societies—societies marked by an absence of shared beliefs, values and behavioural norms and by pervasive mistrust, lack of communication and lack of social cohesion among identifiable subgroups within the total population (Putnam 1993)—a higher level of parent involvement and more effective monitoring and discipline are needed to socialize children successfully. Neighbourhoods high in density, crime and drug abuse but low in cohesion or a sense of control of their own destiny are likely to undermine even many committed families' attempts to raise children successfully (Bronfenbrenner 1985; Garbarino et al. 1992; Richters and Martinez 1993).

We know that abusive parenting, a potent contributor to both internalizing and externalizing psychiatric disorders in children and to delinquency (Ontario Mental Health Foundation 1994), commonly complicates the isolation so common in disadvantaged populations. The alienation can serve to perpetuate ongoing, even if self-imposed, social deprivation, and to insulate such families from social sanctions against abusive behaviour that, in less isolated families, could have a moderating effect. Longstanding isolation is frequently accompanied by increasing depression, resentment and hostility, all of which are associated with higher rates of abusive parenting, psychiatric disorders, school failure and drop-out, and juvenile delinquency (Ontario Mental Health Foundation 1994). Also, in an uncivic society, groups further from the centre of power typically feel marginalized, and the resulting sense of exclusion from society's benefits frequently potentiates alienation, a loss of social cohesion and the rejection of the behavioural norms of the larger society (Steinhauer 1996). When poverty and marginalization are superimposed on each other, as occurs in some of our disadvantaged minorities, it may take considerable personal strength and familial support to achieve resiliency and productivity despite the unfriendly environment.

Many of these factors influence the lives of Aboriginal children and young people living on reserves. Many such communities are multiply disadvantaged, with their inhabitants very much marginalized (Hanvey et al. 1994). Does the degree to which these Aboriginal communities feel isolated and powerless, over and above the psychological scars remaining from an earlier age when children were routinely taken from their families and reserves to be educated in what for them was a foreign culture, account for the high levels of substance abuse, family violence (up to 85 percent), alcoholism (nearly 80 percent) sexual assault and incest in these communities (Canadian Council on Social Development 1987; Griffiths and Yerbury 1995)? We know that substance abuse, delinquency and suicide in Aboriginal children and youth are far above the national average (Vanderburg, Weekes, and Millson 1995; Steinhauer 1996). Yet significant numbers of Aboriginal children, despite often extreme adversity, manage not just to survive but to succeed. Their ability to do so is a tribute to the power of personal resiliency with or without family support.

PROMOTING RESILIENCY IN THE FACE OF DISADVANTAGE: SUCCESS STORIES

Considering the major risks that threaten successful development from conception through adolescence, have any programs demonstrated the ability to neutralize these factors and to protect the potential for significant numbers of children achieving resiliency in spite of disadvantage? Let us recall that even in the face of major stress—be it in the child, the family or the community—other factors may still sustain developmental competence and help the child not just to survive but to rise above adversity.

As in the preceding section, each developmental level is presented in turn.

Goal No. 1: From Conception through Delivery: Interventions to Increase the Number of Healthy Babies Born to Relaxed Mothers.

During this stage, successful interventions will have a proven ability to decrease the number of low- and very low birthweight babies, and/or the number of infants born brain-damaged as a result of maternal substance abuse during pregnancy. Although the goal is to decrease the risk to the health of the baby, in most cases the social stresses and lifestyle problems of the mother will have to be addressed to improve her health and that of the baby.

Conventional prenatal care is *not* the solution to the problems of low birthweight (i.e., growth impairment and preterm delivery). For optimal effectiveness, prenatal care should target the known causes of low birthweight. Smoking cessation programs, which are not emphasized in most prenatal care, are the single component best able to address the highest modifiable contributor to low birthweight and infant mortality. Purely nutritional interventions have only a modest effect on a small subset of women whose babies are at risk for low birthweight (U.S. Department of Health and Human Services 1989). But this does not mean that prenatal care or nutritional programs are not worthwhile.

Women who receive prenatal care do have somewhat fewer low-birthweight babies and lower infant mortality, but it is not clear whether this is because of the prenatal care itself or because those women who use prenatal care tend to be healthier, better educated and more advantaged. We do know that the greatest benefits of prenatal care lie beyond the prevention of low birthweight. These include: the diagnosis and treatment of medical conditions affecting the health of the baby and the mother; the provision of education about pregnancy, labour and delivery for first-time mothers; the linking of poor mothers to valuable medical and social services, including supports for both parents and children whose ability to improve developmental outcomes for low-birthweight babies is proven; and the fact that those mothers who choose to receive prenatal care are more likely to use preventive interventions after the birth of their babies (Bates et al. 1995; Paneth 1995).

Here are two descriptions of quite different prenatal care programs that have demonstrated the ability to produce healthier babies for better prepared and more relaxed mothers. A third, based on a home visiting model, is grouped with other such interventions and is described under Goal No. 2.

The Prevention of Preterm Delivery through Improved Prenatal Care in France

Actions on nonmedical determinants of health – This program first determined through epidemiological studies that women of low socioeconomic status were at higher risk for preterm births and for low-birthweight babies. Then, from an analysis of the principal causes of preterm birth and the preventive techniques available, it reorganized service delivery, evaluating the results and analysing cost-effectiveness.

Education was the key intervention, since the main obstacle to effective prevention was inadequate public understanding stemming from insufficient dissemination of pertinent information. For the program to succeed, doctors and midwives (via journal articles and conferences) and the women them-selves (via the press and television) needed to learn that many preterm births could be prevented by a well-organized approach with both medical and social components. One goal was to alert professionals to identify women with cervical incompetence (a condition increasing the risk for preterm labour) within the first trimester, to ensure:

- women at risk would receive full care with regular examinations to detect signs of risk of preterm labour;
- women at risk would reduce physical exertion and be prescribed rest by having them stop work, and by persuading their husbands or other family members to share household responsibilities;

- a trained midwife would be monitoring women at risk in their homes weekly; and
- highest-risk cases would be admitted to hospital.

Educating women to modify their lifestyle to decrease their risk of preterm labour was central to the program.

Reasons for the initiative – The program was developed to improve prenatal services and reduce preterm births, which—given advances in neonatology that were keeping alive babies who once would have died—were producing many more immature babies weighing less and less at birth. Concern about how many of these children were surviving with variable degrees of disability and the sharp increase in costs for their care prompted the move to develop a coherent and well-coordinated program to decrease preterm births. Since 1945, all pregnant women in France had received a stipend for having at least one prenatal consultation during the first trimester of pregnancy. However, before this intervention, prenatal care before the last month of pregnancy was provided by family doctors who, generally speaking, were not enthusiastic about a new prevention policy. For that reason, the new program was introduced by obstetricians or midwives under a specialist's supervision at outpatient maternity clinics in four areas.

Actors –This program counted on the contributions of French doctors, midwives and public health authorities, and French women at high risk for preterm birth and low birthweight.

Analysis of the results – Results were obtained on four different sets of data. One set (city of Hagenau) showed that the socioeconomically disadvantaged and poorly educated mothers were hardest to involve but benefited most. In the Martinique study, which relied heavily on home-monitoring of high-risk women, the risk of preterm birth in the disadvantaged group was reduced to the same level as the "privileged" group. The authors stress that success was achieved not by using specialists or technology, but by educating midwives and patients.

Replicability of the initiative – Successful replication would require that physicians and Ministries of Health be committed to a program based on the education of doctors and midwives, and on the primary role of women themselves in a prevention policy.

Funding – The program largely paid for itself by a better use of existing government funding for maternal and child health. The major new item was the extensive public education campaign to modify women's opinions of what adequate prenatal care should be.

Evaluation – The nationwide results showed a decrease in preterm deliveries, from 8.2 percent in 1972 to 5.6 percent in 1981. The results were extensively published in professional journals. A cost-benefit analysis led to replication of the program on a national scale by the French government in 1971 (Papiernik 1984; Goujon, Papiernik, and Maine 1984; Papiernik et al. 1985, 1986).

The Montreal Diet Dispensary

Actions on nonmedical determinants of health – The Montreal Diet Dispensary (MDD) is the only working example of a supplementary maternal food program in North America established before the 1970s. The MDD provides nutritional counselling, motivation and food supplements, when needed, to high-risk pregnant women, 62 percent of whom are on social assistance and almost 10 percent of whom are teenagers. The MDD works to break the poverty cycle through a three-pronged program that includes:

- a home visit to establish rapport and begin nutritional assessment;
- education and motivation of clients through ongoing counselling; and
- food supplementation (94 percent of clients receive a litre of milk and an egg a day).

Women are taught that they are eating to feed a baby they have never met. The earlier in pregnancy counselling starts, the better the results. Volunteers play an important role in the program.

Reasons for the initiative – The director, Agnes Higgins, had noted that 80 percent of the mothers seen in public prenatal clinics were poorly nourished entering pregnancy. They were underweight and had low protein intake, an increased risk for teenage mothers especially since underweight mothers need to gain more to nourish and protect the fetus. Poverty, lack of motivation and inaccurate professional advice to underweight pregnant women were thought to be compounding their nutritional problems.

Actors – The key counsellor is a dietitian. The program's success derives from the relationship she establishes with the client in biweekly or, in severe cases, more frequent visits.

Analysis of the results – In a study of more than 1000 women, infants of MDD mothers had significantly higher birthweights than those of high-risk women not enrolled.

Replicability of the initiative – This program is the precursor of U.S. government programs of nutrition supplementation and education for pregnant women. A pilot project, with the MDD helping two local community service centres to apply the MDD method of nutritional counselling, appears promising at 18 months. The national foundation of the March of Dimes was impressed enough to sponsor a series of three-week internships in the program. Participants lauded the program, stressing the importance of its counselling component.

Funding – This private nonprofit corporation is a registered charity with a volunteer board and a tax exemption from both federal and provincial tax authorities. Fifteen percent of its nutrition counselling budget is raised directly from the community; the rest is obtained presumably from the United Way and government sources.

Evaluation – The MDD babies born in 1991 had half the usual evidence of low birthweight expected in a disadvantaged population, with only

4.9 percent weighing less than 2500 g. The cost of the program per pregnancy is about $300. This suggests considerable benefit in terms of reduced morbidity and costs (Wynn and Wynn 1975; Siever and O'Connell 1979; Higgins 1975; Montreal Diet Dispensary 1991).

Goal No. 2. From Birth and for at Least Three Years: Home-Visiting Programs to Support the Mothers of Children at Risk.

Home-visiting programs are an extremely useful way—and, in some cases, the only way—of successfully engaging extremely high-risk and isolated women in programs to reduce low birthweight and prematurity (Goujon, Papiernik, and Maine 1984; Olds et al. 1986a).

During the first three years of a child's life, home-based parent/child support programs also are well suited to decrease abuse and to protect the potential for competence and resiliency of children in high-risk families. At this stage, especially inexperienced parents and those without support systems of their own may accept support from home-visiting programs, or may prefer drop-in community-based child development or parenting centres able to empower them, to combat their isolation, and to help meet their own and their babies' needs. Such programs can also identify any special needs of the child, and when necessary, ensure that these needs are met by initiating and facilitating referral for comprehensive assessment. They may also provide high-quality child care, specialized programs and respite for parents of children with special needs. Descriptions of three such programs that have demonstrated their effectiveness are highlighted below.

Prenatal and Early Infancy Project (Olds)

Actions on nonmedical determinants of health – This is a home-based education program by nurses that went over more than two years. The program encouraged:
- good nutrition;
- decreased smoking;
- decreased alcohol and drug use;
- adequate rest;
- preparation for pregnancy and delivery;
- an understanding of human development, temperament, and infants' socioemotional and cognitive needs;
- enhancement of the woman's informal support network; and links with other services, including prenatal and nutritional supplementation.

Periodic health and developmental screening was also carried out. The nurses visited families an average of 8 times during pregnancy and 23 times from birth to two years. Education directed to the mother's needs at the time made up 83 percent of visiting time.

The program designers recognized that their anticipated outcomes had multiple determinants that had never been studied comprehensively using a rigorous experimental design.

Reasons for the initiative – This project was designed to decrease the number of cases of low-birthweight babies and to improve child health and development, parental functioning, and interaction among mothers who were first-time parents and/or low socioeconomic status and/or single and/or under 19 years of age. The program was delivered in a high-risk, semi-rural community with one of the highest rates of infant mortality and the highest rate of reported and confirmed child abuse in New York State.

Actors – This already classic program and study was carried out by David Olds of the University of Rochester (New York) and a team of researchers and nurses he assembled for the purpose.

Analysis of the results – This project produced many positives, especially for the mothers at greatest risk and those most intensely involved. The visited mothers smoked less, had better home environments, and made better use of childbirth classes, nutritional supplement programs and other services. Young adolescents and smokers gained more weight during their pregnancies and had heavier babies. Mothers who smoked had 75 percent fewer preterm deliveries. Visited mothers were more involved with the babies' fathers, their family, friends and service providers, and were more likely to be accompanied by a supportive person for their delivery. Their infants did better on a standardized developmental test (Bayley 1969), and visited mothers described their babies as happier and more content. Visited mothers were also less likely to abuse their child. This program conclusively shows that a sensitively and comprehensively designed nurse home-visiting program can extend the benefits of clinic-based prenatal care for socially disadvantaged women.

Replicability of the initiative – This program and study could be replicated.

Funding – This research was supported by the Bureau of Community Health Services, the Robert Wood Johnson Foundation and the W. T. Grant Foundation.

Evaluation – This project is the first randomized clinical trial of comprehensive prenatal services to prove that the social and health contexts for child bearing in severely socially disadvantaged families can be improved (Olds et al. 1986a, 1986b).

The Hawaii Healthy Start Program

Actions on nonmedical determinants of health – Since its initiation in 1985 as a demonstration project in one very high-risk community, the Hawaii Healthy Start Program has evolved into a statewide program designed to:
- promote positive parenting;
- enhance parent-child interaction;

- improve child health and development;
- prevent child abuse and neglect;
- link all families to a primary health care provider; and
- assure optimal use of community resources.

Families are identified by paraprofessional 'early identification workers' who review hospital admissions to locate families in the target area. These are then screened using a list of 15 stress indicators. Those families with high stress scores are interviewed by a trained worker and rated using the Family Stress Checklist (Kempe). Ninety-five percent of families rated 'high risk' agreed to be visited. Paraprofessional 'family support workers' meet the high-risk mothers before they leave hospital and visit them weekly for about a year, then monthly, and then four times a year until the child turns five. The frequency of family crises, the quality of parent-child interaction, the ability to use other community resources, and the results of standardized scales help workers decide when to lower the intensity of contact, to refer parents either to the family's assigned primary care provider (doctor or clinic), or to negotiate a referral to one of a range of professional services.

The visits are used to build a trusting relationship, which then serves:
– to provide child development information;
– to improve parenting skills;
– to model child-parent interaction;
– to link the family to a primary health care provider; and
– to refer to and coordinate the use of other social services.

The program has built-in mechanisms to keep staff from burning out; indeed, external reviewers have commented on the unusually high staff morale.

Reasons for the initiative – The Hawaii Healthy Start Program was designed to lower the rates of child abuse and neglect for children four and under in Hawaii from the existing level of 15/1000.

Actors – Hawaii's Healthy Start program was developed by the Hawaii Family Stress Center and carried out by professional early identification workers and paraprofessional family support workers.

Analysis of the results – In 1992, 13,377 families that were screened, assessed and served from July 1987 to July 1991 were compared with con-firmed child abuse and neglect cases and with clients of other home visiting programs. Among the 2193 well-profiled high-risk families in the program, there was no abuse in 99.2 percent of those families served. For the at-risk families that did *not* receive service, the rate of abuse was almost double the state average (29.3/1000). The rate of abuse was only 7.2/1000 in those high-risk families that did receive service, half the state average and less than the rate of abuse in families rated low risk at birth (8.7/1000). There was no further abuse in any of the families already known to child protection services when first assessed by the program. Neglect in program families (1 percent) was half that of families involved with less intensive visiting programs.

Replicability of the initiative – A structured training program trains new teams of five to eight paraprofessionals, supervisors and managers to replicate the program as it expands across the state. An evaluation of the expanded service for the period 1987–1989 reveals outstanding results (99.99 percent non-abuse rate; 99.95 percent nonneglect rate), and has shown that the model is replicable. By 1993, the families of 54 percent of Hawaii's newborns were screened through 13 sites in Hawaii at a cost of roughly $7 million, of which 75 percent is targeted for home visiting.

Funding – The Maternal and Child Health Branch of the Department of Health coordinates the program by purchasing services from seven private agencies. Despite proven success, the program has had trouble obtaining funding, and its proponents stress the need to seek multiple sources of funding—Medicaid, Zero to Three, and National Centre on Child Abuse and Neglect grants—rather than to rely exclusively on government funding.

Evaluation – Families served are compared with the high-risk population not served and with the state average, but there are no random controls. The National Committee to Prevent Child Abuse is close to completing a randomized trial evaluation, and another is planned by the Robert Wood Johnson Foundation (Breakey and Pratt 1991; Fuddy 1992).

Staying on Track

Actions on nonmedical determinants of health – Staying on Track is a community-wide early identification, tracking and referral project designed to track and assess periodically all babies born in the area from birth to 5 1/2 years of age. It was established to:
- enable all children in the community to reach their optimal physical, mental, emotional and social development;
- increase health knowledge and skills in parents and caregivers; and
- allow earlier identification of vision and communication disorders that could potentially undermine a child's education.

Public health nurses visited children and their families in their homes to observe parent-child interaction when the children were one month and six months of age. Other data on child development, parental factors, and sociodemographic information were collected by questionnaires at public health clinics and at schools when the babies were 1 1/2 years, 2 1/2 years, 3 1/2 years, 4 1/2 years and 5 1/2 years of age. As well as tracking and assessing, public health nurses assisted parents with child development problems and distributed parenting information on issues related to infants or preschoolers.

When significant difficulties in children or families were identified, the families received follow-up visits and/or referrals to appropriate local agencies. Almost half the families required additional phone calls, visits or support for feeding problems, depression, lack of resources, need for support, concerns about abuse, family or marital difficulties, and conflict. Some of these problems were minor and the families required only reassurance but others, many of which would not have been identified without the tracking system and assessments, entailed a series of visits or referral to specialized services. An advisory board from local children's service agencies met regularly to locate services for children identified by the tracking system and to coordinate services across agencies.

Reasons for the initiative – Staying on Track was based on the belief that for optimal family and child functioning during infancy and early childhood, supports must be available.

Actors – The Leeds-Grenville and Lanark Health Unit developed the program. The home visitors were public health nurses, backed up by mental health professionals.

Analysis of the results – The program found a surprisingly high proportion—22 percent—of mothers depressed after the birth of an infant. Fifteen percent were significantly depressed, and 15 percent were still depressed six months after the baby was born. The degree of family dysfunction and the number of negative incidents experienced in recent months increased the likelihood of depression. This confirmed Cowan and Cowan's 1992 finding that good communication and effective problem solving before delivery served to protect the mothers from depression. Twenty-six percent of the mothers did not feel supported by their partners at the time of the child's birth, and 29 percent felt overwhelmed by their infant. Twenty-seven percent of mothers rated their infant "below average," a finding that has been associated in the literature with poor outcomes for the child thus designated. When the children were 3 1/2 years old, 25 percent of the mothers rated their offspring as hostile/aggressive, and 22 percent rated them as anxious/fearful. Twenty-one percent of the mothers reported that their child had a significant behaviour problem.

In the final report (Landy et al. 1994), the authors reported on 600 children in three cohorts. They found that the longer a family had been in the program, the greater the improvement in the children's development, in child-parent interaction, and in the parents' sense of competence. The $400 cost per child was compared with the far greater amounts estimated by Schorr (1988) that such children, if not supported, are likely to cost society for remedial education, crime control and social assistance.

Replicability of the initiative – The program could be replicated in other areas.

Funding – Staying on Track was funded for 3 1/2 years by the Health Innovation Fund of the Ontario Premier's Council on Health, Well-Being and Social Justice. Thereafter, the project designers needed to seek additional government funding to extend the project over six years.

Evaluation – As initial funding was only available for 3 1/2 years, a cohort design was used. Since the project was designed to include all children in the community (a universal intervention), there could be no strictly experimental design with random allocation to treatment or control groups. Instead, the authors used a quasi-experimental design comparing time-lagged contrasts between age-equivalent groups (Landy et al. 1994).

Goal No. 3. During the Preschool Years: High-Quality Early Child Care and Education Can Maximize School Readiness and Control over Aggression.

The impact of poverty on health, academic performance and control over aggression can be reduced by high-quality ECCE, which promotes social, emotional and cognitive development, leading to improvements in school performance and a decrease in dropping out (Cameron 1986; MacKillop and Clarke 1989; Bertrand 1993, table 2). Yet poor children are less likely to receive high-quality ECCE, despite their greater need for it (Hayes, Palmer, and Zaslaw 1990; Pence and Goelman 1987).

Table 2
Effects of high- vs. poor-quality early child care and education

High quality	Poor quality
Increased social competence	Decreased social competence
Better language and play development	Poorer language and play development
Better control over aggression	Poorer control over aggression
Increased compliance with adults	Decreased compliance with adults
Fewer behaviour problems in Grade 1 as reported by teacher	More behaviour problems in Grade 1 as reported by teacher
Better learning orientation (the will/skills required to learn)	Poorer learning orientation (the will/skills required to learn)
Better school readiness	Poorer school readiness

Source: Data from Bertrand 1993.

The differences between good- and poor-quality ECCE have been well defined. High-quality ECCE has proven to be one of the most effective supports for resiliency in those children from highly disadvantaged familial and environmental circumstances fortunate enough to receive it (Doherty 1991). Poor-quality child care has all the disadvantages of poor parenting, and can undermine child development so severely that even excellent parenting cannot entirely compensate for it. For that reason, a guarantee of sufficient high-quality affordable ECCE for all Canadian children who need it represents one of the most effective and efficient investments the country could make to support the competence, resiliency and future productivity of disadvantaged children and youth.

The Perry Preschool Project

Actions on nonmedical determinants of health – This project provided a school-based enriched model of high-quality ECCE for multiply disadvantaged preschoolers (ages 3–6 years). The project consisted of high-quality ECCE for the children four half-days per week and a weekly visit by the teacher to the family in their home.

Reasons for the initiative – This began as a local effort in Ypsilanti, Michigan, to improve the poor school performance of disadvantaged children during the 1960s.

Actors – The High/Scope Educational Research Foundation (Ypsilanti, Michigan). The ECCE staff were certified teachers, with six children assigned to each.

Analysis of the results – Although the project is small (the sample for follow-up was just 123 children) and ended in 1967, its long-term follow-up (more than 25 years) with its extensive benefit-cost analysis still make it one of the strongest and most widely recognized longitudinal studies of the ability of high-quality ECCE to foster resiliency in poor and multiply disadvantaged children (see table 3).

Replicability of the initiative – The program, curriculum and research design are well described, making this a replicable program.

Funding – The project was government funded; it generated a benefit-cost ratio of more than 7:1.

Evaluation – The children were randomly assigned to experimental and control groups, with two minor exceptions that are not considered enough to weaken the experimental design. The children were followed up at ages 19 and 27. The program's graduates at age 27 are compared in table 2 with the performance of members of the control group at the same age (Berrueta-Clement et al. 1984; Schweinhart et al. 1993; Barnett 1993).

Goal No. 4. School-Based Programs: Helping Children Succeed in Spite of Disadvantage.

The potential of schools to protect the developmental potential and capacity for resiliency of many disadvantaged children is widely recognized. Four quite different prevention programs will be profiled here. Helping Children Adjust and the Ryerson Outreach are universal programs designed to improve outcomes for all children in the participating schools. Cities in School and the Montreal Longitudinal Study were developed to reduce specific outcomes—dropping out and serious delinquency respectively—in children identified as being at high risk.

Table 3

**Outcomes for graduates of the Perry Preschool Program at age 27
compared with a control group (no preschool)**

Arrests and convictions	Lower by 50%
Five or more arrests through age 27	Lower by 80% (7% vs. 35%)
Teenage pregnancies (and, therefore, chronic dependency)	Lower by 42%
Graduations from high school	Higher by 33%
Average monthly earnings (age 28) • earning $2000/month or more	$1219 • Four times as many (29%)
Own own home	Three times as many
Never on welfare over past 10 years	Twice as many (41% vs. 20%)
Committed to partner/children	Significantly more
Paying taxes	Significantly more
Estimated savings by age 27 for each $1.00 spent on program	$7.16

Please note: Programs marked by an asterisk (*) are ones with extremely promising design and preliminary reports, but ones in which final analysis of the data is not yet complete.

The Ryerson Outreach/Ryerson Community Initiative*

Actions on nonmedical determinants of health – Ryerson Outreach was designed to advance the well-being of the whole child—academically, socially and emotionally—by using a public school as the hub of service for its community with the active collaboration of child health, child mental health, daycare, child welfare and social service professionals serving in a school setting. Before the Ryerson Outreach program, the school operated basically on its own, seeking collaboration with external agencies or professionals on a case-by-case basis only and usually as a last resort. Previously, board of education psychologists and social workers dealt only with the academic and related needs of diagnosed children.

From the beginning of this very low budget program, the mental health consultants worked with the principal, vice-principals and school staff to:
– achieve greater understanding of children's psychosocial needs;
– involve the community as a full partner in the school;

- bridge the gaps that existed between the community, the school and different caregivers, services and programs; and
- make the school an active partner in the development of the surrounding community.

The reaching of a common agenda and the initial phase of the project are well described elsewhere (Chung, Charach, and Ferguson 1993). Social agencies were individually invited to work with the school to provide an improved service for students and families, to help develop the surrounding community, to provide nutritional, mental health and social service supports and, when necessary, improved liaison, and to expand and integrate recreational activities, out-of-school programming and community services.

Catalysts for change were staff concerns about the behaviour and unmet needs of the students; the agreed-on need for a better way for school and social agencies to combine to serve children and families with whom both were involved; and the shrinking of available funding caused by an economy in recession. There was no active resistance, although some school staff remained minimally involved while others participated enthusiastically (Bolton 1996). The vision, energy and commitment of all involved, especially the strong leadership of the principal, were crucial to the success of the program.

Reasons for the initiative – The project grew out of a desire to improve academic and social outcomes and the quality of life for children in a school in a poor, high-density, high-crime, high–drug abuse, multicultural neighbourhood in inner city Toronto. The project was intended to replicate James Comer's use of consultee-centred consultation by mental health professionals in a school setting (Comer 1985, 1988).

Actors – The project began with the Hincks Children's Mental Health Centre and the Children's Aid Society of Metropolitan Toronto donating the services of a child psychiatrist and a social work supervisor for one half-day a week to work in the school with the principal and staff. All three organizations were founding members of the Sparrow Lake Alliance (Steinhauer 1992), which brought the project together.

Analysis of the results – A survey of the teachers' opinions about changes (based on 32 returns in 1993 and 44 in 1995) is summarized in table 4. More teachers feel that students with special needs are being identified earlier, and that the gap between the identification of student needs and the delivery of help has shortened over the last two years.

Staff, however, express some concerns about their communication with, and the support they receive from, the administration compared with two years ago (Ryerson Community Outreach 1995). This may reflect a change in the style of the new principal who came to the school and the project just two years ago, but may also result from changes following from deteriorating economic conditions, and a general decrease in teacher morale not confined to this project. The prevention literature notes that, frequently,

Table 4
Highlights from the Ryerson Teacher Survey

Variable	1993	1995
Number/severity of conduct problems outside the classroom has decreased	17%	44%
Amount/severity of vandalism has decreased	17%	48%
Respect shown to teachers has increased	13%	39%
Respect shown to other students has increased	7%	41%
Respect shown school property has increased	13%	47%
Average proportion of class reported as frequently absent	13%	5%
Percentage of teachers who believe that students with special needs are being identified earlier	37%	57%

innovative prevention projects collapse when a charismatic leader leaves. This project, however, has improved its results since the originating principal retired.

Replicability of the initiative – This project will be replicated in five schools in the City of North York in September 1996, with the Ryerson principal serving as an advisor.

Funding – This is an extremely low budget project, with costs shared between the school board and the social agencies that donated the services of their staff. For one year, the Ontario Ministry of Community and Social Services funded a community worker. This funding has been withdrawn, and replacement funding is being sought in the private sector.

Evaluation – So far, the evaluative component of the program has been based on responses to a staff questionnaire. The evaluation component of this adaptation of the work of Comer in the schools of New Haven, Connecticut is currently being extended and made more rigorous through, for example, the inclusion of more objective data and the incorporation of randomization into the design. The North York replication will use the strengthened evaluation protocol and will include comparison schools in the experimental design.

Helping Children Adjust*

Actions on nonmedical determinants of health – This project was designed to compare the effectiveness of distinct types and combinations of interventions at improving the behavioural adjustment, interpersonal competence (social skills), and academic performance of public school students. It specifically targeted: troublesome or persistent antisocial behaviour that is oppositional and/or aggressive; and passive, submissive, withdrawn and overly compliant behaviour that may involve victimization. It aims to reduce the number of current behaviour problems, as well as the number of future problems. The top 10 percent of students identified in teacher and parent questionnaires were defined as "at risk" for project purposes. The project involves students between kindergarten and Grade 3 in more than 60 schools under 11 school boards across Ontario over a five-year period. One of these boards dropped out after the first year. Begun in 1990–1991, the project is now in its fifth year.

Project schools are randomly selected to become intervention sites. Each board receives a full mix of interventions that are, for the most part, built on existing resources in the school. Schools not yet selected for intervention serve as comparison sites in the interim. About the same number of children are assigned to each program. All principals, teachers and primary division students in the study schools participate. The programs include:
- a classwide social skills/behaviour management program (CSSP) combined with a parent management training program (PMT);
- an academic support program (ASP); and
- no program.

All three programs are being tested alone and in combination with others, but so few parents (less than 15 percent) used the PMT that it was soon dropped.

Reasons for the initiative – This school-based primary prevention program grew out of concern about the 8.3 percent of children between ages 4 and 11 identified by the Ontario Child Health Study (Offord et al. 1989) as having persistently troublesome externalizing behaviours, and out of concern for children who are excessively compliant.

Actors – The design was developed and the project conducted by a team from McMaster University headed by Dr. David Offord and Dr. Michael Boyle.

Analysis of the results – Final results are not yet available. This project is still going on, so that the evaluation of the data is not yet complete. It is included because of the rigour of the evaluation process.

Of the eight schools that participated in the CSSP program in the first year of the study, four have expressed interest in continuing beyond the formal commitment period. Allowing teachers to modify program components to fit their particular style increases the rate of continuation. Preliminary results reported in September 1994 (after the third year) noted interesting profiles for children who had changed schools during the program and for those whose parents did use PMT. Most teachers and a smaller majority of parents considered the CSSP and the ASP helpful, but teachers complained about the planning time and paper work involved in combined interventions.

Four schools out of 42 did not comply with the experimental design over the first four years of the study. In most cases, these failures were due to insufficient support, such as lack of resources at the board level (e.g., to cover all personnel costs associated with program delivery) or a negative administrative response at the school level (disappointment with program assignment or concern about how much time program implementation would take from teachers). The principal's enthusiastic support was crucial to success. It is possible the demands on staff to carry out a protocol handed down from above contributed to some of the negative responses.

Replicability of the initiative – The project design and research protocol are very clearly described and could be replicated.

Funding – Total cost and resources—$4 million over six years—were shared by three ministries (Health, Education, and Community and Social Services) and the school boards involved.

Evaluation – The experimental design is comprehensive, with randomized assignment of programs to the participating schools. An economic analysis will compare the cost of each intervention yielding significant improvements with the dollar savings resulting from the decreased use of special services (Boyle et al. 1994).

Cities in Schools

Actions on nonmedical determinants of health – Cities in Schools (CIS) develops community partnerships that bring resources from business, social agencies, foundations and volunteer organizations into schools to serve young people at risk of dropping out of high school. Such youth, often struggling under the weight of multiple social, economic and emotional problems, receive a program that is highly personal, accountable and coordinated. The CIS program uses small teams of caring adults working within the school to provide a highly supportive learning experience and lower the stress of social and emotional problems. Academic guidance is provided by teachers and volunteer tutors during school hours, and a service coordinator hired by the program arranges necessary social supports (e.g., financial, housing, job counselling, social counselling, health care, in-school tutoring).

Reasons for initiative – Cities in Schools, Inc. is the United States' largest nonprofit organization devoted to preventing school dropout. Pilot projects in two North York schools were set up in 1989. The organization quotes the Conference Board of Canada that decreasing the dropout rate to 10 percent by the year 2000 would save Canada $20 billion.

Actors – This is a replication of a program that has been operating in the United States for more than 30 years. The volunteers, teachers and social agency staff who provide the school-based services are described above.

Analysis of results – The program claims it can lower the dropout rate, increase the high school graduation rate, give at-risk students the skills needed in the work force, and thereby increase Canada's productivity and competitiveness. The pilot projects in North York claim to have retained in school 75 percent of the 259 students enrolled in the program.

Replicability – The North York experience shows that the program can be replicated successfully. The CIS manual entitled *The Cities in Schools Context: Concept and Strategy* contains an extremely concrete and readable description of the program and why it works, along with an unusually clear and thoughtful analysis of the procedure for and barriers commonly encountered in community mobilization.

Funding – The North York Pilot program relied for two-thirds of its funding ($1700/student) on a government grant that has since been cancelled. The other third, which the organization is working to expand, is from the corporate sector, social service agencies (which assign staff to the target schools), and the board of education (which contributes the teachers). The corporations contribute cash donations, part-time and summer jobs, computers, direct involvement as volunteer mentors, tutors and board members. The North York program is currently vulnerable because of the loss of government support.

Evaluation – CIS has an obvious outcome measure—the number of participants who do not drop out or who drop back in and stay in—and has been operating for 30 years. The retention rate in North York was 75 percent over five years (Cities in Schools, undated; Cities in Schools—North York 1995).

Montreal Longitudinal-Experimental Study of Disruptive Kindergarten Boys

Actions on nonmedical determinants of health – The study began in 1984 by assessing the behaviour of all (1037) boys in kindergarten in the 53 Franco-phone schools in the most disadvantaged neighbourhoods of Montreal. A random sample of highly disruptive kindergarten boys was enrolled in an intensive prevention program; there were two randomly allocated comparison groups of similar boys. The prevention program, starting at the end of Grade 1 and lasting two years (ages 7 to 9), included home-based parent training and school-based social skills training for the boys. Using assessments, direct observations and questionnaires, the study followed the entire sample of boys, their families and their friends annually from age 10 to 16 years.

Reasons for the initiative – To understand the development of violent behaviour in boys and to identify ways to prevent deviant development.

Actors – A team from the Research Unit on Children's Psychosocial Maladjustment, University of Montreal, headed by Dr. Richard Tremblay.

Analysis of results – The risk of being among the 8 percent most delinquent between ages 10 and 14 was nine times greater for kindergarten boys rated aggressive by two or more teachers than for those never rated aggressive. Boys rated aggressive by only one teacher were five times likelier to become delinquent than those never rated aggressive. The following forms of kindergarten behaviour (apart from aggression) were used to predict delinquent behaviour from ages 10 to 13: hyperactivity in kindergarten (best predictor); lack of anxiety (next best); and lack of altruistic behaviour. Having all three quadruples the risk for severe delinquency in early adolescence, but the strongest protective factor—the presence of altruistic behaviour—in itself decreases the level of risk by 80 percent. The association of individual characteristics of the boys in kindergarten was stronger with substance abuse by age 13 than was having deviant peers in preadolescence (see also Kellam 1990). Boys treated by the program had only half as many serious school adjustment problems up to age 15 (22 percent vs. 44 percent), and from ages 10 to 15 the treated boys reported fewer delinquent behaviours than those not treated. The more aggressive boys were also less likely to achieve to their age level in school.

Replicability of the initiative – The clear description of both the intervention and the research protocols suggest that the only barrier to replication would be financial.

Funding – Funding came from federal, provincial and municipal government agencies.

Evaluation – This is a seminal model for a selected preventive intervention with boys at high risk for serious delinquency and school failure as indicated by their kindergarten behaviour (Tremblay et al. 1995).

Goal No. 5. Programs Designed to Mobilize Disadvantaged Neighbourhoods: Transforming Them from Negative to Positive Influences That Support Successful Development.

Better Beginnings, Better Futures*

Actions on nonmedical determinants of health –This major research-prevention program is reaching 4000 families with young children at risk, up to the age of eight, in seven urban and five First Nations communities. It is designed to:

- promote cognitive, emotional and social development in children;
- prevent cognitive, emotional, social and behavioural problems in children; and
- increase the ability of high-risk communities to support healthy and competent child development.

All programs involve the community extensively in all aspects of the program, and in integrating existing and new services for children. One project has 19 people on staff and is training 16 community members who will remain in the community after the project is completed. Each community chooses a focus on infant, preschool or ecological primary school programs, which will continue for four to five years, but 85 percent of the funds must be spent on one of these, while the rest are discretionary. Each project respectfully mirrors the language and cultural traditions of its community.

Programs are designed:
- to strengthen children, through:
  - home visiting by community members to decrease the isolation of unsupported high-risk mothers,
  - before- and after-school latchkey care, and
  - support for classroom teachers;
- to strengthen families, by inviting parents to contribute any way they can (e.g., at daycare centre)
  - because "when they feel respected, they bloom",
  - and through support groups for isolated mothers (e.g., Take a Break groups; Parent to Parent groups for parents of older children); or
- to strengthen communities.

Reasons for the initiative – Better Beginnings is a comprehensive attempt to promote healthy development and prevent developmental problems in young children living in disadvantaged communities, and to help disadvantaged families and communities provide for their children.

Actors. – This project was funded by Ontario's ministries of Community and Social Services, Health, and Education, with additional funding from the federal Department of Indian and Northern Affairs and the Secretary of State.

Analysis of the results – The final results and analysis of this project have not yet been published. The researchers will follow these children for approximately 25 years, to see if they do better than children from comparable communities. Although the project is not yet complete, some valuable lessons have already been learned by the end of the fourth year.

Parents and community members are effectively participating in planning, implementing, steering and evaluating. Services are being integrated and the quality of programming is being upgraded and tailored to what the communities define as their needs. Effective home-visiting, enhanced child care, and ecological primary school programs are now in place. There is increased neighbourhood pride, the children are less stressed, more cooperative, and better clothed and fed, and parents, teachers and project staff are working together on the children's behalf. More parents are being trained, and they are dealing with their own children better.

On the other hand, there is clearly a limit to what local service integration can do while funding for services remains segmented. Also, service integration without genuine community involvement may be worse than no integration at all. It is clear that for success, there must be 50 percent volunteers/parents/community members on each major committee, enough to reflect the true diversity of each neighbourhood. The community must truly share power in all major decisions, such as job descriptions, spending and research questionnaires, rather than leaving decisions to core staff or an elite board of directors.

Replicability of the initiative – Since both the model and the research protocols are clearly described, the project could be replicated if funding was made available

Funding – The project received $7 million a year for five years from the ministries listed above.

Evaluation – The project found enormous resistance to research. People in these communities felt stigmatized, second class and researched to death without benefit to themselves or their children while their neighbourhoods continued to deteriorate. They saw the demand that they take part in research as blackmail to get necessary services that the middle class gets for free. As a compromise, the project hired site researchers living in or near the communities and set up local research committees with the power to modify forms, or veto research that they considered patronizing or irrelevant. Final results have not yet been analysed. (Ontario 1993; Peters and Russell 1993).

Growing Together*

Actions on nonmedical determinants of health – To serve multiproblem families while keeping central the needs of young children, Growing Together offers a multimodal intervention program of: 20 different services for individuals; family therapy; 14 different group programs; and seven community approaches. Workers with the program visit families after a baby is born and assess their needs and level of risk. Based on this information, families are offered a variety of services ranging from health promotion through intensive parent-infant therapy to less intensive family support, and a variety of initiatives including advocacy, entrepreneurial activities and such community development activities as outreach, community mobilization and others chosen by the residents.

Project staff are building a partnership with the community. They hope to:

- optimize the attachments, health, cognitive ability, language and social skills, school readiness, adjustment (home and school), and competence of the community's children from birth to age five;
- meet the emotional and therapeutic needs of psychiatrically disordered parents, severely dysfunctional families and substance abusers, thereby helping them develop the knowledge, skills, and stability needed for sound parenting; and
- help the parents use social services better, and build a sense of community cohesion, mutual aid, support, ownership and control needed to make the community a safe one for its residents.

Reasons for the initiative – This project was designed to improve the health, well-being and development of infants, young children and their families living in an apartment complex where one-third of the families have eight or more risk factors. Four or more factors constitute a serious risk for developmental failure. One obstacle to overcome was the sheer magnitude of the problems faced by members of the community and the damage that would be done by such an environment. The average income in the complex is only half of the city average. Only 27 percent of the families speak English in the home and interpreters were needed to translate the 18 languages used by the population. Another problem was opposition from senior public health officials to public health nurses participating in the home visits that are at the heart of the program, and to their investing so much time and energy in a single community.

Actors – Growing Together is sponsored by the Hincks Centre for Children's Mental Health, the Toronto Department of Public Health, with funding from the Invest in Kids Foundation.

Analysis of the results – Growing Together is still in its early stages, and its largely qualitative evaluation protocol is still being developed. As a result, only anecdotal evidence as to its effectiveness is available at this point. It did, however, receive the Peter Drucker Canadian Foundation Award for Innovation in the Nonprofit Sector in 1995.

Replicability of the initiative – The Invest in Kids Foundation plans to replicate the program in other sites in Canada in 1996–1997. If the replications are true to the philosophy of the original, each will have its own individual character through responding to the will of the community it serves.

Funding – A significant problem in obtaining funding has been the sensitivity of the program to individual needs, which, while essential to the integrity of the design, has made it harder to satisfy the conventional criteria set down by potential funders. Although its financing is not yet secure, it is not known whether the Invest in Kids Foundation will continue funding this original program as it expands the program to other Canadian cities.

Evaluation – Problems in designing the research protocol have been the high degree to which the program is tailored to meet the needs of individual children and families, and the conviction that it is unethical, in so needy a population, to assign residents randomly to experimental or control groups (Growing Together 1996).

IMPLICATIONS FOR POLICY

Currently, at a conservative estimate, the health, mental health, competence and future productivity of at least one in four of Canada's children and youth are being compromised by psychiatric disorders, school failure, and antisocial and violent behaviour. Also, at a time when cutbacks in employment opportunities and services are greatly increasing pressure on all but the wealthiest and most secure families, health and social service are being cut back, overcrowding and undermining both the mainstream and specialized services so badly needed by many children and families.

If we fail to help vulnerable families meet the needs of their children, especially while the windows of opportunity remain open (some of the most important of which close within the first two or three years of life), both the children whose healthy development, competence and future productivity we will have undermined and Canadian society will pay the price for the rest of those children's lives (Carnegie Corporation of New York 1994; Keating 1992; Promotion/Prevention Task Force 1996; Begley 1996). The following changes in policy *at all levels of government* will help protect the potential for resiliency of a significant number of children whose prospects would otherwise be blighted.

1. The elimination of child poverty is an excellent long-term investment, one that deserves the highest national priority.

This is crucial, not only because of Canada's existing commitment as a signatory to the *United Nations Convention on the Rights of the Child*, but also because we will pay later—and much more—for our failure to protect our children from poverty. As documented in this paper, poverty and its associated risk factors at least double the risk for most major disorders that undermine children's competence and potential. This is unacceptable for Canada as well as for its children. We, as a nation, end up paying more for medical care, remedial education, psychiatric and social services, crime control, and social assistance. We also pay through the deterioration of our social capital, with an increasingly uncivic society with unacceptably high levels of crime and violence, and through the waste of the potential productivity on which Canada's future, including its competitive edge, depends.

2. The protection of children's—and especially disadvantaged children's—developmental potential must become an integral part of economic policy at all levels of government.

Until this is so, roughly one in four of our children and youth will come off the developmental assembly line as "seconds". At a time when social policy is being made by ministers of finance, we must realize that this country has two deficits—one economic, the other social. These two deficits are inextricably intertwined, as New Zealand has demonstrated, and any attempt to correct one at the expense of the other will, ultimately, lead to aggravation of first the other, and then both.

3. At a time of diminishing resources, a high priority should be given to protecting the development of children and youth.

The quality of care that a child receives in the first three years of life is the single most important factor (excepting genetics) influencing that child's future development, health, mental health and productivity. Support for the healthy development of children should be a cornerstone of policy at all levels of government. It is easier, cheaper and more effective to get children off to a good start than to redirect them once they are already on a trajectory toward mental illness, delinquency, dropping out and chronic dependency. Those children who fail to rise above the constraints of disadvantage will continue to be a burden rather than an asset to society throughout their entire lives. It is in Canada's interest—as much as in theirs—to ensure that all children's families have the social supports needed to protect their developmental potential.

4. To achieve this goal, all levels of government should adopt and give high priority to a broadly based, comprehensive, integrated, long-term, research-based policy supportive of child development from conception through infancy, through the preschool years, through to school completion and a successful transition to the workplace.

Such a policy will require integration among policies at all levels of government, between all ministries that affect the lives of children; Justice, Immigration and Indian Affairs have just as important a role in such a policy as do Health and Human Resources. Such a policy will recognize the excellent investment in Canada's future, in both human and economic terms, represented by programs like those profiled in this paper.

Programs particularly deserving of support include those that:
- are population-based;
- derive from and respond to a clear analysis of the problem they are addressing; and
- are designed to promote health (assist development) across the life span, e.g., through prenatal supports; home visiting; ECCE; school-based programs and community mobilization programs that are:
  • research-based, in that they apply to or build on what is known, but are prepared to adapt what is known to the needs of the population being served, and
  • accountable, and have an evaluative component, but one that does not stifle the need for creativity and flexibility on the part of truly innovative service providers (see Schorr 1988, summarized in Steinhauer 1993).

5. Each level of government should commit a prescribed percentage of its revenues (1 percent) to programs that support the healthy development of children.

As we continue to adjust the service system in response to economic constraints, preference should be given to health promotion and prevention programs that:

- support isolated or at-risk mothers-to-be and new mothers through home-visiting programs for all mothers of newborns, including a prompt identification of, and ongoing involvement with, those at risk for neglecting or abusing their babies. Good models are Hawaii's Healthy Start Program and the Olds Prenatal and Early Infancy Project. As an incentive, consider Health Canada's estimated cost of supporting an abused child over a lifetime: $1 million (Children's Aid Society of Metropolitan Toronto 1995).
- provide a continuum of developmental supports similar to the model projects profiled in this chapter for parents of children at all ages;
- increase the availability of sufficient, affordable high-quality ECCE for children in families where both parents must work to avoid poverty— this should be a national priority; and
- increase funding and give priority to culturally sensitive, respectful community mobilization programs, to help them develop a sense of community, and to provide environmental support for families raising young children in high-risk areas.

6. We need a community-based strategic planning process to focus community attention on the human and economic costs of the failure to protect the development of vulnerable children and their families, especially in the first three years of life.

Much of the public opposition to ECCE and to rational, effective and efficient ways of dealing with young offenders is strongly rooted in ignorance and frustration (Ekos Research Associates 1995). People need to know what works, why it works, what will happen if we ignore disadvantaged children's developmental needs, and why the promotion of healthy child development, especially for children of disadvantaged families, makes such sense in both human and economic terms. An informed public will be more supportive of children and their developmental needs.

7. As part of this process of public education, we need to persuade the community to begin to look at children as the Europeans do— as a shared natural resource that represents society's future—rather than as most North Americans do—as solely the responsibility of their parents.

The world of the 1990s is very different from the world of the 1950s,'60s and '70s. The effect of change on family structure and functioning, and the fact that many will need assistance from society as they struggle to raise their children in increasingly difficult times, is not widely appreciated. We need our political leaders to educate the public about child poverty, ECCE and delinquency.

8. We need to establish a single base to coordinate funding for family-centred programs to strengthen families with infants and toddlers.

Innovative service providers like the initiators of the success stories described in this paper waste far too much time shopping around for funds to keep their programs viable. They are often at the mercy of funding agencies whose rigid criteria, if met, would undermine the effectiveness of the program. Growing Together is a good example of a program whose major design strengths made it harder to obtain funding. As stated in Recommendation 4, accountability should not stifle creativity or flexibility.

9. We need a national standard for social supports and services.

The change to the Canada Health and Social Transfers represents a particular threat to Canada's neediest children and their families. Not only are transfer payments being cut, but the reduced cash transfers will go primarily to the established institutions—medicare, postsecondary education—while the social assistance and social services needed to support the development of disadvantaged children and youth and their families are left out in the cold (Steinhauer 1995b).

There is a need for—and room for—well-designed cuts in some areas of social spending, but choices about where to cut should be governed by research, not ideology or public pressure (Steinhauer 1995b). But there will be no agreement on a national standard for social supports and, in the absence of one, several provinces are already turning their backs on those children and families most in need of help. There is rising opposition to national standards by many provincial governments, but if the federal government abdicates its constitutional responsibility to level the playing field (i.e., by abandoning vertical and horizontal equity), it will be ignoring what a recent poll says Canadians consider most unique about being Canadian (Gregg 1995). A positive and informed campaign to protect what Canadians clearly value might be one of our strongest weapons in the war to hold the country together.

10. We need to increase public awareness of the importance of social capital and the diminishing status of civility in our society, and to mobilize as many individuals and groups as possible to begin rebuilding the social fabric.

Dr. Paul Steinhauer *is a professor of psychiatry at the University of Toronto and a staff psychiatrist at the Hospital for Sick Children. A child psychiatrist, he has been a practicing family therapist since 1962, and for twenty years was director of postgraduate training in the Division of Child Psychiatry, University of Toronto. He has conducted research and published in the areas of family therapy, foster care, education in child psychiatry and, most recently, mental health promotion. He was the founding president of the Canadian Academy of Child Psychiatry and currently chairs two large coalitions—Sparrow Lake Alliance (www.sparrowlake.org) and Voices for Children (www.voices 4children.org)—working to promote greater health, competence, and productivity for Ontario's children, and for a better use of limited professional resources to improve outcomes for children.*

BIBLIOGRAPHY

ALLEN, M. C., DONOHUE, P. K., and DUSMAN, A. E. 1993. The limit of viability—Neonatal outcome of infants born at 22 to 25 weeks' gestation. *New England Journal of Medicine* 329: 1597–1601.

AVARD, D., and CHANCE, G. 1994. Editorial in *Journal of the Canadian Medical Association*. Quoted by D. CRANE. *Toronto Star*, Aug. 23, p. B-2.

AVISON, W. R. 1994. *Single Parenthood, Poverty and the Health of Mothers and Children: A Stress Process Analysis*. University of Western Ontario. Quoted in B. WATTIE (1996). *Statement of Concern* (revised). Toronto: Child Mental Health Committee of the Canadian Mental Health Association, Ontario Division.

BALDWIN, A. L., BALDWIN, C., and COLE, R. E. 1990. Stress-resistant families and stress-resistant children. In *Risk and Protective Factors in the Development of Psychopathology*, eds. J. ROLF, A. MASTEN, D. CICCHETTI, K. NEUCHTERLEIN and S. WINTRAUB. Cambridge: Cambridge University Press. pp. 257–280.

BARNES, G. M., and FARRELL, M. P. 1992. Parental support and control as predictors of adolescent drinking, delinquency and related problem behaviors. *Journal of Marriage and the Family* 54: 763–776.

BARNETT, W. S. 1993. Benefit-cost analysis of preschool education: Findings from a 25-year follow-up. *American Journal of Orthopsychiatry* 63: 500–508.

BARR, L. 1993. *Basic Facts on Canada, Past and Present*. Ottawa (ON). Statistics Canada publication: Catalogue no. 89–516.

BATES, A. S., FITZGERALD, J. F., DITTUS, R. S., and WOLINSKY, F. D. 1995. Risk factors for underimmunization in poor urban infants. *Journal of the American Medical Association* 272: 1105–1109.

BAUMRIND, D. 1989. Rearing competent children. In *Child Development Today and Tomorrow*, ed. W. DAMON. San Francisco: Jossey-Bass. pp. 349–378.

BAYLEY. 1969. *Scales of Infant Development*. Cleveland (OH): The Psychological Corporation.

BEARDSLEE, W. R. 1989. The role of self-understanding in resilient individuals: The development of a perspective. *American Journal of Orthopsychiatry* 59: 266–278.

BEARDSLEE, W. R., SALT, P., PORTERFIELD, K., ROTHBERG, P. C., VAN DER VELDE, P., SWATLING, S., HOKE, L., MOILANEN, D. L., and WHEELOCK, I. 1993. Comparison of preventive interventions for families with parental affective disorder. *Journal of the American Academy of Child and Adolescent Psychiatry* 32: 254–263.

BEGLEY, S. 1996. Your child's brain. *Newsweek*. Feb. 19. 54–62.

BENARD, B. 1991. *Fostering Resiliency in Kids: Protective Factors in the Family, School and Community*. Portland (OR): Northwest Regional Educational Laboratory.

BERRUETTA-CLEMENT, J. R., SCHWEINHART, L. J., BARNETT, W. S., EPSTEIN, A. S., and WEIKART, D. P. 1994. *Changed Lives: The Effects of the Perry Preschool Program on Youths through Age 19*. Monographs of the High/Scope Educational Research Foundation. Ypsilanti (MI): High/Scope Press.

BERTRAND, J. 1993. *Employers, Unions and Child Care*. Toronto: Ontario Coalition for Better Child Care.

BIEDERMAN, J., ROSENBAUM, J. F., HIRSHFELD, D. R., FARAONE, S. V., BOLDUC, E. A., GERSTEN, M., MEMINGER, S. R., KAGAN, J., SNIDMAN, N., and REZNICK, J. S. 1990. Psychiatric correlates of behavioral inhibition in young children of parents with and without psychiatric disorders. *Archives of General Psychiatry* 47: 21–26.

BOLTON, C. 1996. Personal communication.

BOYLE, M. H., OFFORD, D. R., RACINE, Y., CUNNINGHAM, C., and HUNDERT, J. 1994. *Helping Children Adjust: A Triministry Project. Annual Report. Year 3 of Implementation.* Hamilton (ON): Department of Psychiatry, McMaster University. Mimeographed document circulated by Helping Children Adjust investigators.

BREAKEY, G., and PRATT, B. 1991. Healthy growth for Hawaii's "Healthy Start": Toward a systematic statewide approach to the prevention of child abuse and neglect. *Zero to Three* 11 (April): 16–22.

BRONFENBRENNER, U. 1985. Freedom and discipline across the decades. In *Ordnung und Unordnung* (Order and disorder), eds. G. BECKER, H. BECKER, and L. HUBER. Weinheim, Germany: Beltz Verlag. pp. 326–339.

BYRNE, C., BROWNE, G., ROBERTS, J., EWART, B., SCHUSTER, M., UNDERWOOD, J., FLYNN-KINGSTON, S., RENNICK, K., GAFNI, A., WATT, S., ASHFORD, Y., and JAMIESON, E. 1996. *Interim Report for When the Bough Breaks and Benefiting the Beneficiaries of Social Assistance.* Working Paper 96-2. System-Linked Research Unit. Hamilton (ON): Health and Social Service Utilization, McMaster University.

CAMERON, V. 1986. *The Benefit-Costs of Preschool Child Care Programs: A Critical Review.* Prepared for the Special Committee on Child Care. Ottawa: Government of Canada. Unpublished. Located in Library of Parliament.

CAMPBELL, S. B. 1995. Behaviour problems in preschool children: A review of recent research. *Journal Child Psychology and Psychiatry and Allied Disciplines* 36: 113–149.

CANADA. PARLIAMENT. HOUSE OF COMMONS. STANDING COMMITTEE ON HEALTH AND WELFARE, SOCIAL AFFAIRS, SENIORS AND THE STATUS OF WOMEN. 1992. *Fetal Alcohol Syndrome: A Preventable Tragedy.* Unpublished.

CANADIAN BROADCASTING CORPORATION. 1995. The Remaking of New Zealand. Program on series *Ideas.* Toronto: CBC Radio Works. October 26 and 27.

CANADIAN COUNCIL ON SOCIAL DEVELOPMENT. 1987. *Native Crime Victims Research.* Ottawa: Unpublished working paper.

CANADIAN INSTITUTE OF ADVANCED RESEARCH. 1991. *The Determinants of Health.* CIAR publication no. 5. Toronto: The Canadian Institute of Advanced Research.

CAPALDI, D. M., and PATTERSON, G. R. In press. Interrelated influences of contextual factors on antisocial behavior in childhood and adolescence for males. In *Psychopathy and Antisocial Personality: A Developmental Perspective*, eds. D. FOWLES, P. SUTKER, and S. GOODMAN. New York: Springer Publications.

CARNEGIE CORPORATION OF NEW YORK. 1994. *Starting Points: Meeting the Needs of our Youngest Children.* Waldorf (MD): Carnegie Corporation.

CHILDREN'S AID SOCIETY OF METROPOLITAN TORONTO. 1995. *Government Cutbacks to Children's Services: The Issues and Their Impact.* (This internal report quotes the figure, but does not reference it.)

CHOMITZ, V. R., CHEUNG, L. W. Y., and LIEBERMAN, E. 1995. The role of lifestyle in preventing low birthweight. *The Future of Children* 5: 121–138.

CHUNG, R. C. Y., CHARACH, A., and FERGUSON, L. R. 1993. Ryerson Outreach: A school-based collaboration from policy to practice. Unpublished.

CICCHETTI, D., ROGOSCH, F. A., LYNCH, M., and HOLT, K. D. 1993. Resilience in maltreated children: Processes leading to adaptive outcomes. *Development and Psychopathology* 5: 629–647.

CITIES IN SCHOOLS. n.d. *The Cities in Schools Context: Part One: Concept and Strategy.*

CITIES IN SCHOOLS–NORTH YORK. 1995. *Annual Report 1994–1995.* Mimeographed copy obtainable from 44 Appian Drive, North York, ON M2J 2P9. Phone: (416) 395-8090, Fax: (416) 395-3710.

COLEMAN, J. S., and HOFFER, T. 1987. *Public and Private Schools: The Impact of Communities.* New York: Basic Books. pp. 90–91.

COMER, J. P. 1985. The Yale-New Haven Primary Prevention Project: A follow-up study. *Journal of the American Academy of Child Psychiatry* 24: 154–160

————. 1988. Educating poor minority children. *Scientific American* 259: 42–48.

COWAN, C. P., and COWAN, P. A. 1992. *When Partners Become Parents*. New York: Basic Books.

DANIELI, Y. 1994. Resilience and hope. *Children Worldwide* 21: 47–49.

DAVEY SMITH, G., BARTLEY, M., and BLANE, D. 1990. The Black Report on socioeconomic inequalities on health ten years on. *British Medical Journal* 301: 373–377.

DEMBO, R., WILLIAMS, L., WOTHKE, W., SCHMEIDLER, J., and BROWN, C. H. 1992. The role of family factors, physical abuse, and sexual victimization experiences in high-risk youths' alcohol and other drug use and delinquency: A longitudinal model. *Violence and Victims* 7: 649–665.

DODGE, K. A., PETTIT, G. S., and BATES, J. E. 1994. Socialization mediators of the relation between socioeconomic status and child conduct problems. *Child Development* 65: 649–665.

DOHERTY, G. 1991. *Factors Related to Quality in Child Care: A Review of the Literature*. Toronto: Ontario Ministry of Community and Social Services.

EGELAND, B., CARLSON, E., and SROUFE, A. 1993. Resilience as process. *Development and Psychopathology* 5: 517–528.

EKOS RESEARCH ASSOCIATES. 1995. *Rethinking Government '94: An Overview and Synthesis*. Ottawa: Ekos Research Associates, Inc. pp. 16–18.

FERGUSSON, D. M., HORFWOOD, L. J., and LYNSKEY, M. T. 1992. Family change, parental discord, and early offending. *Journal of Child Psychology and Psychiatry and Allied Disciplines* 33: 1059–1075

FINE, S. B. 1991. Resilience and human adaptability: Who rises above adversity? *The American Journal of Occupational Therapy* 45: 493–503.

FISHER, D. G. 1985. *Family Relationship Variables and Programs Influencing Juvenile Delinquency*. Ottawa: Solicitor General of Canada.

FOX, N., KIMMERLY, N. L., and SCHAFER, W. D. 1991. Attachment to mother/attachment to father: A meta-analysis. *Child Development* 62: 210–225

FUCHS, V. R., and REKLIS, D. M. 1994. *Mathematical Achievement in Eighth Grade: Interstate and Racial Differences*. NBER Working Paper no. 4784. Stanford (CA): NBER. Obtainable from NBER, 204 Junipero Serra Blvd., Stanford, CA 94305.

FUDDY, L. J. 1992. *Hawaii Healthy Start Successful in Preventing Child Abuse*. Mimeograph. Honolulu: Loretta J. Fuddy, 741 A Sunset Avenue, HI 96816.

GABEL, S., and SHINDLEDECKER, R. 1993. Characteristics of children whose parents have been incarcerated. *Hospital and Community Psychiatry* 44: 656–660.

GARBARINO, J., DUBROW, N., KOSTELNY, K., and PARDO, C. 1992. Resilience and coping in children at risk. In *Children in Danger: Coping with the Consequences of Community Violence*. San Francisco: Jossey-Bass. (A joint publication in the Jossey-Bass social and behavioral science series and the Jossey-Bass education series.) pp. 100–114.

GARCIA-COLL, C., KAGAN, J., and REZNICK, J. S. 1984. Behavioural inhibition in young children. *Child Development* 55: 1005–1019.

GARMEZY, N. 1991a. Resiliency in children's adaptation to negative life events and stressed environments. *Pediatric Annals* 20: 462–466

————. 1991b. Resiliency and vulnerability to adverse developmental outcomes associated with poverty. *American Behavioral Scientist* 34: 416–430.

————. 1993. Children in poverty: Resilience despite risk. *Psychiatry* 56: 127–136.

GARMEZY, N., and MASTEN, A. 1991. The protective role of competence indicators in children at risk. In *Perspectives on Stress and Coping*, eds. E. M. CUMMINGS, A. L. GREENE and K. H. KARRAKEI. Hillsdale (NJ): Erlbaum Associates. pp. 151–174.

GOODYER, I. M. 1990. Family relationships, life events and childhood psychopathology. *Journal of Child Psychology and Psychiatry* 31: 161–192.

GOUJON, H., PAPIERNIK, E., and MAINE, D. 1984. The prevention of preterm delivery through prenatal care: An intervention study in Martinique. *American Journal of Obstetrics and Gynecology* 155: 939–946.

GREGG, A. 1995. Poll result quoted in A quiet passion. *Maclean's*, 1 July, 8–15.

GRIBBLE, P., COWEN, E., WYMAN, P., WORK, W., WANNON, M., and RAOOF, A. 1993. Parent and child views of parent-child relationship qualities and resilient outcomes among urban children. *Journal of Child Psychology and Psychiatry and Allied Disciplines* 34: 507–519.

GRIFFITHS, C. T., and YERBURY, J. C. 1995. Understanding Aboriginal crime and criminality: A case study. In *Canadian Criminology*, eds. M. A. JACKSON and C. T. GRIFFITHS. Toronto: Harcourt Brace and Co. pp. 383–397.

GROWING TOGETHER. 1996. Mimeo obtainable from Growing Together, 260 Wellesley Street E., Suites 103 and 104, Toronto, ON M4X 1G5.

HACK, M., TAYLOR, H. G., KLEIN, N., EIBEN, R., SCHATSCHNEIDER, M. A., and MERCURI-MINICH, B. S. 1994. School-age outcomes in children with birthweights under 750 g. *New England Journal of Medicine* 331: 753–759.

HANVEY, L., AVARD, D., GRAHAM, I., UNDERWOOD, K., CAMPBELL, J., and KELLY, C. 1994. *The Health of Canada's Children: A CICH Profile*. 2nd ed. Ottawa: Canadian Institute of Child Health.

HAYES, C., PALMER, J., and ZASLOW, M. Eds. 1990. *Who Cares for America's Children: Child Care Policy for the 1990s*. Washington (DC): National Academy Press.

HENGGELER, S. W., and BORDUIN, C. M. 1990. *Family Therapy and Beyond: A Multisystemic Approach to Treating the Behavior Problems of Children and Adolescents*. Pacific Grove (CA): Brooks/Cole. (Out of print, but available from the Family Services Resource Center, Department of Psychiatry and Behavioral Sciences, Medical University of South Carolina, Charleston, SC 29425-0742.)

HERTZMAN, C., FRANK, J., and EVANS, R. 1990. *Heterogeneities in Health Status*. CIAR internal document no. 3C. Toronto: Canadian Institute for Advanced Research.

HEWLETT, S. A. 1991a. Mainstream kids and the time deficit. Chapter in *When the Bough Breaks: The Cost of Neglecting Our Children*. New York: Harper Perennial. pp. 77–123.

———. 1991b. *When the Bough Breaks: The Cost of Neglecting Our Children*. New York: Harper Perennial. pp. 110–118.

HIGGINS, A. C. 1975. Nutritional status and the outcome of pregnancy. *The Journal of the Canadian Dietetic Association* 37: 17–35.

HINCHEY, F. S., and GAVELEK, J. R. 1982. Empathic responding in children of battered women. *Child Abuse and Neglect* 6: 148–153.

HIRSHFELD, D. R., ROSENBAUM, J. F., BIEDERMAN, J., BOLDUC, E. A., FARAONE, S. V., SNIDMAN, N., REZNICK, J. S., and KAGAN, J. 1992. Stable behavioral inhibition and its association with anxiety disorder. *Journal of the American Academy of Child and Adolescent Psychiatry* 31: 103–111.

INSTITUTE OF MEDICINE. 1985. *Preventing Low Birth-Weight*. Washington (DC): National Academy Press.

JACOBSON, F. W., and FRYE, K. F. 1991. Effect of maternal social support on attachment. Experimental evidence. *Child Development* 62: 572–582.

JAFFE, P., WOLFE, D. A., WILSON, S., and ZAK, L. 1986. Similarities in behavioral and social maladjustment among child victims and witnesses to family violence. *American Journal of Orthopsychiatry* 56: 142–146.

JONES, M. B., and OFFORD, D. R. 1989. Reduction of antisocial behaviour in poor children by non-school skill development. *Journal of Child Psychology and Psychiatry and Allied Disciplines* 30: 737–750.

KAGAN, J., REZNICK, J. S., and SNIDMAN, N. 1987. The physiology and psychology of behavioural inhibition in children. *Child Development* 58: 1459–1473.

KAUFMAN, J., COOK, A., ARNY, L., JONES, B., and PITTINSKY, T. 1994. Problems defining resiliency: Illustrations from the study of maltreated children. *Development and Psychopathology* 6: 215–229.

KEATING, D. P. 1992. *Developmental Determinants of Health and Well-Being in Children and Youth*. Working paper prepared for the Premier's Council on Health, Well-Being and Social Justice. Toronto.

KELLAM, S. 1990. *Perspectives on Identifying and Explaining Resilience.* Address to the Fifth Family Research Consortium, June 1–4. Monterey, California. Unpublished.

KOCHANSKA, G. 1991. Patterns of inhibition to the unfamiliar in children of normal and affectively ill mothers. *Child Development* 62: 250–263.

KRAMER, M. S. 1987. Determinants of low birthweight: Methodological assessment and meta-analysis. *Bulletin of the World Health Organization* 65: 663–737.

LANDY, S., PETERS, R. DeV., ALLEN, A. B., BROOKS, F., and JEWELL, S. 1994. Evaluation of "Staying on Track": An early identification, tracking, intervention referral system for infants, young children and families. *IMPrint* 9: 18–19.

LAST, C. G., HERSEN, M., KAZDIN, A. E., FINKELSTEIN, R., and STRAUSS, C. C. 1987. Comparison of DSM-III separation anxiety and overanxious disorders: Demographic characteristics and patterns of comorbidity. *Journal of the American Academy of Child and Adolescent Psychiatry* 26: 527–531.

LEWIS, D. O., SHANOK, S. S., GRANT, M., and RITVO, E. 1983. Homicidally aggressive young children: Neuropsychiatric and experiential correlates. *American Journal of Psychiatry* 140: 148–153.

LOEBER, R., and KEENAN, K. 1995. Developmental pathways in boys' disruptive and delinquent behaviour. *Youth Update* 13: 4–5.

LUTHAR, S., and ZIGLER, E. 1992. Intelligence and social competence among high-risk adolescents. *Development and Psychopathology* 4: 287–299.

LUTHAR, S. S., DOERNBERGER, C. H., and ZIGLER, E. 1993. Resilience is not a unidimensional construct: Insights from a prospective study of inner-city adolescents. *Development and Psychopathology* 5: 703–717.

MACKILLOP, B., and CLARKE, M. 1989. *Safer Tomorrows Begin Today.* Ottawa: Canadian Council on Children and Youth.

MAGNUSSON, D., KLINTEBERG, D., and STATTON, H. 1991. *Autonomic Activity, Reactivity, Behavior and Crime in a Longitudinal Perspective.* Report no. 738. Stockholm (Sweden): Department of Psychology, Stockholm University.

MAIN, M., and GOLDWYN, R. 1984. Predicting rejection of her infant from mother's representation of her own experience: Implications for the abused-abusing intergenerational cycle. *Journal of Child Abuse and Neglect* 8: 203–217.

MANASSIS, K., and BRADLEY, S. 1994. The development of childhood anxiety disorders: Toward an integrated model. *Journal of Applied Developmental Psychology* 15: 345–366.

MANASSIS, K., BRADLEY, S. J., GOLDBERG, S., HOOD, J., and SWINSON, R. P. 1994. Patterns of attachment in mothers with anxiety disorders and their children. *Journal of the American Academy of Child and Adolescent Psychiatry* 33: 1106–1113.

MANNUZZA, S., KLEIN, R. G., BESSLER, A., MALLOY, P., and LAPADULA, M. 1993. Adult outcome of hyperactive boys: Educational achievement, antisocial behaviour, and psychiatric status in adulthood. *Archives of General Psychiatry* 50: 565–576.

MARMOT, M. G., KOGEVINAS, M., and EVANS, R. 1987. Social/economic status and disease. *Annual Review of Public Health* 8: 111–135.

MATTHEWS, F. 1993. *Youth Gangs.* Ottawa: Brighter Futures (Health Canada), Solicitor General of Canada and Department of Justice.

MATTOX, W. R. 1990. The family time famine. *Family Policy* 3:2. See also MATTOX, W. R. 1991. The parent trap: So many bills, so little time. *Policy Review* 55: 6–13.

MCCORMICK, M. C., GORTMAKER, S. L., and SOBOL, A. M. 1990. Very low birthweight children: Behavior problems and school difficulties in a national sample. *Journal of Pediatrics* 117: 687–693.

MCCUBBIN, H. I., MCCUBBIN, M. A., and THOMPSON, A. I. 1992. Resiliency in families: The role of family schema and appraisal in family adaptation to crises. In *Family Relations: Challenges for the Future*, ed. T. H. BRUBAKER. Newbury Park (CA): Sage Publications. pp. 153–177.

MELTZER, L. J., LEVINE, M. D., KARNISKI, W., PALFREY, J. S., and CLARKE, S. 1984. An analysis of the learning style of adolescent delinquents. *Journal of Learning Disabilities* 17: 600–608.

MESSER, S. C., and BEIDEL, D. C. 1994. Psychosocial correlates of childhood anxiety disorder. *Journal of the American Academy of Child and Adolescent Psychiatry* 33: 975–983.

MINDE, K. 1980. Bonding of parents to premature infants: Theory and practice. In *Parents-Infants Relationships*, ed. P. M. TAYLOR. Monographs in Neonatology Series. New York: Grune and Stratton. pp. 291–313.

MONTREAL DIET DISPENSARY. 1991. *111th Annual Report, 1990–1991*. Montreal: Montreal Diet Dispensary.

MOORE, T., PEPLER, D., MAE, R., and KATES, M. 1989. Effects of family violence in children: New directions for research and intervention. In *Intervening with Assaulted Women: Current Theory, Research and Practice*, eds. B. PRESSMAN, G. CAMERON, and M. ROTHERY. Hillsdale: Lawrence Erlbaum Associates. pp. 75–92.

NATIONAL CENTER FOR YOUTH WITH DISABILITIES. 1991. *CYDLINE reviews: Vulnerability and Resiliency: Focus on Children with Disabilities*. Minneapolis (MN).

OFFORD, D. R., BOYLE, M. H., FLEMING, J. E., MUNROE BLUM, H., and RAE GRANT, N. I. 1989. The Ontario Child Health Study: Summary of selected results. *Canadian Journal of Psychiatry* 34: 483–491.

OLDS, D. L., HENDERSON, C. R., TATELBAUM, R., and CHAMBERLIN, R. 1986a. Improving the delivery of prenatal care and outcomes of pregnancy: A randomized trial of nurse home visitation. *Pediatrics* 77: 16–28.

OLDS, D. L., HENDERSON, C. R., CHAMBERLIN, R., and TATELBAUM, R. 1986b. Preventing child abuse and neglect: A randomized trial of nurse home visitation. *Pediatrics* 78: 65–78.

ONTARIO. MINISTRY OF COMMUNITY AND SOCIAL SERVICES. 1993. *Better Beginnings, Better Futures: 1993 Progress Report, Description and Lessons Learned*. Toronto: Queen's Printer for Ontario.

ONTARIO MENTAL HEALTH FOUNDATION. 1994. *Ontario Health Survey: Mental Health Supplement*. Toronto: Ontario Ministry of Health. Figs. 10–14, pp. 12–14.

PANETH, N. S. 1995. The problem of low birthweight. *The Future of Children* 5:19–34.

PAPE, B., BYRNE, C., IVASK, A., KUCZINSKI, L., MALLETTE, C., BROWNE, G., and RAE GRANT, N. 1996. *Analysis of the Impact of Affective Disorders on Families and Children*. Submitted to Strategic Fund for Children's Mental Health, Health Canada, Ottawa.

PAPIERNIK, E. 1984. Proposals for a programmed prevention policy of preterm birth. *Clinical Obstetrics and Gynecology* 27: 614–635.

PAPIERNIK, E., BOUYER, J., YAFFE, K., WINISDORFFER, G., COLLIN, D., and DREYFUS, J. 1986. Women's acceptance of a preterm birth prevention program. *International Journal of Obstetrics and Gynecology* 22: 339–343.

PAPIERNIK, E., BOUYER, J., DREYFUS, J., COLIN, D., WINISDORFFER, G., GUEGEN, S., LECOMTE, M., and LAZAR, P. 1985. Prevention of preterm births: A perinatal study in Haguenau, France. *Pediatrics* 76: 154–158.

PEDERSEN, W. 1994. Parental relations, mental health and delinquency in adolescence. *Adolescence* 29: 975–990.

PENCE, A., and GOELMAN, H. 1987. Silent partners: Parents of children in three types of day care. *Early Childhood Research Quarterly* 2: 108–118.

PERRY, B. D. In press. Incubated in terror: Neurodevelopmental factors in the "Cycle of Violence". In *Children, Youth and Violence: Searching for Solutions*, ed. J. D. OSOFSKY. New York (NY): Guilford Press.

PETERS, R. De V., and RUSSELL, C. C. 1993. *Better Beginnings, Better Futures Project: Model, Program and Research Overview*. Toronto: Queen's Printer for Ontario.

PHILP, M. 1995. Studies roll back rosy view of divorce. *Globe and Mail*, 15 July.

PREVENTION AND CHILDREN COMMITTEE. 1995. *A Compendium of Approaches from across Canada*. Ottawa (ON): The National Crime Prevention Council.

PROMOTION/PREVENTION TASK FORCE, SPARROW LAKE ALLIANCE. 1996. *The Primary Needs of Children: A Blueprint for Effective Health Promotion at the Community Level.* Ottawa: The Caledon Institute of Social Policy.

PUTNAM, R. 1993. *Making Democracy Work.* Princeton (NJ): Princeton University Press.

RAE-GRANT, N. 1991. Primary prevention. In *Child and Adolescent Psychiatry: A Comprehensive Textbook,* ed. M. LEWIS. Baltimore: Williams and Wilkins. pp. 918–929.

RAINE, A., VENABLES, P. H., and WILLIAMS, M. 1990. Relationships between central and autonomic measures of arousal at 15 and criminality at age 24 years. *Archives of General Psychiatry* 47: 3–7.

REEVES, J. C., WERRY, J. S., ELKIND, G. S., and ZAMETKIN, A. 1987. Attention deficit, conduct, oppositional, and anxiety disorders in children. II: Clinical characteristics. *Journal of the American Academy of Child and Adolescent Psychiatry* 26: 144–155.

REICH, W., EARLS, F., FRANKEL, O., and SHAYKA, J. J. 1993. Psychopathology in children of alcoholics. *Journal of the American Academy of Child and Adolescent Psychiatry* 32: 995–1002.

RESNICK, M. D., HARRIS, L. J., and BLUM, R. W. 1993. The impact of caring and connectedness on adolescent health and well-being. *Journal of Paediatrics and Child Health* 29 (suppl. 1): S3–S9.

RICHARDSON, J. L., DWYER, K., MCGUIGAN, K., HANSEN, W. B., DENT, C., JOHNSON, C. A., SUSSMAN, S. Y., BRANNON, B., and FLAY, B. 1989. Substance abuse among eighth-grade students who take care of themselves after school. *Pediatrics* 84: 556–566.

RICHTERS, J. E., and MARTINEZ, P. E. 1993. Violent communities, family choices, and children's chances: An algorithm for improving the odds. *Development and Psychopathology* 5: 609–627.

RODGERS, B. D. 1989. Substance abuse in pregnancy. *The Add-On Journal of Continuing Medical Education* 38: 6865–6871.

ROSS, D. P., SHILLINGTON, E. R., and LOCHHEAD, C. 1994. *The Canadian Fact Book on Poverty– 1994.* Ottawa (ON): Canadian Council on Social Development.

RUBIN, K. H. 1982. Social and social-cognitive developmental characteristics of young isolated, normal and sociable children. In *Peer Relationships and Social Skills in Childhood,* eds. K. H. RUBIN, and H. S. ROSS. New York: Springer-Verlag. pp. 353–374.

RUSH, D., and CASSANO, P. 1983. Relationship of cigarette smoking and social class to birthweight and perinatal mortality among all births in Britain, 5–11 April 1970. *Journal of Epidemiology and Community Health* 37: 249–255.

RUTTER, M. 1979a. Invulnerability, or why some children are not damaged by stress. In *New Directions in Children's Mental Health,* ed. S. J. SHAMSIE. New York: Spectrum. pp. 53–75.

———. 1979b. Protective factors in children's responses to stress and disadvantage. In *Primary Prevention of Psychopathology,* eds. M. W. KENT, and J. E. ROLF. Hanover (NH): University Press of New England. pp. 49–74.

RUTTER, M., and QUINTON, D. 1984. Parental psychiatric disorder effects on children. *Psychology Medicine* 14: 853–880.

RUTTER, M., MAUGHAN, B., MORTIMER, P., and OUSTON, J. 1979. *Fifteen Thousand Hours: Secondary Schools and Their Effects on Children.* Cambridge (MA): Harvard University Press.

RYERSON COMMUNITY OUTREACH. 1995. Key findings of the Ryerson Teacher Survey: Changes between 1993 and 1995. Mimeographed sheet. Copy obtainable from author.

SCHNEIDER, J., GRIFFITH, D., and CHASNOFF, I. 1989. Infants exposed to cocaine in utero: Implications for developmental assessment and intervention. *Infants and Young Children* 42: 25–36.

SCHORR, L. 1988. *Within Our Reach: Breaking the Cycle of Disadvantage.* New York: Doubleday.

SCHWEINHART, L. J., BARNES, H. V., WEIKART, D. P., BARNETT, W. S., and EPSTEIN, A. S. 1993. *Significant Benefits: The High/Scope Perry Preschool Study through Age 27.* Ypsilanti (MI): High/ Scope Press.

SCRIVENER, L. 1994. Why we all spend more time at the office…"Slaves" of the '90s caught in job world. *Toronto Star,* 11 December.

SHEPPARD, J. A., and KASHANI, J. H. 1991. The relationship of hardiness, gender, and stress to health outcomes in adolescents. *Journal of Personality* 59: 747–768.

SHIONO, P. H., and BEHRMAN, R. E. 1995. Low birthweight: Analysis and recommendations. *The Future of Children* 5: 4–18.

SHIONO, P. H., KLEBANOFF, M. A., GRAUBARD, B., BERENDES, H. W., and RHOADS, G. G. 1986. Birthweight among women of different ethnic groups. *Journal of the American Medical Association* 255: 48–52.

SIEVER, A., and O'CONNELL, P. 1979. *Urban Health.* Montreal: The Montreal Diet Dispensary. pp. 31–34.

SINNEMA, G. 1991. Resilience among children with special health care needs among their families. *Pediatric Annals* 20: 483–486.

STEINHAUER, P. D. 1992. The Sparrow Lake Alliance. *The Canadian Child Psychiatric Bulletin* 1: 24–27.

———. 1993. Primary prevention strategies for disadvantaged populations. In *The Health Needs of Disadvantaged Children and Youth: Ninth Canadian ROSS Conference in Paediatrics*, eds. M. COX and J. DORVAL (page 19 speaks to this point directly). Montreal: Ross Laboratories. pp. 15–27.

———. 1995a. The effect of growing up in poverty on developmental outcomes in children: Some implications of the revision of the social security system. *Canadian Child Psychiatry Bulletin* 4: 32–39.

———. 1995b. *The Canada Health and Social Transfer: A Threat to the Health, Development and Future Productivity of Canada's Children and Youth.* Ottawa: Caledon Institute of Social Policy.

———. 1996. *Model for the Prevention of Delinquency.* Ottawa: The National Crime Prevention Council.

STEINHAUER, P. D., SANTA-BARBARA, J., and SKINNER, H. 1984. The process model of family functioning. *The Canadian Journal of Psychiatry* 29: 77–88.

SYLVA, K. 1994. School influences on children's development. *Journal of Child Psychology and Psychiatry* 35: 135–170.

THAPAR, A., and McGUFFIN, P. 1995. Are anxiety symptoms in childhood heritable? *Journal of Child Psychology and Psychiatry* 36: 439–447.

TREMBLAY, R., PIHL, R. O., VITARO, F., and DOBKIN, P. L. 1994. Predicting early onset of male antisocial behaviour from preschool behaviour. *Archives of General Psychiatry* 51: 732–739.

TREMBLAY, R. E., KURTZ, L., MASSE, L. C., VITARO, F., and PIHL, R. O. 1995. A bimodal prevention program for disruptive kindergarten boys: Its impact through mid-adolescence. *Journal of Consulting and Clinical Psychology* 63(4): 560–568.

TREMBLAY, R. E., ZHOU, R. M., GAGNON, C., VITARO, F., and BOILEAU, H. 1991. Violent boys: Development and prevention. *Forum on Corrections Research* 3: 29–35.

TURNER, S. M., BEIDEL, D. C., and COSTELLO, A. 1987. Psychopathology in the offspring of anxiety disordered patients. *Journal of Consulting and Clinical Psychology* 55: 229–235.

U. S. DEPARTMENT OF HEALTH AND HUMAN SERVICES, PUBLIC HEALTH SERVICE EXPERT PANEL ON THE CONTENT OF PRENATAL CARE. 1989. *Caring for Our Future: The Content of Prenatal Care.* Washington (DC): DHHS.

VANDERBERG, S. A., WEEKES, J. R., and MILLSON, W. A. 1995. Early substance abuse and its impact on adult offender alcohol and drug problems. *Forum on Corrections Research* 7(1): 14–16.

VANIER INSTITUTE OF THE FAMILY. 1994. *Canadian Families* (brochure). Ottawa: Vanier Institute of the Family.

WATKINS, S. C., MENKEN, J. A., and BONGAARTS, J. 1987. Demographic foundations of family change. *American Psychological Review* 52: 346–358.

WEISSMAN, M. M., GAMMON, G. D., JOHN, K., MERIKANGAS, K. R., WARNER, V., PROSOFF, B. A., and SHALOMSKAS, D. 1987. Children of depressed parents: Increased psychopathology and early onset of major depression. *Archives of General Psychiatry* 44: 847–853.

WERNER, E. E. 1984. Resilient children. *Young Children* 40: 68–72.

WIDOM, C. S. 1989. The cycle of violence. *Science* 244 (14 April): 160–166.

WILLIAMS, P. G., WIEBE, D. J., and SMITH, T. W. 1992. Coping processes as mediators of the relationship between hardiness and health. *Journal of Behavioral Medicine* 15: 237–255.

WOLIN, S. J., and WOLIN, S. 1993. *The Resilient Self.* New York: Villard Books/Random House.

WYNN, M., and WYNN, A. 1975. *Nutritional Counselling in the Prevention of Low Birth-Weight: Some Conclusions about Ante-Natal Care Following a Visit to Canada.* London: Foundation for Education and Research in Child Rearing.

Prevention of Child Abuse and Neglect

DAVID A. WOLFE, PH.D.

Professor of Psychology and Psychiatry
University of Western Ontario

SUMMARY

Key Conclusions Related to Determinants of Health

Children are most often maltreated early in infancy, when their parents first assume the role of caring for them, and during early childhood, when parents face the task of socializing them. Abuse or neglect of a child also often accompanies instability or disruption in the family, or the family's prolonged detachment from social supports and services.

Preventing child abuse and maintaining healthy families therefore requires the promotion of positive child-rearing methods and healthy parent-child relationships. This can be achieved in a manner that is congruent with the needs of each family and community and responsive to situational and developmental changes in the parent-child relationship.

Interventions with parents of maltreated children were once based on an individual-focused, pathology model. Gradually, the model has given way to a more holistic, environmental one, with a growing emphasis on the importance of the parent-child relationship and its context. At the same time, the orientation toward treatment has shifted from one of deviance to one that recognizes the vast number of stress-creating factors that impinge on the developing parent-child relationship.

Although we can now identify many of the early indicators that presage the transition of families toward child abuse and neglect, our child welfare systems do not use such knowledge to assist families at risk. Most services to families with abused or neglected children favour protection of the child over treatment for the family. This use of resources fails the larger number of parents who are at risk of abusing or neglecting their children and who would benefit from early intervention. Generally, a family's first contact with the system is precipitated by a "crisis".

While treatment models have greatly improved and have contributed to better outcomes, practitioners remain torn between acting on promising research findings and serving immediate needs for child protection and welfare.

Current theories of child maltreatment favour promoting parental competence and reducing the burden of stress on families. Proponents of these theories conclude that early intervention services should be designed and implemented with a view to enhancing:

– parents' knowledge of child development and the demands of parenting;
– parents' ability to cope with stress related to caring for small children;
– parent-child attachment and communication;
– parents' knowledge of home management; and
– families' access to social and health services.

These theorists also maintain that services should help families reduce or redistribute their child care burden.

Interventions that seek to reduce child abuse and neglect among high-risk parents and children have developed considerably in the past two decades. According to the literature:

* *Intensive group interventions and home visits that provide support and instruction in child management and/or child cognitive stimulation improve parents' attitudes and behaviours and enhance maternal adjustment.*
* *Programs that provide consistent (not necessarily lengthy), child development-focused interventions improve both children's cognitive abilities and their behavioral adjustment.*
* *Family support programs improve general maternal functioning.*
* *Compared with less intensive services, multidimensional programs—those offering an array of services, as parents require, over a longer period—for higher-risk families are worth the additional effort and expense.*

Overall, one- to three-year, personalized programs, e.g., those that offer home visits, are most successful in achieving the desired outcomes, and are especially successful with higher-risk individuals. Parents' need for support, parenting instruction and access to resources seems to be fulfilled by the personalized nature of the home visitor approach.

One success story in the field of child maltreatment prevention is the ongoing work of David Olds, which began in the late 1970s in upstate New York. Subjects are first-time parents who also possess one or more of the risk factors for child abuse; i.e., they are teenaged, single, or poor. The program offers varying degrees of child care services to participants, as well as prenatal and postnatal home visits by a nurse who provides child development education and refers the client to appropriate resources.

Interventions seek to capitalize on the mother's strengths and abilities, rather than merely to assess her deficits. This translates into an empowerment strategy, in which each woman receives help in understanding and meeting her own needs, as well as those of her newborn child. She is taught the skills necessary to enhance her relationship with her child and to further her own self-development.

The initiative addresses several psychological, social and economic determinants of health; mothers improve their understanding of child health and development and change their expectations about their own development. The program enhances self-efficacy in the mothers by developing their strengths and confidence. Health workers form close, therapeutic ties with the mother and other family members during pregnancy, building effective relationships with their clients by focusing on the strengths of family members and addressing issues of concern them. Family stressors are identified, and families are given help obtaining health and human services, including financial assistance, subsidized housing, family counselling, nutritional supplementation, clothing, furniture and adequate medical care.

The program has been replicated in three U.S. cities, and a similar program is being tested in Hamilton, Ontario. The evidence to date suggests that the results are replicable in different settings, although variations in local environments should be carefully reviewed before a program site is selected. The program developers emphasize that understanding better how to manage variations in local environments to ensure that the essential elements of the program are reproduced is an important consideration in the dissemination of this method.

Policy Implications

Children at developmental risk due to conditions that accompany child maltreatment need positive relationships with adults. These relationships provide the teaching opportunities that prevent developmental harm and promote healthy adaptation. Children who are maltreated are generally denied the opportunities for guidance that are most apt to produce forward movement; they live in conditions of high stress and benefit from few resources. Such high-stress, low-support social environments deserve the highest priority in social policy making; the children in these environments are least likely to tolerate maltreatment or further developmental interference. The prescription for the prevention of child abuse and neglect offered in this paper is based on an ethic of inclusion and support, rather than one of mere interception and protection. Such an approach assumes that the primary needs of children and families (and a reduction in the incidence of child maltreatment), are well served through supportive communities and neighbourhoods. Success requires diligent planning and action to ensure that communities and families receive support at the optimal time. Achieving the desired results will not be easy. It will involve a reversal of powerful social trends within neighbourhoods at highest risk and in the nation as a whole.

Federal government policy should therefore stimulate initiatives that are:
- *sufficiently intensive and diverse to provide communities with the support and resources necessary to put into place comprehensive, neighbourhood-based, child-centred and family-focused programs; and*
- *sufficiently flexible that such efforts can be adapted to meet the needs and capitalize on the strengths of rural, urban, cultural and ethnic communities in various regions of the country, including Aboriginal communities.*

New policies should also reflect programmatic emphases on child abuse and neglect across many different federal and provincial agencies, with the intent of fostering involvement by different professional groups, administrators and practitioners.

A major research initiative should be established that can be carried out by provincial and regional centres.

Funding structures should be simplified to permit the development of neighbourhood-based, child protection and family support efforts through a unified interagency plan.

Policies should favour a movement toward universal voluntary prenatal and neonatal home visits. The first step in such a plan would be the funding of numerous, coordinated pilot projects with sufficient funding to permit both outcome and impact evaluations on diverse sectors of the population. Such projects should seek to determine what is needed (at a federal level), to establish and administer a national, home visitation system.

A national strategy should:
- *strengthen and support urban, suburban and rural neighbourhoods in ways that meet the needs of children and families;*
- *reorient service delivery to make it as easy to provide child maltreatment prevention services to families as it currently is to remove children from their homes and place them in foster care;*
- *further develop public health and health promotion approaches to the prevention of child abuse and neglect;*
- *develop programs that provide child development and parenting information that is easily understood, practical, and accessible to present and prospective parents; and*
- *undertake a comprehensive analysis of the total cost of child maltreatment across all government agencies and the savings achieved by home visitation programs.*

Since many of the factors that result in child maltreatment affect the health and functioning of the majority of families, a national strategy should address the causes of child abuse and neglect from a public health perspective, rather than through tertiary intervention.

TABLE OF CONTENTS

KEY CONCLUSIONS FROM THE LITERATURE

Definition and Prevalence of Child Abuse and Neglect

An adequate definition of child abuse and neglect is essential to research on the etiology and course of child maltreatment, and is central to the entire system of detection, prevention and service delivery to problem families. Communities must identify those children and families in need of help, while educating all community members in acceptable and unacceptable forms of child rearing. However, despite public outcry and disdain for child maltreatment, efforts to define child abuse and neglect have been fraught with controversy, and resultant definitions have proven inadequate. The controversy exists in part because the nature of child maltreatment requires that its definition be applied with considerable discretion.

Child abuse is so complex an issue that both professionals and the public have difficulty determining what is and is not acceptable treatment of children by caregivers. Consequently, actions to address child abuse have vacillated in response to public sentiment, highly publicized cases, new legislation and promising treatment methods. Both legal definitions and research definitions of *physical abuse* have made considerable effort to include much detail about the types of physical evidence that constitute abuse, the behaviours that characterize an abused child, and the pervasive and longstanding psychological and developmental consequences of inadequate (i.e., abusive, neglectful, inappropriate), child rearing (Mash and Wolfe 1991).

These gains notwithstanding, different definitions of maltreatment have emerged in the past 20 years. They have been refined to reflect the needs of organizations, community agencies, researchers or legislators. Municipalities and states, for example, often adopt a definition that focuses largely on evidentiary criteria to facilitate prosecution of an offender or state action on behalf of a child. Treatment providers, on the other hand, may weigh other criteria more heavily in determining what they consider to be an act of abuse or neglect.

Child maltreatment is broadly defined as *the physical or mental injury, sexual abuse or exploitation, negligent treatment, or maltreatment of a child under the age of 18 years by a person (including any employee of a residential facility or any staff person providing out-of-home care), who is responsible for the child's welfare.* The behaviour must be avoidable and non-accidental. This general definition separates abuse into two categories:

- moderate injury or impairment not requiring professional treatment but remaining observable for a minimum of 48 hours; and
- serious injury or impairment involving a life-threatening condition, long-term impairment of physical capacities, or treatment to avoid such impairments.

Based on these general criteria, *physical abuse* usually includes scalding, beatings with an object, severe physical punishment, slapping, punching and kicking; acts constituting *neglect* include deficiencies in caretaker obligations, such as failure to meet the educational, supervisory, shelter and safety, medical, physical, or emotional needs of the child, as well as physical abandonment.

Prevalence data related to the nature and description of unsubstantiated, suspected and substantiated reports of child maltreatment were analyzed by the former Institute for the Prevention of Child Abuse in Toronto, based on the Ontario Incidence Study of Reported Child Abuse and Neglect (Trocme et al. 1994, OIS). A sample of 2,950 family intake cases was randomly drawn from a total population of 53,000 open cases across Ontario in 1993. Two-thirds of the cases in the sample (1,898) had been opened for investigation of suspected abuse or neglect, involving a total of 2,447 children. These data offer an interesting comparison to U.S. data, as well as insights into the associated characteristics of these families.

The data show that the incidence of child maltreatment in the United States is about double the rate in Canada (43/1,000 vs. 21/1,000). This difference reflects a rate of investigations for neglect in the United States that is about double the rate in Canada; this may be a function of the higher rates of poverty in the United States, as well as the more limited social services and medical and education programs available to many U.S. families (Trocme et al. 1994). Moreover, the Ontario child welfare system deals with fewer, and less serious, cases of child maltreatment than its U.S. counterparts, according to descriptive information provided to state and provincial organizations in both countries (Trocme et al. 1994).

Causes of the Problem

Children are most often maltreated early in infancy, when their parents first assume the role of caring for them, and during early childhood, when parents grapple with the task of socializing the child. Abuse or neglect of a child also often accompanies instability or disruption in the family, or the family's prolonged detachment from social supports and services (Milner, in press). This is because child abuse and neglect are *relational disorders*, problems that result from a "poor fit" of the parent, child and environment (Cicchetti et al. 1988). Parents' failure to provide nurturing, sensitive and supportive caregiving is a fundamental feature of both forms of maltreatment. Moreover, the parents' inadequacy and/or excessive harshness is a primary cause of the child's future developmental problems, precipitating the recurrence of violence across generations (National Research Council 1993).

Notwithstanding the critical role of the parent, there is now a well-established consensus that child abuse and neglect do not stem from any single risk factor or cause. On the contrary, the literature supports the view that a combination of factors—individual, family, environmental and socio-cultural—increase the risk of harm to the child, while protective mechanisms can thwart the process. Recent models that seek to explain physical abuse and neglect have focused on the nature of the parent-child relationship (e.g., Bugental 1993; Crittenden and Ainsworth 1989; Milner 1993), and the factors that influence the normal formation of a healthy, child-focused relationship (Cicchetti et al. 1988). The major environmental, family and individual factors are described briefly below.

Psychological Factors

The majority of abusive and neglectful parents were raised in multiproblem families, where they were exposed to traumatic or negative childhood experiences such as family violence and instability (Wolfe 1985). As adults, they often are incapable of managing stress, and tend to avoid social contacts they perceive as potential sources of stress. Because these parents have had inadequate or inappropriate exposure to positive parental models and supports (in the present and the past), and may have limited intellectual and problem-solving skills (e.g., the inability to make appropriate decisions in a child-rearing situation), they may find child rearing a difficult and unpleasant responsibility (Wolfe 1987). Moreover, abusive or neglectful parents often report symptoms indicative of health and coping problems, which further impair their ability to function effectively as parents. Thus, low levels of competence (i.e., interpersonal positiveness, social skill, and accurate observation and judgment in the parental role), characterize a large percentage of parents who have been reported for child maltreatment (Wolfe 1985).

Studies on the psychological characteristics of abusive and high-risk parents have led to other important conclusions; although abusive parents may not suffer from psychiatric illness, they are more likely to have limited learning abilities and/or immaturity problems that can contribute to child maltreatment. These parents show problems related to emotional arousal, and control of anger and hostility; they react swiftly to provocation by the child (Vasta 1982). Abusive and neglectful parents also show limited or inappropriate child-rearing patterns and skills, including inadequate child stimulation. For example, abusive parents use mainly negative teaching techniques with their young children, rather than offering encouragement and positive attention (Burgess and Conger 1978).

Abusive and neglectful parents also have inaccurate and inappropriate expectations of children generally, and of their child in particular. This reflects the finding that parents' attitudes and beliefs about child rearing are often more parent-focused than child-focused, resulting in a discrepancy between what the parent expects from the child and what the child is capable of doing (Azar et al. 1984).

Finally, parents' lifestyles and habits are known to influence the developing parent-child relationship (Harrington et al. 1995). For example, problems related to the use of alcohol or drugs, criminal behaviour and limited support systems are common among abusive parents, and these problems serve further to interfere with the delivery of intended social and community services (Cohen and Densen-Gerber 1982).

Interadult conflict, another important, suspected antecedent to abuse, has received considerable attention in recent studies. Marital disharmony and violence are significantly associated with higher rates of severe violence towards children. (In approximately 40 percent of families where adult partners are violent toward one another there is also violence toward a child at some point during a given 12-month period (Straus et al. 1980).) Concurrently, recent findings in the marital and child clinical literature have documented the relationship between adult conflict and increased child behaviour problems (Hennessy et al. 1994). This latter finding is not surprising, since the escalation of emotional arousal and/or physical aggression that accompanies conflicts between adults can easily carry over to interactions with the child; the child may be caught in the "cross fire" between his parents (or other adults in the home), or he may precipitate a marital conflict by creating stress for either or both parents. (For example, he may disobey mother, claiming that father gave permission.) Later, the child may be injured when he attempts to interrupt the parents' fighting, escape from the situation, or continue with routine activities (Jaffe et al. 1990).

Child behaviour is also a major trigger of abusive episodes, underscoring the importance of helping parents to develop effective child-rearing skills and knowledge at an early stage. Evidence suggests that incidents of child abuse are most often precipitated by child behaviour that is challenging to deal with, but not uncommon (Herrenkohl et al. 1983). In such contexts, child behaviour such as crying may cause anger and tension in the adult, resulting in aggression against the child. Incidents of *physical abuse* are most often associated with such child behaviours as refusal, fighting and arguing, and accidents, as well as the child's immoral, dangerous, or sexual behaviour. Circumstances preceding incidents of *neglect* are characterized more by chronic adult inadequacy (including refusing to meet family needs, inadequate supervision of children, parents' lack of knowledge, inappropriate use of medical facilities, unsafe home environment and a parent's dangerous behaviour), than by child behaviour (Herrenkohl et al. 1983).

Socioeconomic Factors

Children from low-income, disadvantaged families are vastly over-represented among victims of child abuse and neglect, both in the United States (Pelton 1978) and Canada (Trocme et al. 1994). It is not surprising, therefore, that research has largely confirmed the relationship between child maltreatment and socioeconomic stress. Unemployment, restricted opportunities for work and education, family violence and/or instability, and other kinds of disadvantage often associated with lower social class membership (e.g., inadequate housing and privacy; high noise and pollution levels), have all emerged as major socioeconomic factors influencing rates of child abuse in North America. Thus, although child maltreatment is not exclusively a function of socioeconomic status, poverty and financially related stress are important factors.

Many researchers who study families of abused or neglected children describe these families as highly stressed by their living conditions and personal problems. Poverty and material hardship may accompany child maltreatment, but they do not explain it. Low-income families tend also to be isolated from appropriate supports and resources (Thompson 1994); they often lack peer groups or close friends, and adequate daycare or housing. These factors play an indirect, yet significant, role in the early formation and healthy establishment of a positive parent-child relationship.

Social and Cultural Context

The maltreatment of children is most common in multiproblem homes, where poverty, parent psychopathology, parent alcoholism and family dysfunction have a major influence on child development (National Research Council 1993). As noted above, socioeconomic disadvantage, marital distress, domestic violence and family conflict seem to characterize many of the families in child maltreatment caseloads (Wolfe 1987). Such disadvantage plays an important, yet inconclusive, causal role in child maltreatment, since most disadvantaged families are neither abusive nor neglectful.

Families with inadequate resources face a greater degree of stress and confusion than those with better access to resources. This may influence child maltreatment. For example, a recent review of accidental and non-accidental child injuries identified poverty, family chaos and unpredictability, household crowding, and frequent residence changes as factors in both unintentional child injury and child maltreatment cases (Peterson and Brown 1994). These findings support the argument that the risk of multiple forms of maltreatment rises with the number of such stressors.

One of the commonly noted features of abusive and neglectful parents is their social isolation (Thompson 1994). Such parents often lack significant social *connections* with the extended family, a neighbourhood, a community and social agencies capable of providing needed assistance (Korbin 1994). As a result, abuse and neglect are difficult to detect, and community agents who could promote healthy parent-child relationships are less likely to be influential. Added to the problem of social isolation is the possibility that certain cultural factors (e.g., child-rearing practices, geographical distinctions, kinship systems, etc.), may enhance or reduce the risk of child abuse and neglect.

Determinants of Healthy Parent-Child Relationships

The parent-child relationship and its context are today considered to be of primary importance in the promotion of healthy families and the prevention of child abuse and neglect (Cicchetti et al. 1988; Martin 1990). Accordingly, theorists and practitioners have gradually abandoned a deviance/disease orientation toward the treatment of child abuse and neglect, and adopted an approach that takes stock of the many factors that impinge on the developing parent-child relationship. The shift toward a more process-oriented, contextual approach to child abuse and neglect favours the promotion of parents' competence and the reduction of burdens on families (Melton and Barry 1994).

Determinants of healthy parent-child relationships include:
- parents' knowledge of child development and the demands of parenting;
- the ability of parents to cope with the stress of caring for small children and to enhance child development through age-appropriate stimulation and adequate attention;
- the ability of families to form normal parent-child attachments and to establish positive early patterns of communication;
- parents' knowledge of home management, including basic financial planning, proper shelter and meal planning;
- opportunities to reduce the burden of child care and to share it among men and women; and
- access to social and health services.

Although some families possess these attributes, others require early assistance and resources to acquire them (from Wekerle and Wolfe 1993).

Families at high risk of child maltreatment have benefitted from advances in service delivery derived from an understanding of the factors described above. The literature reveals that (from Wekerle and Wolfe 1993; Wolfe and Wekerle 1993):
- Fairly intensive group and home visit interventions, providing support to parents and instruction in child management and/or child cognitive stimulation, improve parents' attitudes and behaviour and enhance the adjustment of new mothers.
- Consistent (but not necessarily lengthy), child development–focused interventions improve both child cognitive ability and behavioral adjustment.
- Family support programs improve general maternal functioning and personal adjustment overall; and

- Compared with less intensive services, multidimensional programs— those offering an array of services, as parents require, over a longer period—for higher-risk families are worth the additional effort and expense.

During the past 15 years, several programs have been designed to strengthen the early parent-infant relationship by helping new parents face the challenge of child rearing. Most of these projects used medical professionals and/or hospital facilities and staff to serve participants; many also offered home visits that began either prenatally (generally in the third trimester), or soon after childbirth. A consultation model, in which parenting issues were explored in a supportive and unstructured way, was usually used, rather than a didactic, parent education or infant-focused curriculum.

Wekerle and Wolfe (1993) have noted that one- to three-year, personalized programs (e.g., those that offer home visits) are most successful in achieving the desired outcomes, and are especially successful with higher-risk individuals. Parents' need for support, parenting instruction and access to resources seems to be fulfilled by the home visitor approach.

The following success story illustrates this approach.

SUCCESS STORY

Overview

One of the greatest success stories of child maltreatment prevention is the ongoing work of David Olds that began in the late 1970s in upstate New York. (He is now at the Kempe Centre for Child Abuse Prevention in Denver.) Targets of his research were first-time parents who also possessed one or more of the risk factors for child abuse—they were poor, teenaged, or single. The program offered varying levels of child care services to participants, as well as prenatal and postnatal home visits by a nurse, who provided child development education and referred clients to appropriate resources.

The program has studied and followed two large samples of mothers to date: 400 from the Elmira, New York trial and 1,138 from the Memphis, Tennessee trial. The families received an average of 9 prenatal and 23 postnatal visits, depending on the needs of each family. The intervention was comprehensive and broad-based. Mothers were taught how to maintain their physical health, create a safe and sensitive caregiving environment, and make decisions about their own education, career and future family planning.

Actions on Nonmedical Determinants of Health

Values Underlying the Project

The prevention of child maltreatment and associated developmental disorders depends in large part on the mother's ability to adapt to the demands of her role as parent, both during her pregnancy and in the early years of the child's life. Moreover, the formation of a healthy, adaptive parent-child relationship is one of the most important contributors to normal child development; it is also a powerful deterrent to child maltreatment, child behaviour disorders, and intergenerational patterns of violence and abuse. The project designers believed that a mother's psychological resources directly influenced her ability to be a competent parent. They therefore sought to provide mothers with opportunities to increase their knowledge, skills, and confidence in their ability to raise a child and achieve personal goals. The importance ascribed to the mother's psychological resources by the project designers is further reflected in interventions that seek to capitalize on the mother's strengths and abilities, rather than merely to assess her deficits; each woman is taught the skills necessary to further her own self-development and enhance her relationship with her child.

Because fathers were generally absent in the high-risk families studied, their role has not been addressed. Recent critiques have noted this lacuna (Phares and Compas 1992).

Actions on Psychological Determinants of Health

Several strategies have been developed or strengthened to promote the health and success of the emerging parent-child relationship. These actions seek to help mothers improve their understanding of child health and development and change their expectations about their own development. They also seek to enhance self-efficacy in the mothers by developing their strengths and confidence.

To help the pregnant woman gain a better understanding of child health, the home visitor provides her with detailed information on the effects of prenatal weight gain, nutrition, rest, smoking, alcohol use and illegal drug use on her child, her family and herself. After childbirth the educational program focuses on information about common health problems, the demands of infant caregiving, and how to address them. To help women improve their own life course development, home visitors provide educational materials on such topics as birth control and meeting educational goals while caring for children.

To enhance the self-efficacy of new mothers, interactions are designed to create an expectation of personal accomplishment and to reinforce it. First, home visitors encourage mothers to learn by doing, and offer positive reinforcement for things done well, as when a mother identifies and responds appropriately to her infant's needs or removes a safety hazard. Second, small, surmountable problems are addressed in ways that increase the chances of successful performance. The approach, known as "solution-focused therapy", is based on a competence model of problem solving that seeks to help clients repeat successful behaviours rather than eliminate or alter problem behaviours. The method places clients at the centre of the process, recognizing that they are experts on their own lives and that, with help from health professionals, they can find solutions to their problems. Finally, health workers seek to establish a caring relationship with their clients, increasing the effectiveness of role modelling and reducing clients' anxiety.

Actions on Social Determinants of Health

Home visitors establish close, therapeutic ties with the mother and other family members during pregnancy, building effective relationships with their clients by focusing on the strengths of family members and addressing issues of concern them. Because the development of such relationships takes time, home visits begin well before the baby is born and continue for 2 1/2 years.

Actions on Economic Determinants of Health

During the first few visits, the home visitor identifies family stressors, assesses the family's needs, and connects the family with needed health and human services; families are given help obtaining financial assistance, subsidized housing, family counselling, nutritional supplementation, clothing, furniture and proper medical care.

Home visitors thus provide a crucial link between mothers and the community-based professionals and services that strengthen a family's resources and enhance its ability to cope. Mothers are also assisted in finding vocational training programs or other services needed to promote independence. In some instances formal service providers, such as schools and child welfare agencies, have taken a punitive stance toward young women in the program; some school principals have sought to bar pregnant women or parents of young children from attending school because of past behaviour. Home visitors have worked with local schools to mend relations, or have sought alternative sources of education and training for their clients.

Reasons for the Initiative

Dr. Olds' approach to preventing child maltreatment was based on the realization that many of the most pervasive, intractable and costly problems faced by parents and children are a *consequence of adverse maternal, health-related behaviours*, including poor prenatal care, dysfunctional infant caregiving and stressful environmental conditions that interfere with parental and family functioning. These factors result not only in child abuse and neglect, but are also associated with infant mortality, low birthweight, childhood injuries, youth violence and poor economic self-sufficiency.

Moreover, such problems are most common among children born to poor, teenaged, or single parents, or to women who have children in rapid succession. Although many social and cultural factors have a bearing on the health and social functioning of children and youths, a significant portion of their problems are attributable to their parents' behaviour during pregnancy and early infancy. A person's ability to be a good parent is often compromised by his own experience of childhood abuse or neglect, psychological immaturity or depression, stressful living conditions, and inadequate social supports.

Accumulating scientific evidence suggests that it is possible to improve the outcomes of pregnancy, enhance parents' abilities to care for their children, and reduce welfare dependency, by providing programs of pre-natal and early childhood home visitation. But despite such evidence, no program had previously attempted to provide all these components in a manner that was sensitive to the needs and abilities of different families, and for a long enough duration to permit lasting change. Dr. Olds' research team sought to provide the missing services.

Meanwhile, advances in the theory and methods of health promotion helped the research team elaborate its methodology. For instance, the program design profited from developments in health education, a four-step process that involves:
- helping the client recognize that a particular behaviour will lead to a desired health outcome;
- teaching the client how to execute the behaviour;
- convincing the client that he can carry out the behaviour successfully; and
- motivating the client to value the outcomes enough to maintain the new behaviour patterns.

While health education has focused predominantly on the first two steps, the program designed by Dr. Olds combined all four steps in an effort to promote self-efficacy.

Actors

In the late 1970s a team of researchers and health care professionals based at Cornell University developed a home visitation program for mothers at risk of child abuse. The original team consisted largely of psychologists, nurses, social workers and physicians. The project received start-up financial supported from the community, as well as the state and federal governments. Supporters recognized the need for services to high-risk families to prevent the onset of chronic, recalcitrant patterns of abuse, neglect and other negative health outcomes.

Participants in the program now number in the thousands. There are three program sites: Elmira, New York; Memphis, Tennessee; and Denver, Colorado. The participants are primiparous women, 85 percent of whom are either low income, unmarried, or teenaged. Large numbers are Caucasian, African American, or Hispanic in all three sites, and findings related to the unique needs and outcomes of these diverse groups will be available in future evaluations. The program is implemented by trained, B.A.-level nurses, who visit the home of each family during the woman's pregnancy and at bimonthly intervals for two years after the birth of the child.

Analysis of the Results

Child Maltreatment and Developmental Course

Evidence from ongoing research evaluations find the initiative successful in reducing general domains of risk for the development of delinquency, crime and violence (Olds et al. 1986; Olds et al. 1994; Olds et al., in press; Robinson et al., in press). These findings include reduced maternal substance abuse during pregnancy (with probable corresponding reductions in neuro-developmental impairment of the fetus), reduced incidence of child mal-treatment, reductions in family size, fewer closely spaced pregnancies, and reduced incidence of chronic welfare dependency.

Each of these factors has been shown in other research to increase the risk of conduct disorders, delinquency, crime and youth violence; the rela-tionship is even clearer when more than one factor is present (Patterson et al. 1989).

The findings—reduced rates of state-verified cases of child maltreatment and health care encounters for injuries and ingestions—indicate that the program has reduced the rates of dysfunctional caregiving. In the Elmira trial, the rate of verified child maltreatment in the *comparison group* was 10 percent overall, and 19 percent among those individuals who possessed all three risk factors used for recruitment (poor, unmarried teens). By con-trast, the rates of maltreatment in the intervention group (those visited by nurses during pregnancy and during the first two years after the birth of the child), was 4 percent overall and 4 percent for the poor, unmarried teens.

During the two-year period after the program ended, children from nurse-visited families were much less likely to be seen in the physician's office for injuries, ingestions, or social problems and they had 35 percent fewer visits to the emergency department. The pattern of results was very similar in the Memphis trial, again suggesting that the nurse-visited parents were more attentive and more attuned to their children's needs and created safer home environments for them. In-home observations during a two-year follow-up of the Elmira sample (through the child's fourth year of life), found the nurse-visited women more involved with their children and more adept at choosing appropriate forms of child punishment and stimulation than women in the control group (Olds et al., in press).

Maternal Life Course Factors

The program substantially benefitted the life course development of its participants. During the first four years after the birth of a first child, clients of the program had rates of subsequent pregnancy 43 percent lower than women in the comparison sample. Moreover, their participation in the workforce was 84 percent higher, and welfare dependency was significantly lower than in the comparison group.

It is worth noting that these findings continue across a 15-year follow-up of the Elmira sample. (This follow-up is currently 75 percent complete.) The findings are considered preliminary until all data have been analyzed, but results to date strongly suggest that the life-course trajectories of the low-income families served by the program are shifting in important ways that may reduce the children's later exposure to negative peer influences and relationship violence.

The factors most likely responsible for the success of this program (apart from the commitment and hard work of the research team) are largely social. Although financial support to families was important, it appears that the social connections that women acquired through the home visits enhanced the development of the emerging parent-child relationship. The positive outcomes are probably most attributable to the program's supportive, competency enhancement approach.

Replicability of the Initiative

Initiated in Elmira, New York, the program described above is being replicated in two other U.S. cities; a similar trial is in progress in Hamilton, Ontario. The evidence to date suggests that the results are replicable in different settings, although variations in local environments (e.g., the degree of political support, involvement of the health care community, availability of community resources), should be carefully reviewed. (See Policy Implications, below.) The program developers emphasize that understanding better how to manage variations in local environments to ensure that the essential elements of the program are reproduced is an important consideration in the dissemination of this method.

Funding

This program has been funded largely through state trust funds for children and by the National Institute of Mental Health in the United States. Competitive research and demonstration grant applications were peer reviewed and required repeated renewal for continued funding. Staff were paid according to local salary levels.

During one of the trials a nursing shortage nearby caused hospitals to raise nurses' salaries; many of the home-visiting nurses left the program in favour of more highly paid employment. This change in staff had a significant impact on the families (i.e., gains shown among families who continued with the same nurse throughout were greater than those shown among families who changed home visitors).

Evaluation

This project is among the most thoroughly evaluated studies of the impact of early home visitation and intervention. The evaluation was conducted by the research team, with monies received through competitive grant funding. The results (presented in the section above), have been published in peer-reviewed journals since the early 1980s, and a special edition of the *Journal of Community Psychology*, highlighting the growth and results of the project, will appear in 1997.

The evaluation of the project includes longitudinal and cross-sectional components, as well as process and outcome evaluations. The evaluation design is thus arguably one of the most rigorous and state-of-the-art currently available. Established measures of infant development and behaviour and of maternal adjustment and behaviour are taken at regular intervals, and the longitudinal nature of the study allows for a subsequent analysis of growth and change over time. This design also permits the determination of what methods work for whom, because it involves large samples of families with diverse social, cultural and psychological backgrounds. These latter analyses must await data from the long-term follow-up of the samples in all three U.S. sites; however, by assessing current trends, it is possible to draw preliminary conclusions about the impact of the program on women who initially presented with the greatest need. (See Analysis of the Results, above.)

Finally, the ongoing impact evaluation suggests that there will be gains for the larger community. In particular, Olds examined the impact of the program on families' use of other government services, and the corresponding cost. Olds reports that the program cost U.S.$3,173 for 2 1/2 years of intervention. Government savings were calculated as the difference in spending on other government services between the intervention group and the comparison group. By the time their first child was four years old, low-income families who had been visited by a nurse during pregnancy and through the second year of the child's life cost the government U.S.$3,313 *less* per family than did their counterparts in the comparison group (Olds et al. in press).

Evidence of burnout, per se, was not described in the evaluation of the program. On the contrary, nurses who had worked in more traditional social and health care services in their communities anecdotally reported increased job satisfaction.

POLICY IMPLICATIONS

The Vision

We can surmise on the basis of existing research that child abuse and neglect are multiply caused phenomena that follow somewhat predictable "stages". Although the initial stage of maltreatment is relatively benign, insensitive or inadequate parent-infant interactions can quickly escalate into abuse or neglect. Moreover, the parent's failure to deal effectively with the demands of child rearing early on (due to lack of resources, support, or competence, or because of overwhelming levels of stress), can lead to increased pressure on the parent-child relationship, and a concomitant increase in the probability of abusive behaviour. The goals of child abuse prevention, therefore, should be:
  - to increase parents' ability to cope with external demands and provide for the developmental and socialization needs of the child; and
  - to reduce the stress that families experience.

Healthy socialization practices that are responsive to changes in situation and child development buffer the child against stressful or negative influences in the child's environment; such practices also reduce the parents' need to rely on power-assertive methods to control their children, or to ignore children's needs.

Given the important role that supportive communities and neighbourhoods play in meeting the primary needs of children and families, child maltreatment prevention strategies should be guided by an ethic of inclusion and support, rather than one of mere interception and protection. Such an approach is consonant with the Canadian tradition of voluntarism and mutual assistance, although it has seldom been applied to child protection. Implementing this vision will require diligent planning and action to ensure that communities and families receive support at the optimal time. Achieving the desired results will not be easy. It will require a reversal of powerful, social trends within neighbourhoods at highest risk and in the nation as a whole.

The Strategy

The Role of the Federal Government

While action by the federal government is by itself insufficient to bring about the major social transformations needed to ensure that children receive appropriate protection and assistance, the necessary changes are impossible without federal policy reform. Basic, comprehensive services for at-risk children and their families—as well as the associated changes in assistance at provincial and community levels—must be established through federal reform and with federal guidance.

To this end, the federal government's role in reducing the incidence of child abuse and neglect in Canada should be to stimulate programs that are:

- sufficiently intensive and diverse to provide communities with the support and resources necessary to put into place comprehensive, neighbourhood-based, child-centred and family-focused programs; and
- sufficiently flexible that such efforts can be adapted to meet the needs and capitalize on the strengths of rural, urban, cultural and ethnic communities in various regions of the country, including Aboriginal communities. Such flexibility should allow for changes in the state of the art as the strategy is tested and evolves.

New policies should also be created to reflect programmatic emphases on child abuse and neglect across many different federal and provincial agencies, with the intent of fostering involvement by different professional groups, administrators and practitioners.

A major research initiative should be established that can be carried out by provincial and regional centres.

Funding structures should be simplified to permit the development of neighbourhood-based child protection and family support efforts through a unified interagency plan.

Policies should favour a movement toward universal voluntary pre-natal and neonatal home visitation. The first step in such a plan would be the funding of numerous coordinated pilot projects with sufficient funds to permit both outcome and impact evaluations on diverse sectors of the population. *Such projects would not seek to reaffirm the (already well-established) efficacy of home visitation in preventing child maltreatment;* rather, they would seek to determine what is needed (at a federal level), to establish and administer a national, home visitation system.

The National Strategy

As Dr. Olds' research illustrates, neighbourhoods and communities are the real locus of efforts to reduce the incidence of child abuse and neglect; yet such action must be guided and supported by other levels of government. A national strategy to prevent child maltreatment should promote community involvement and participation in child protection and healthy child development. General principles of such a strategy are outlined below.

A national strategy should strengthen and support urban, suburban and rural neighbourhoods in ways that meet the needs of children and families.

There appears to be an inverse relationship between social class and reliance on neighbourhood resources; many poor families and individuals are more dependent on local resources than their middle-class counterparts. Yet, middle-class policymakers and professionals tend to underestimate the importance of neighbourhoods to disadvantaged families.

Many families who maltreat children are trapped in deteriorating neighbourhoods that attract antisocial elements of the population, while repelling and displacing functional families. Neighbourhood revitalization requires the coordination of economic investment, social services, political mobilization and law enforcement (Barry 1994). Communities will need to advocate for resources to preserve and enhance their neighbourhoods, especially low-income neighbourhoods. *It is time to start paying as much attention to the environment for humans as we do to the environment for fish and wildlife.*

The value and cost benefit of in-home services is well supported in the literature. Home visits, in particular those begun prior to the onset of maltreatment, benefit both children and mothers, and reduce child abuse and neglect. In general, such services should provide training that dispels parents' misperceptions and corrects false expectations about the abilities of young children; parents should be offered alternatives to physical punishment and taught prosocial, developmentally relevant activities they can engage in with their children.

Service delivery should be reoriented to make it as easy to provide child maltreatment prevention services to families as it currently is to remove children from their homes and place them in foster care.

The child welfare system is currently designed primarily to protect children, rather to than assist families. This use of resources fails the significant number of parents who are at risk of losing control with their children and who could benefit from early intervention. Policymakers must acknowledge that intervention after the fact is seldom satisfactory for the child, the family, or the community.

Moreover, there is often a large gap between what families need by way of treatment and what is delivered to them in practice. Help should be more easily available to a family before a crisis or tragedy occurs.

While child protection and child welfare require firm guidelines and legal authority, child development is enhanced by family stability, continuity of caregivers, and a supportive family and community. Positive relationships with their parents provide children with the learning opportunities that prevent developmental harm and promote their healthy adaptation. Children who are maltreated are also, generally, denied the opportunities for guidance that are most apt to produce forward movement; they live in conditions of high stress and benefit from few resources. Such high-stress, low-support social environments deserve the highest priority in social policy making; the children in these environments are least likely to tolerate maltreatment or further developmental interference.

Public health and health promotion approaches to the prevention of child abuse and neglect are promising strategies that merit further development.

A national strategy should not undermine existing treatment and early intervention services. Rather it should take a broader, more structural approach. Government fiscal incentives, for example, should favour prevention and treatment rather than detection, investigation and foster care placement. Health promotion policy should address two primary needs: 1) The need of all families for some degree of support and education (an strategy of "enhancement", rather than interception); and 2) the need to maximize each child's developmental strengths through child-centred stimulation that involves primary caregivers.

In conjunction with health promotion efforts, program development should focus on providing child development and parenting information that is easily understood, practical and accessible to all present and potential parenting populations.

In particular, attention should be directed to societal influences that play a role in child abuse and neglect, especially in circumstances where families are exposed to health risks, conflict, and the negative effects of poverty. Such a cross-cultural perspective on child maltreatment prevention would redirect the focus away from individuals and families towards societal and cultural conditions that attenuate or exacerbate family problems. Policy planners also need to advocate for the establishment of "minimum standards of care" in their own communities, taking into account the cultural diversity of the community and the disproportionate share of child care responsibility borne by women.

A variety of other factors also influence the willingness and ability of parents to participate in early intervention initiatives. But the use of appropriate educational materials, Indigenous health care providers, child-focused activities and models of intervention that emphasize on individual strengths rather than weaknesses is currently impeded by the value our society places on family autonomy and privacy. *Child maltreatment must be seen as a collective problem of the neighbourhood, not simply as a problem of individual parents and families.*

Empowering the most needy communities remains a challenge. Neighbourhoods most in need of family and social support programs to reduce the incidence of child maltreatment are generally composed of individuals least likely to define themselves in ways that facilitate such efforts. Special investments in high-stress, low-resource communities are needed.

Specifically:

The needs of ethnic minorities merit further attention.

Research is needed to identify the special risks and strengths of specific cultural and ethnic groups, and to plan services that are sensitive to ethnic and cultural differences. Although there is a general lack of research on maltreated children of ethnic and minority communities, adequate information exists to recommend the implementation and evaluation of culturally relevant intervention and prevention methods.

Young adults, especially teenaged parents, represent a sizeable proportion of child maltreatment reports, yet they typically receive less than adequate assistance.

Prevention services for youth could help them acquire the attitudes and knowledge to help them recognize and develop healthy relationships; education programs could focus on practical skills for noncontrolling conflict resolution. Prevention programs that seek to educate low- and high-risk adolescents about such issues as control and power in relationships, sexual and physical violence, and family and child-rearing values merit development and evaluation in schools, communities and service agencies (Wolfe et al. 1995).

An economic analysis of child maltreatment that includes all relevant government agencies should be undertaken to better assess the true cost to society of child maltreatment and the savings that home visitation programs achieve.

No single health care organization or branch of government can justify, on cost recovery grounds, investing in the full cost of home visitation services. There is therefore little incentive for single agencies or health care organizations to fund these types of programs, even though the potential cost savings to government or society as a whole are considerable. Moreover, the cost of remediating serious problems related to inadequate child rearing is prohibitive, while spending on prevention services not only prevents child abuse, but benefits individuals and communities in other ways as well. Further analyses are needed to confirm these conclusions.

Finally, there is evidence that the cost of providing services for the neediest families may be reduced by better preparing parents for their child-rearing role, and by having a wider range of appropriate services available. Such an intervention model requires staff who are trained to assist families when they need help, rather to detect problems and intervene after the fact. Staff need to be sensitive to individual, community and cultural preferences, as well as the socioeconomic factors that constrain the majority of disadvantaged families. Staff must also be willing to accept their clients' limitations and respect their cultural differences.

While this approach requires more and earlier investment in family development, it promises to deliver better results for less money than the current, reactive system.

Since many of the factors that result in child maltreatment affect the health and functioning of the majority of families, a national strategy should address the causes of child abuse and neglect from a public health perspective, rather than through tertiary intervention.

A national strategy should not undermine existing efforts at treatment and early intervention; instead, it should be designed to approach the problem of child maltreatment from a broader, more structural perspective.

To this end:

- *Attention must be directed toward educating the public and policymakers and building coalitions with relevant political constituencies if an early intervention/prevention initiative is to gain broad support.*
- *Effective communication strategies must be developed to promote the program at the grassroots, community and legislative levels.*

CONCLUSIONS

Ideally, a national strategy should be comprehensive and begin on several fronts at once. However, the reality of child protection and our lack of prior investment in health promotion for children and families make it unrealistic to expect the required level of coordination and backing from different levels of government. Thus, the question "What is the best plan?" must be rephrased as "What can we do with what we have?" and "Where do we start?"

Clearly, the answer varies widely among government departments, public health agencies and nongovernmental organizations. Each policymaker, legislator, administrator and agency director should harness the resources that are most easily available and seek to integrate his efforts with those of others who have similar goals and responsibilities. It is best to start from the bottom, seeking the views of residents and community leaders about how their neighbourhoods might be made better places to live and to raise children in safety (Barry 1994).

Evidence based on replicated trials of home visits to disadvantaged parents shows that programs that are comprehensive, intensive and of long duration improve the outcomes of pregnancy and early child rearing and reduce the risks of welfare dependency, conduct disorders and violence. Although the programs are expensive, preliminary data indicate that the long-term cost of failing to provide service exceeds the initial investment.

Even among children and youth who have grown up with violence, major shifts in their ability to relate to others can and do happen. When a person's behaviour shifts from coercive to cooperative—and such shifts are the exception rather than the rule—the change is often attributable to the influence of healthy, non-violent individuals, such as teachers, foster parents and grandparents, and the strength and resources of the child or youth (e.g., intelligence, good schools and other learning opportunities).

Given its prevalence, child maltreatment can be compared to other major threats to public health, such as AIDS, childhood diseases, poverty and unsafe homes. Therefore, it makes sense in the long run to address the causes of this problem from a public health perspective, rather than through tertiary intervention.

Evidence of the effectiveness of such a preventative model can be found in reports from Scandinavian countries. Sweden, Finland and Denmark all have nationwide programs that resemble the family support programs being explored in the United States. In addition, these countries have the benefits of universal insurance, free tuition for academic and vocational training, paid educational leave to upgrade skills, yearly cash allowances for each child under age 16 and for nonworking mothers for six months during pregnancy, maternal child health services, subsidized primary health care and other benefits. Pransky (1991) summarized the results of these benefits:

- 95 percent of pregnant mothers start prenatal care before the end of the fourth month, compared with less than 85 percent in the United States and Canada;
- Fewer than 4 percent of mothers are under the age of 20 at the time of their first birth, compared with 10 percent in the United States, and 26.6 percent in Canada;
- Infant deaths from respiratory disease range from 22 to 67 per 100,000, compared with 107/100,000 in the United States and 20/100,000 in Canada;
- Prevalence of mild mental retardation is 8 to 10 times lower than in the United States and Canada; and
- Rates of child abuse are about eight times lower than in the United States and about four times lower than in Canada.

Moreover, health care expenditures in Scandinavian countries range from 7 to 10 percent of gross national product; Canadian expenditures are comparable at 9.7 percent. In the United States, these expenditures total 11 percent. These comparative costs should figure prominently in a cost-benefit analysis of the North American approach to child rearing and family problems. For example, based on U.S. statistics (no Canadian figures are currently available):

- It cost approximately U.S.$19 billion nationwide in 1987 to assist families that were started by teenagers;
- Nearly 66 percent of daughters of single women eventually go on welfare;
- Providing high-quality, prenatal care for high-risk infants costs, on average, almost twice as much as care for normal, low-risk infants (Pransky 1991).

Despite their doubts, communities, agencies and professionals occasionally acknowledge that prevention has some appeal over treatment alone. This appeal is supported by two facts. First, there will never be sufficient numbers of trained professionals, police, or prisons to meet the mental health and criminal justice needs of most communities. Secondly, current interventions in the areas of mental health, child welfare and criminal justice that seek to remove at-risk children or dangerous persons in an effort to restore balance are simply not very effective.

These facts lend appeal to strategies that seek to enhance competence, adaptiveness and other positive conditions.

Although prevention programs are, in general, desirable and effective, some programs are more successful than others. Reviews of the literature reveal components of programs that show particular success. In general, prevention programs are most effective when they target high-risk individuals *before* they become involved in risky behaviours, and offer them high-quality programs that are firmly ground in theory; in addition, the more integrated and comprehensive the program is in relation to the community and the target population, the more likely it is to show success. Problems usually come in packages, and programs that acknowledge this reality and incorporate it into their programming tend to be more successful.

Finally, we need to ask whether our communities are being forced to adopt a *crisis management* approach to child and family needs, and whether we would prefer proper planning and access to opportunities for assistance during critical transitional periods.

Child welfare laws are designed solely for protection. This means service providers are often forced to wait until the last possible moment before attempting to intervene. Meanwhile, many families at risk remain un-detected. Notable exceptions to this pattern include some aspects of medicine, education and other services destined for the healthy, non-problematic majority of the population. Professionals who work with troubled children or at-risk parents, on the other hand, are too often left with a task that cannot be handled well under the current system and with the resources available. Interventions are too little and come too late, and service providers routinely suffer stress, burnout and fatigue from "putting out fires".

A conceptual shift is needed that acknowledges the contribution of each member of society and the benefit of encouraging families to assume their responsibilities, rather than punishing them for failure. Rather than focusing on efficiency, costs, safety, protection, or deviance, current theory in the fields of health and mental health favours health promotion strategies and programs that encourage positive change, offer opportunities and promote people's competence to achieve their health potential. This perspective speaks to the importance of attaining a balance between the abilities of the individual (or groups of individuals) and the challenges and risks of the environment.

The effects of this conceptual shift on the health care field will be far reaching; the new model will change how individuals think about health, how daily life is organized and experienced, how social resources are allocated, and how other social policy decisions are made. Such an approach offers much promise for the field of mental health and the future of children and youth.

David A. Wolfe, *Ph.D., is a professor of psychology and psychiatry at the University of Western Ontario and a founding member of the Center for Research on Violence Against Women and Children in London, Ontario. As the former director of research for the Institute for the Prevention of Child Abuse in Toronto, he became involved in the development of policy and research aimed at the prevention of violence, which led to the beginnings of the Youth Relationships Project. His books include* Child abuse: Implications for child development and psycho-pathology *(1987) and* Preventing physical and emotional abuse of children *(1991). He is also coauthor of* Children of battered women *(1991),* Youth relationships manual: A group approach with adolescents for the prevention of woman abuse and the promotion of healthy relationships *(1996) and* Alternatives to violence: Empowering youth to develop healthy relationships *(1997).*

BIBLIOGRAPHY

AZAR, S. T., ROBINSON, D. R., HEKIMIAN, E., and TWENTYMAN, C. T. 1984. Unrealistic expectations and problem-solving ability in maltreating and comparison mothers. *Journal of Consulting and Clinical Psychology* 52: 687–691.

BARRY, F. 1994. A neighbourhood-based approach: What is it? In *Protecting Children from Abuse and Neglect: Foundations for a New National Strategy*, eds. G. B. MELTON and F. D. BARRY. New York: Guilford. pp. 14–39.

BUGENTAL, D. B. 1993. Communication in abusive relationships: Cognitive constructions of interpersonal power. *American Behavioral Scientist* 36: 288–308.

BURGESS, R. L., and CONGER, R. 1978. Family interactions in abusive, neglectful, and normal families. *Child Development* 49: 1163–1173.

CICCHETTI, D., TOTH, S., and BUSH, M. 1988. Developmental psychopathology and incompetence in childhood: Suggestions for intervention. In *Advances in Clinical Child Psychology*, eds. B. B. LAHEY and A. E. KAZDIN. New York: Plenum. 11: 1–77.

COHEN, F. S., and DENSEN-GERBER, J. 1982. A study of the relationship between child abuse and drug addiction in 178 patients: Preliminary results. *Child Abuse and Neglect* 6: 383–387.

CRITTENDEN, P. M., and AINSWORTH, M. D. S. 1989. Child maltreatment and attachment theory. In *Child Maltreatment: Theory and Research on the Causes and Consequences of Child Abuse and Neglect*, eds. D. CICCHETTI and V. CARLSON. Cambridge: Cambridge University Press. pp. 432–463.

HARRINGTON, D., DUBOWITZ, H., BLACK, M. M., and BINDER, A. 1995. Maternal substance use and neglectful parenting: Relations with children's development. *Journal of Clinical Child Psychology* 24: 258–263.

HENNESSY, K. D., RABIDEAU, G. J., CICCHETTI, D., and CUMMINGS, E. M. 1994. Responses of physically abused and nonabused children to different forms of interadult anger. *Child Development* 65: 815–828.

HERRENKOHL, R. C., HERRENKOHL, E. C., and EGOLF, B. P. 1983. Circumstances surrounding the occurrence of child maltreatment. *Journal of Consulting and Clinical Psychology* 51: 424–431.

JAFFE, P., WOLFE, D., and WILSON, S. 1990. *Children of Battered Women*. Thousand Oaks (CA): Sage.

KORBIN, J. 1994. Sociocultural factors in child maltreatment. In *Protecting Children from Abuse and Neglect: Foundations for a New National Strategy*, eds. G. B. MELTON and F. D. BARRY. New York: Guilford. pp. 182–223.

MARTIN, B. 1990. The transmission of relationship difficulties from one generation to the next. *Journal of Youth and Adolescence* 19: 181–199.

MASH, E. J., and WOLFE, D. A. 1991. Methodological issues in research on physical child abuse. *Criminal Justice and Behaviour* 18: 8–29.

MELTON, G. B., and BARRY, F. D. 1994. Neighbors helping neighbors: The vision of the U. S. Advisory Board on Child Abuse and Neglect. In *Protecting Children from Abuse and Neglect: Foundations for a New National Strategy*, eds. G. B. MELTON and F. D. BARRY. New York: Guilford. pp. 1–13.

MILNER, J. In press. Characteristics of abusive parents. In *Child Abuse: New Directions in Prevention and Treatment across the Lifespan*, eds. D. A. WOLFE, R. MCMAHON, and R. De V. PETERS. Thousand Oaks (CA): Sage.

MILNER, J. S. 1993. Social information processing and physical child abuse. *Clinical Psychology Review* 13: 275–294.

NATIONAL RESEARCH COUNCIL. 1993. *Understanding Child Abuse and Neglect*. Washington (DC): National Academy Press.

OLDS, D., HENDERSON, C. R., and KITZMAN, H. 1994. Does pre-natal and infancy nurse home visitation have enduring effects on qualities of parental caregiving and child health at 25 to 50 months of life? *Pediatrics* 93: 89–98.

OLDS, D., HENDERSON, C., CHAMBERLIN, R., and TATELBAUM, R. 1986. Preventing child abuse and neglect: A randomized trial of nurse home visitation. *Pediatrics* 78: 65–78.

OLDS, D., PETTITT, L. M., ROBINSON, J., ECKENRODE, J., KITZMAN, H., COLE, B., and POWERS, J. In press. The potential for reducing antisocial behaviour with a program of prenatal and early childhood home visitation. *American Journal of Community Psychology.*

PATTERSON, G. R., DeBARYSHE, B. D., and RAMSEY, E. 1989. A developmental perspective on antisocial behaviour. *American Psychologist* 44: 329–335.

PELTON, L. H. 1978. Child abuse and neglect: The myth of classlessness. *American Journal of Orthopsychiatry* 48: 608–617.

PETERSON, L., and BROWN, D. 1994. Integrating child injury and abuse-neglect research: Common histories, etiologies, and solutions. *Psychological Bulletin* 116: 293–315.

PHARES, V., and COMPAS, B. E. 1992. The role of fathers in child and adolescent psychopathology: Make room for Daddy. *Psychological Bulletin* 111: 387–412.

PRANSKY, J. 1991. *Prevention: The Critical Need.* Springfield (MO): Burrell Foundation.

ROBINSON, J. L., EMDE, R. N., and KORFMACHER, J. In press. The role of emotional development in the home visitation program model. *American Journal of Community Psychology.*

STRAUS, M. A., GELLES, R. J., and STEINMETZ, S. 1980. *Behind Closed Doors: Violence in the American Family.* Grand City (NY): Doubleday/Anchor.

THOMPSON, R. A. 1994. Social support and the prevention of child maltreatment. In *Protecting Children from Abuse and Neglect: Foundations for a New National Strategy,* eds. G. B. MELTON and F. D. BARRY. New York: Guilford. pp. 40–130.

TROCME, N., McPHEE, D., KWAN TAM, K., and HAY, T. 1994. *Ontario incidence study of reported child abuse and neglect.* Toronto: Institute for the Prevention of Child Abuse.

VASTA, R. 1982. Physical child abuse: A dual-component analysis. *Developmental Review* 2: 125–149.

WEKERLE, C., and WOLFE, D. A. 1993. Prevention of child physical abuse and neglect: Promising new directions. *Clinical Psychology Review* 13: 501–540.

WOLFE, D. A. 1985. Child-abusive parents: An empirical review and analysis. *Psychological Bulletin* 97: 462–482.

———. 1987. *Child Abuse: Implications for Child Development and Psychopathology.* Thousand Oaks (CA): Sage.

WOLFE, D. A., and WEKERLE, C. 1993. Treatment strategies for child physical abuse and neglect: A critical progress report. *Clinical Psychology Review* 13: 473–500.

WOLFE, D. A., WEKERLE, C., REITZEL-JAFFE, D., and GOUGH, R. 1995. Strategies to address violence in the lives of high-risk youth. In *Ending the Cycle of Violence: Community Responses to Children of Battered Women,* eds. E. PELED, P. G. JAFFE, and J. L. EDELSON. Thousand Oaks (CA): Sage. pp. 255–274.

Decreasing Child Sexual Abuse

CHRISTOPHER BAGLEY, PH.D.,
AND WILFREDA E. THURSTON, PH.D.

Faculty of Social Work and Faculty of Medicine
The University of Calgary

SUMMARY

Evidence suggests that sexual abuse of children is common in Canadian society; thus, many children have already experienced sexual abuse and deserve support to prevent further abuse or sequelae. Children at risk should be protected from ever experiencing sexual abuse. Children rely on adults for policy implementation; however, a sizeable proportion of the adult population may have impaired social, emotional or physical health as a result of their own experiences of childhood abuse, including sexual abuse. This is especially true of mothers, and little research has been done on the impact of abuse they suffered as children on their responses to their children.

There are many weaknesses in research and service responses to childhood sexual abuse (CSA), and this is understandable: the issue has usually been viewed as a personal clinical problem and has only recently begun to be redefined as a social health problem. The frequency, type and source of abuse, as well as outcomes, vary for girls and boys. The long-term sequelae depend on other family and social factors around the child; therefore, severity of abuse does not seem directly correlated to outcome, although increased duration is predictive of more ill effects. It is also clear that ill effects can result from ill-conceived interventions rooted in moral outrage or punitive goals. Reporting, assessment and evidence collection can be detrimental for the child. Assessments should cover abuse and neglect in addition to sexual abuse, but medical examinations are not recommended as standard procedure. The search for risk factors with high predictive value appears pointless; for instance, disordered patterns of communication; mental illness; having a stepfather; parentification; poverty; and alcohol abuse are some factors associated with increased risk.

An understanding of sequelae of abuse must be grounded in models of normal childhood development, vulnerability, resiliency and cultural norms. Somatic disorders, dissociation, eating disorders, borderline personality and deliberate self-harm are found in CSA victims more often than in nonvictims, but only a minority of CSA victims will experience these extreme problems; for example, few CSA victims become prostitutes, but most adolescent female and male prostitutes are CSA survivors. Similarly, most adolescents who act out in seemingly antisocial or conduct-disordered ways are survivors of CSA, but this etiology is most often overlooked. Outreach to teen prostitutes has had limited success, and, in fact, few programs for treatment of CSA have been rigorously evaluated.

By far the most common form of prevention program is school-based education; thus, prevention of CSA has been placed almost entirely on the shoulders of children. The most common approaches are fundamentally flawed in theoretical basis, message and unintended outcomes. Furthermore, there is no evidence of primary prevention. Stepfathers and adolescent boys at risk of becoming abusers have received little attention; in fact, there is scant research on abusers. Other foci for prevention emerge from findings on adult survivors (e.g., a warm, loving, accepting and sexually open family can minimize harms; families with equitable power relations are less likely to have abuse; victim blaming undermines emotional and social health; memories can be suppressed; simple disclosure to a supportive person is therapeutic; and CSA cannot be confronted meaningfully without considering the spectrum of violence against women, including sexual assault, date rape, sexual harassment and wife abuse).

Policy development depends on a cycle of setting agendas, identifying solutions, selecting options, and implementing policies. Two federal committees helped create a policy agenda around CSA; however, this has faltered, and the National Forum on Health may help in revisiting and revitalizing this agenda. Once prevention is accepted by a community with committed leadership, effective holistic programs can be implemented, as illustrated by the Alkali Lake Band example; however, it takes time to complete the policy cycle and see success. Some exemplary policy options have been tested in Canada and await broader dissemination. Court preparation has been shown by the London Family Court to reduce anxiety for children, but it also has therapeutic benefits such as preventing males from becoming abusers. The Sexual Behaviour Clinic in Kingston has provided evidence of successful therapy for offenders. Since few cases go to court and incarceration is an expensive solution not often favoured by victims, prevention of recidivism through treatment is an important option. Furthermore, treatment may be identified for men who are at risk of offending. The Quebec model offers another alternative for protection of children, coordinated assessment and treatment; and alternatives to incarceration. The York Region Abuse Program provides an example of a coordinated multisectoral approach to treatment and prevention that builds community capacity and involves survivors in self-help and mutual aid. Community capacity building is effective, but the End the Silence project illustrates that social change is not easily attained and that the participation of especially vulnerable populations must be given particular attention. Finally, not all members of communities will support efforts to eradicate CSA, and policy implementation may encounter resistance from a variety of sources.

Prevention of CSA and its sequelae would benefit from action based on the population health concept. Policies and interventions must address the social and economic environment; the physical environment; personal health practices; individual and community capacity and coping skills; and development of effective health services. The interrelatedness of policies at the levels of primary, secondary and tertiary prevention should be made explicit. This report concludes with several policy recommendations.

TABLE OF CONTENTS

Decreasing the amount of sexual abuse experienced by Canadian children is fundamental to the national goal of "achieving health for all" (Epp 1986). Childhood sexual abuse (CSA) is an experience with different short- and long-term health impacts, depending on the resilience of the child, his family and the community, which is partly determined by socioeconomic status (SES). Untreated CSA can decrease the SES of the victim, thereby affecting other health issues. CSA has rarely been viewed from a population health perspective (Hertzman 1994; Marmor et al. 1994; Marmot 1994). In a population health model, CSA prevention would involve more than individually focused interventions or development of more professional health services. We will use the Framework for Population Health (Health Canada 1994) to guide our discussion of CSA prevention and also draw on experience in both population health promotion and clinical care. The following review is based on about 1,500 studies published between 1979 and 1995 (Bagley and Thurston 1989, 1996a, 1996b).

PREVALENCE AND HEALTH OUTCOMES OF CHILD SEXUAL ABUSE

Ideally, random community surveys give complete population figures for the prevalence and long-term social and psychological sequelae of CSA. Few surveys can obtain a response rate of more than 75 percent, which is statistically acceptable but provokes the question, Why do some people decline to be interviewed about their childhood and family history? Two sources of bias are possible: troubled individuals who welcome the opportunity to talk to an interviewer about a history of CSA; and troubled individuals who do not wish to talk about traumatic early experiences.

    1. Canadian studies using a conservative definition of CSA (unwanted, repeated sexual assaults involving physical contact) indicate that about 7 percent of females and about 5 percent of males will have been sexually abused by the age of 16. Long-term contact abuse of this type is associated with the greatest health impairment, particularly when CSA coexists with physical and emotional abuse. Children with poor self-esteem before suffering CSA (reflecting emotional and/or physical abuse) are least able to get help when CSA begins. Although CSA can occur in any type of family, there is a statistical trend for a higher incidence of CSA in economically poor families. Women from families in which CSA has occurred tend to marry earlier and have less satisfactory sex lives, less satisfactory marital partners, and higher rates of divorce than women from families in which CSA has not occurred. CSA survivors, both men and women, also have fewer educational and occupational achievements when class of origin is controlled.

    2. The studies reviewed indicate that the sequelae of CSA and associated family problems, such as physical and emotional abuse, family disruption and parental absence, constitute an important public health problem because

of the links (probably causal) of these family problems to failure to achieve personal and educational potential, and adult health conditions, including unwanted pregnancy, sexually transmitted disease, chronic health conditions involving physical pain, psychiatric disorders, sexual problems, suicidal behaviour, substance abuse.

3. The long-term sequelae of physical and emotional abuse often resemble the sequelae of sexual abuse. When different types of abuse are combined, outcomes for the adult are appreciably poorer. It has been difficult to isolate CSA as a sole cause of negative outcomes (except for bulimia and suicidal behaviour), and the most viable model seems to be that in which other types of abuse, family disruption and social factors potentiate and interact with the negative effects of CSA.

4. All studies indicate that fewer than 10 percent of abused children ever tell anyone about CSA while they are children or adolescents, and that those who tell adults are often not believed or are blamed for the abuse.

5. Girls are most often abused by a family member; boys by someone outside the nuclear family. Males apparently suffer less long-term harm from abuse than females; nevertheless, they manifest a significantly higher prevalence of suicidal behaviour in adulthood. This might be linked to doubts over sexual identity arising from male-on-male abuse and to movement into the role of abuser.

6. U.S. studies give contrasting accounts of CSA in community samples of adult women. Russell (1986) argues that long-term CSA, usually involving a father or stepfather, is followed by very negative adjustments in about 33 percent of cases. In contrast, Kilpatrick (1992) argues that only about 6 percent of CSA victims have very negative outcomes as adults; moreover, these negative outcomes may be related to the reactions of others in conjunction with the abuse itself. Society's desire to punish offenders may, paradoxically, harm victims.

7. One important U.S. study (Moeller, Bachmann and Moeller 1993) found that 53 percent of white, middle-class women had experienced at least one incident of physical, emotional or sexual abuse in childhood; 19 percent had experienced two of these types of abuse; and 5 percent had experienced all three types. CSA was twice as likely to be associated with another type of abuse as it was to occur in the absence of physical or emotional abuse. The three types of abuse seem to act in an additive way to cause greater emotional and physical harm to adult women. Although "milder" forms of CSA may have no direct effect on health in the presence of emotional and/or physical abuse, frequent acts of intercourse imposed on a girl over many years can have a powerfully negative effect on the developing identity of an adolescent woman. Suicidal behaviour, depression and bulimia are particularly linked to this kind of CSA.

8. Despite these findings, about 50 percent of women who have endured intrusive CSA over several years do not, as adults, have mental health

impairments, defined as mental health problems that interfere with daily functioning. This may be attributed to individual resilience and to supportive family factors.

REPORTING, ASSESSMENT AND EVIDENCE COLLECTION

The research reviewed in this section indicates a system of *role conflict*: conflict between the roles of the abused (or allegedly abused) child and the roles of child protection workers, therapists, police, prosecutors and parents, including even an abusing parent to whom the child and the rest of his family are still bonded. Added to these competing and conflicting roles are the roles of most of the moral guardians of modern society. When roles are in conflict, it is all too easy to lose sight of the needs of the child. Some careful, methodologically exact studies in this field should advise caution in addressing CSA. The better the studies, the more we realize that there are no certainties. Many children are not seriously damaged by the actual CSA, some are hurt by intervenors and by the criminal trial, and some are hurt by the community's failure to respond at all. Many children who are examined and tested following CSA do not manifest abnormalities of action, thought or emotion when compared with "normal" children; however, this does not preclude long-term consequences. Punitive enterprises to satisfy the moral outrage of communities and interest groups may damage the child as well as the alleged offender.

    1. False or mistaken CSA accusations are rare—between 3 and 8 percent of all cases. They may occur in the context of a bitter custody battle or when a parent is psychotic or mentally ill. However, mistaken (rather than malicious) allegations of CSA constitute around 60 percent of all cases investigated by child protection workers, highlighting how few cases are officially investigated and suggesting that child protection workers have a biased perception of CSA.

    2. Questioning a child about CSA to gather evidence for a criminal trial can frighten and even injure the child. Repeated interrogation about the abuse may result in blunting of affect. The delay between revelation and criminal trial, often more than a year, is usually fraught with anxiety for the child and the parents and can interfere with the beginning of therapy. This is also the time when the offender awaiting trial is more likely to attempt or commit suicide. Offender suicide may compound the victim's feelings of guilt.

    3. The process of interviewing and testing children who have alleged CSA is difficult. Most abused children (abuse verified by perpetrator confession) exhibit neither psychiatric symptoms nor abnormality on psychological tests. Anatomically correct dolls may be useful in therapy, but they are unreliable in a criminal investigation: most children who have suffered CSA do not behave abnormally when handling these dolls, and a

proportion of children who have not suffered CSA manifest behaviour that seems sexually explicit when they handle those dolls. Special skill is needed in interviewing children with developmental disabilities, for whom the risk of abuse is four times as high as it is for children without developmental disabilities.

4. Family Court and criminal prosecution can be effective threats in efforts to persuade the offender to leave the family home.

5. Professionals involved in assessing alleged CSA victims should also seek information on physical and/or emotional abuse in the parents' families of origin, problems in family roles, patterns of communication, other family violence, social networks, and social supports. A focus limited to CSA may fail to capture the source of a child's disturbed behaviour.

6. In reviewing literature on medical assessments, we reach two conclusions. First, children should be examined by a paediatric gynaecologist only for medical reasons, not to gather legal evidence or proof. Medical examinations are often traumatic for the child, and they are unlikely to produce evidence because, after 72 hours has elapsed, signs of gross intrusions may have been obliterated by the natural ability of the anogenital area to heal rapidly. Second, a specially trained, female health professional is the best person to conduct a medical examination when it is needed.

FAMILY FACTORS IN UNDERSTANDING, PREVENTING AND TREATING CHILD SEXUAL ABUSE

The study of the family interactions and emotional climates and interchanges that precede, accompany and follow the sexual, emotional and physical abuse of children presents researchers and clinicians with major and sometimes paradoxical challenges.

1. It is unusual for CSA to occur in nuclear families independently of other types of abuse, including excessive, frequent physical punishment and/or frequent cruel remarks and comments addressed by adult to child, as well as emotional and physical neglect. The child's psychological adjustment and long-term coping skills are most likely to be damaged by physical abuse and neglect combined with emotional abuse and neglect. CSA is hard to detect when preceded by other kinds of abuse and neglect. In the absence of other types of abuse and in the context of a family in which emotional bonding and support exist, CSA imposes less harm on a child, and the harm does not seem to last as long, provided that the child is not blamed for causing the abuse and is offered emotional and social support after the abuse.

2. CSA occurs more often than by chance in nuclear families with disordered patterns of communication, tension of interchange, mental illness or alcoholism in a parent, and distorted roles, such as expecting a child to perform duties (e.g., cooking, child care, earning money) that are normally

adult tasks. This is "parentification," and it may include CSA. When a girl in such a situation tries, in adolescence, to end an incestuous relationship, the adult will try to stop her because he is more emotionally and physically dependent on her than she is on him. This role transition is crucial, but if a girl is not accused of seducing her father and is accepted and supported by her mother and community, the long-term outcome for her is likely to be good.

3. In the worst-case scenario, a girl is beaten frequently; is raped frequently; is hurt repeatedly if she resists; suffers emotional cruelty from her abuser and other family members; is blamed for lying or causing the abuse; is ejected from her home, sometimes with the connivance of child welfare workers or is simply pushed out or runs away; and is then sexually revictimized. This victim will suffer profound identity problems, and sexual adjustment problems and self-blame are likely to follow.

4. Families in which CSA occurs are similar in dynamics to families in which interactions are distorted by an adult alcoholic member. Therapists are advised to consider the possibility that alcohol dysfunction and CSA occur together in families.

5. It is difficult to untangle the effects of physical, emotional and sexual abuse. Children who have experienced physical and/or emotional abuse but no CSA often have as many adjustment problems as CSA children from families with similar characteristics. Some studies indicate that the effects of different kinds of abuse are additive, while others present findings indicating an interactive effect, i.e., the combination of CSA with physical and emotional abuse is powerfully negative in a way not predicted by an additive model.

6. The nature of the abusive acts, the duration of the abuse, and the relationship of the abuser to the victim (father, other family member, person external to the family) predict some of the variance in negative outcomes for victims. Most children do not reveal family sexual abuse (incest) to individuals outside their family; however, close relatives often learn or are told about incest. A supportive and sympathetic reaction, especially from the mother, is crucial for the recovery and maintenance of the victim's health. The reaction of the social network, including other family members, is critical in both the short and long term.

7. Several studies have identified subtypes of incestuous families, such as families marked by affectional erotic exchange; families marked by the cruel exercise of despotic, male power with multiple kinds of abuse and multiple victims; and polyincestuous extended families with multiple kinds of incest between different nuclear families across and between generations.

8. The possibility also exists that the "kind" or "gentle" seduction of a child, as a form of affectional interchange, may cause no immediate harm. Paradoxically, health, social service, legal, and victim-oriented interventions

in this type of abuse may cause more harm than the abuse itself by arousing guilt and self-doubt and by applying diagnostic models that are sexist or classist.

9. Early interaction of a father with his infant child may create a biosocial process that inhibits incest, but stepfathers and common-law husbands must find other methods to restrain themselves from sexual involvement with their acquired children. Stepfathers are at least five times more likely to abuse a child in their household than biological fathers. The rate of biological father incest in Canada is less than 1 percent.

10. Several schools of family therapy have been developed for treating incestuous families. The humanistic model of Giarretto (1981) is best known, and evaluations indicate largely positive outcomes for reconstituted families. The system of therapy developed by Larson and Maddock (1995) has the strongest theoretical base but has yet to be evaluated fully. Bentovim's model (1988) is well described, and evaluations of it have found that child welfare systems often fail to support or cooperate in therapy, many families drop out of therapy, and girls of families resistant to treatment may be revictimized.

Most family therapy models include legal compulsion for abusers to cooperate in therapy in return for nonprosecution or suspended sentences. Incestuous fathers have been characterized as weak, egocentric, selfish, and lacking empathy for or insight about the psychological confusion of their child victim; therefore, an incestuous family should not be reconstituted unless the mother supports her victimized daughter strongly and the father admits guilt and expresses remorse. Unfortunately, this compels many mothers to make an invidious choice: between her daughter (and divorce and poverty) and her husband (and continuing the comparative prosperity of marriage). Family therapy models continue to be criticized for failure to incorporate power differentials and other socioeconomic forces such as the lower status of women.

11. Girls who are not supported by their mothers or who are disbelieved or blamed by other family members are often unable to stay at home or to return home. A follow-up study indicates that about 20 percent of girls regretted disclosing incest and often had poorer mental health than at revelation. This was linked to lack of maternal support and to repeated, harrowing interrogations by medical, legal and social work systems that provided little social and emotional support.

CLINICAL AND TREATMENT ISSUES FOR SEXUALLY ABUSED CHILDREN

Clinical studies of children who have experienced sexual abuse are usually based on referrals to hospitals, mental health clinics and therapy programs. It is likely such children are probably the most-damaged CSA victims; thus, although the findings of many clinical studies are important, they should not be generalized to all sexually abused children. Some of the studies summarized in this section did not use standardized measures of adjustment or measures with established reliability and validity. Also, many studies did not use control or comparison groups. We have noted some of these studies in our review because of their clinical insights and their hypotheses for further research.

1. CSA (often combined with other forms of abuse) can undermine healthy identity development in profound ways, leaving the chronically abused child without a strong sense of competence in performing the roles of adult life and sometimes confused about psychosexual identity.

2. "Sexual abuse syndrome," per se, does not exist. Studies that compare adolescents who were victims of chronic CSA before adolescence with adolescents who had not been abused suggest that around 25 percent of adolescent CSA victims manifest serious problems. The nature of these problems may depend on other factors, such as individual vulnerability, temperament, and other experiences of emotional and physical abuse. The most distinctive disturbed behaviours of CSA victims are traumatic sexualization and sexual acting out (e.g., sexual promiscuity). Somatic disorders, dissociation, eating disorders, borderline personality, and deliberate self-harm are also found in CSA victims more often than in nonvictims, but only a minority of CSA victims will exhibit these extreme problems.

3. Many clinical, evaluative and descriptive studies are atheoretical, but some excellent conceptual articles have begun to appear, such as those by Finkelhor (1995), Putnam and Trickett (1993), Bukowski (1992) and others. These studies stress that an understanding of CSA must be grounded in accounts of normal child development, vulnerability and resiliency at different ages, and the different impacts of various kinds of trauma.

4. There is a dearth of systematic follow-up studies of treatment for CSA victims. Studies with randomized, untreated controls are difficult to undertake, but many studies have not even attempted to obtain comparison groups. The more methodologically exact studies of CSA show that other forms of abuse and neglect contribute to negative outcomes, as do the reactions of others after the abuse is revealed and involvement in legal proceedings. Failure to address the etiological complexity of negative outcomes has meant that taxonomies are based on individual characteristics and cannot be replicated from study to study.

5. Children from economically deprived backgrounds and from single-parent families seem to be more likely to experience more than one type of abuse and have poorer outcomes. It is not clear, however, whether these children and families are simply more prone to official intervention and research. Rates of abuse may be lower in some cultures (e.g., sexually conservative Asian groups). The lives of many urban North American children are sexualized through peer group participation; this might make them more vulnerable to CSA; and, paradoxically, the normative sexuality of childhood could make them less vulnerable to the long-term effects of CSA.

MOTHERS OF VICTIMS

When CSA is revealed, the mother's support is crucially important to the victim; therefore, the absence of studies of the mother's role is disquieting. We seem to have gone from blaming mothers for CSA to relative silence on mothers and their needs, in comparison with the mass of literature on other aspects of CSA.

The published reports indicate that a mother is caught in a dilemma when she realizes that the man who supported her economically and, frequently, dominated her life has extended a cruel hand in abusing her children. If the mother is a CSA survivor, the shock of this realization may evoke painful memories from her own unhealed psyche and bring on a mental health crisis of her own. American studies indicate that, when CSA is revealed, up to 25 percent of mothers do not accept that their daughters are victims. This is especially likely when the child revealing abuse is a teenager and when intercourse has taken place. Often such girls are removed to foster care or group homes, and their long-term adjustment is poor. Even the mother who supports her child spends many unhappy months (along with her child) waiting for the trial process to begin.

The sparse literature on mothers of victims gives the distinct impression, which must be investigated in further studies, that an adolescent who is rejected by her mother when she reveals an incestuous relationship is almost certain to experience long-term mental and other health problems. Mothers from disorganized families of low social status often have difficulty negotiating through the maze of services that should offer support and protection. Without social support and attention to pressing issues such as financial support, mother and adolescent will attend therapy intermittently if at all, and both will be vulnerable to revictimization. It is a cruel fact that such adolescents might have better health outcomes if they keep incest secret.

SEXUAL ABUSE PREVENTION EDUCATION FOR CHILDREN

Several writers argue that since CSA is prevalent and victims rarely receive adequate treatment when they reveal abuse, sexual abuse prevention should be an important strategy. Few disagree with this idea, but how prevention is to be achieved is open for debate. Most child sexual abuse prevention programs (CSAPPs) focus on education for children between 4 and 12 years old. These programs have positive aspects, but there are many serious problems with the common approaches. Frequently, children learn little about CSA prevention concepts and seem to be able to acquire only certain concepts; however, these ideas can be long lasting. Some children can learn concepts of bodily integrity and improper use of authority.

Criticisms of CSAPPs with policy implications are as follows:

1. CSAPPs rarely address cultural diversity, which should be part of the program's theoretical framework. Furthermore, educating children should be only part of a multidisciplinary, community-based approach to prevention. Children with special needs, such as latchkey children, who are vulnerable in the period between the end of school and when parents return home, must be considered.

2. Few teachers are trained to handle the tasks surrounding CSAPPs, such as helping a child who reveals abuse following a program.

3. Several writers comment on the lack of sex education in CSAPP programs, a fact that paedophiles note with approval, since the definition of sexual abuse is unclear. Conservative parents often discourage sex education for children in elementary school, frequently because of church policies.

4. Similarly, programs rarely include moral messages about CSA. Although most programs stress a child's right to bodily integrity and to refuse "bad touches," the idea that an adult has no right to involve a child sexually is rarely emphasized. Also, programs do not address the possibility that a sexually ignorant child may receive "good touches" from a skilled paedophile.

5. Preparing CSAPP packages is a multimillion dollar industry in the United States, but most such materials have not been tested or evaluated. Widespread use of such programs may make teachers complacent, giving them the mistaken idea that, in using a packaged CSAPP, they have done everything necessary to prevent CSA. There is great variation in the way teachers use CSAPP packages and no evidence that they actually prevent abuse or are worth what they cost.

6. CSAPPs are often used inappropriately with younger children, children from cultural minorities, and children with special cognitive needs. Ideally, programs should be tailor-made for each age and gender. Several writers suggest that CSAPPs rarely work for children younger than seven, who usually cannot understand or retain CSA-prevention information. Some children are "repeat failures" in longitudinal studies of knowledge gains following CSAPPs. These children tend to have poor cognitive skills and low self-esteem. Unfortunately, these children may be most at risk of CSA. Boys and girls need different types of CSAPPs. Boys are likely to be approached in a gender-specific way by potential molesters, who are usually male, and appeals to masculinity or machismo may be made. Many boys feel that innate toughness is a natural defence against CSA, failing to understand the variety of approaches used by the determined paedophile.

7. Programs rarely address the gaps between knowledge, attitudes, beliefs and behaviour. The few CSAPPs that include role play have promising results. However, a case study indicates that an employee in one elementary school was able to involve 22 children in a "sex ring" although they had all watched a CSAPP video.

8. There is a strong case for addressing prevention education efforts to adolescents, who may be tempted to abuse children and sexually assault peers. "Date rape" and the victim-to-abuser cycle in adolescence are key problems that could be addressed by educational programs on sexual etiquette, sex roles, and the harmful effects of rape and sexual abuse.

9. Bullying is an issue that designers did not foresee but that children raise in CSAPPs. Children often construe bullying as a violation of bodily integrity and, therefore, as an example of "bad touch."

10. Many writers agree that CSAPPs concentrate too much on CSA by strangers and by people from outside the family and fail to clarify the actual meanings and implications of incest. This reflects, in part, inhibitions about casting fathers in the role of potential abusers and, in part, the parental coyness and pressure that also prevent CSAPPs from including specific sex education topics. CSAPPs have failed to address the issue of family dynamics in which a child will endure CSA to satisfy natural needs for affection, love, attachment and dependence that are not otherwise met.

11. Studies note some negative effects of CSAPPs on children such as increased anxiety and fear of strangers, aversion to affectionate and innocent touching by family members, mistaken accusations of CSA based on a misunderstanding of program messages, and refusal to accept the "bad touch" involved in disciplinary measures such as spanking.

12. Some CSAPPs urge children to "fight back" when approached by a potential abuser. This is dangerous advice: a national U.S. study produced evidence that fighting back can elicit counter-aggression, especially when the abuser is a stranger.

13. CSAPPs imply that CSA is a sudden assault that a child can recognize, understand and avoid. Programs fail to address how many abusers create or use the child's emotional dependence on and attachment to the abuser. Abusive touches are often peripheral and gradual, desensitizing the child to the abuse inherent in these touches. Such gentle seduction often gives children "the yes feeling."

More fundamental critiques, which argue that CSAPP programs should be abandoned until fundamental questions and problems are addressed, are the following:

1. By concentrating on CSAPPs, we effectively make children responsible for preventing CSA themselves. This is neither right nor fair. This criticism is linked to the false assumption that CSAPPs can protect children from CSA and that, once a child has viewed a CSAPP video, CSA issues can be safely shelved.

2. There is no evidence that any school education program has prevented a single case of CSA. In theory, the widespread use of CSAPPs should reduce the overall incidence of CSA as measured by repeated surveys of young adults. No such studies are available, and other studies indicate an increase.

3. The "good touch, bad touch" message of many CSAPPs represents a fundamental conceptual flaw. Children are usually powerless in their families and must endure frequent, unpleasant physical touches ranging from slaps to beatings, which are unfortunately legal in Canada. Until society prohibits physical punishment as well as sexual exploitation of children, such CSAPPs are doomed to fail.

4. CSAPPs are dangerous because they give teachers, parents and children the false idea that problems of sexual abuse can be avoided by screening a video.

5. Offenders have given useful information about their own patterns of behaviour that could be incorporated into CSAPPs. Many paedophiles become family friends to gain access to a child. Hard-pressed single mothers are particularly likely to be entrapped by men who seek sexual access to their children. Children with good self-esteem and good communication with stable parents are much less likely to be sought out or ensnared by a paedophile. Offenders report that a child who has been physically and/or emotionally abused by a parent is a prime target for sexual abuse.

6. The money and effort directed to ineffectual CSAPPs for elementary school children should be directed toward adolescents, who are both potential victims and potential offenders, and to potential adult offenders. Cogent arguments have been made for family life education and programs to support father-infant bonding (a natural deterrent to sexually abusing one's child) and for advising stepfathers of the dangers of sexual involvement with the children in their acquired families.

7. Although there is no systematic evidence on how many children reveal abuse after CSAPPs, what exists suggests that the number of children who reveal CSA after a prevention program is much smaller than the number of sexually abused children indicated by adult recall studies. Many abused children have very low self-esteem and may feel guilt or despair if they cannot reveal abuse to their teacher after a CSAPP.

8. The CSAPP messages—"listen to your feelings," "choose the good touch," and "your body is your own"—are unrealistic. Indeed, determined paedophiles can easily expoit the child who has been told to choose the good touch for his body, a body that only the child has the right to allow others to touch. Voluntary sexual touching gives adults good feelings; this is true for children too.

9. In the United States, programs to persuade adolescents to postpone sexual relations and thus to avoid pregnancy and sexually transmitted diseases, have failed dismally. The same may prove true of CSAPPs.

ADOLESCENT VICTIMS: MENTAL HEALTH, DELINQUENCY, RUNAWAY BEHAVIOUR, PROSTITUTION AND THE VICTIM-TO-ABUSER CYCLE

Studies of adults show that many men begin their sexually deviant activities in adolescence. This is a crucial time for intervention and treatment, since adult paedophiles are difficult to detect or treat and may assault hundreds of victims. In this section, we also review studies of complete populations of high school students. These studies are significant because they are likely to achieve more complete profiles of populations (at least up to the age of 16) than are available from studies of postsecondary students or adult communities. School-based studies indicate not only the prevalence of current and past sexual abuse causing extreme stress to young adolescents, but also the adverse health effects on adolescents associated with other family stressors.

1. Adolescent girls are at risk of various types of forced sexual encounter, the most prevalent being date rape, but rape by strangers and by family members also occurs. Adolescent girls rarely report rape to any authority. After sexual assault, these victims are often fearful, anxious and depressed for the rest of their teenage years. Girls who live in economically depressed neighbourhoods are more at risk of rape. Teenage sexual assailants tend to be in their midteens, and a national American study indicated that they come from all ethnic groups. Youths who rape tend to be outside the mainstream of teenage life and are often generally delinquent. These findings challenge the designers of prevention-education programs for schools: teenage girls must be advised of risky situations, and teenage boys must learn that sexual assault is cruel and hurtful and can cause victims long-term psychological harm.

2. Several Canadian and American studies of young adolescent prostitutes indicate that both males and females have very high rates of CSA (about 70 percent) before leaving home and becoming entrapped in street life. Their families of origin are often outwardly respectable but are marked by high rates of alcoholism in parents and by emotional as well as sexual and physical abuse of children. For adolescents, street life involves drug addiction and exploitation at the hands of pimps. Outreach services have limited success with this group.

3. Adolescents who sexually assault younger children are often social isolates, with internalized symptoms such as anxiety, depression and suicidal feelings. They frequently come from families marked by alcoholism and emotional abuse and, very often, are survivors of sexual abuse. Early neurological problems may also be associated with sexual offending by adolescents. Many adolescent males who enter the victim-to-abuser cycle come from emotionally neglectful or abusive homes and have experienced "traumatic bonding" with their own abuser. For these adolescents, treatment

must involve accepting responsibility for their sexual assaults and reframing assault as a desperate attempt to achieve some sense of personal power.

4. Self-completion measures can be used to identify sexually victimized adolescents. About 9 percent of Canadian students come from homes marked by emotional, physical or sexual abuse, or two of the three types, or all three, with dysfunctional and often alcoholic parents; the adolescent children are often depressed and suicidal and have markedly low self-esteem. Policies do not acknowledge the roots of deviant behaviour and, therefore, tend to blame victims. About 15 percent of adolescents in Canadian child care facilities and child welfare populations display signs of dissociative personality, reflecting a history of severe physical and sexual abuse. Wolfe, Sas et al. (1994) observed that about 40 percent of female delinquents and many male delinquents referred to the London Family Court Clinic disclose a history of serious sexual abuse. "The majority of these adolescents saw their own abusive experiences as unresolved. They harboured great emotional pain, and believed their situations had been handled poorly by those responsible for their care" (p. 2). This "system-induced trauma" is a form of blaming victims of CSA who act out in the community: they are punished when they act out in antisocial or conduct-disordered ways.

5. Normal adolescents have to make major identity transitions based on physical, social and psychological changes in their status. The sexually mature adolescent will recapitulate early experiences in a newly formed identity. Sexually abused adolescents may find this process difficult, be socially isolated, and end up with an identity fixated in a stage of guilt and sexual acting out. Identity fixation may be an important factor in assaultive behaviour in males and defeated promiscuity in females. Pregnant teens are particularly likely to be survivors of CSA or rape.

6. One important Canadian study has found that abused youth did not define the abuse situation the way professionals saw alleged sexual abuse. For youth, abuse takes place when the events cause emotional hurt or harm. This phenomenological perspective implies that adolescents should be listened to carefully during abuse investigations and treatment.

ADULT SURVIVORS: PSYCHOLOGICAL OUTCOMES AND THERAPEUTIC INTERVENTION

Many of the studies reviewed in this section report very negative adult outcomes of CSA. It is important to remember, however, that not all victims have adult outcomes as serious as those the survivors described in clinical studies have. Research based on people going to hospitals, clinics and general practitioners with specific psychological and physical problems is, by definition, concerned with those most damaged by abuse. Nevertheless, these individuals are very important and require effective, skilled, informed intervention. The long-term psychological harm experienced by a significant number of CSA victims emphasizes that prevention strategies for all types of child abuse must be improved. We note a dearth of studies of male survivors relative to the known incidence of sexual victimization of male children. We found no available systematic studies of the small number of abusers (about 5 percent) who are adult women. The studies reviewed point to the following conclusions:

1. Chronic, severe physical and emotional abuse in childhood can also interfere with the child's healthy attachments and developing sense of identity. Emotional and physical abuse and disorders of family interaction often precede and accompany CSA, contributing to or exacerbating its effects. It is difficult to establish the causal significance of CSA in later adjustment problems without controlling for other family and developmental factors. When this is done, CSA appears to have a causal connection with adult suicidality, sexual adjustment problems, eating disorders, dissociation, and psychosomatic complaints such as chronic pelvic pain and gastrointestinal symptoms. For males, suicidality, substance abuse and chaotically ordered aggression may be causally linked to CSA.

2. Surprisingly few studies have found any direct link between adult mental health problems and who the abuser is (e.g., father), what happened in the abuse (e.g., fondling, intercourse), and when abuse began. The crucial element seems to be the combination of secrecy in a family climate of disordered communications and attachment processes; emotional or physical abuse or both; and the shame and guilt felt by the victim.

3. The victim's social and family environment is crucial: a warm, loving, accepting and sexually open family can minimize the harmful results of CSA. Likewise, a family and social network that accepts the victim without blame after CSA is revealed can contribute to good health in the victim.

4. Revictimization (e.g., a girl is victimized in her family and is later subjected to serious sexual assault by other family members or by people outside the family) is associated with poor prognosis, often associated with overwhelming feelings of self-blame and powerlessness, including movement into learned helplessness and attachments to abusive men. This cycle of victimization is likely to occur in children from families in which CSA coexisted with emotional or physical abuse of the child or both, alcoholism or mental illness in a parent, and disordered types of parent-child attachment. Therapy for adult survivors must address these pathological parent-child interactions and family climates before the serious harm wrought by CSA can be addressed. Such individual therapy can prepare the adult survivor for group therapy.

5. Various group therapy models, often in combination with individual therapy, can successfully reduce social isolation and feelings of guilt. Female therapists are most effective for both female and male survivors.

6. CSA and its association with physical and emotional abuse may be associated with dissociative personality states. However, positive dissociation

(the ability to detach from abuse without entering a self-hypnotic trance) is associated with good prognosis for victims. Downward comparisons (comparisons with those less fortunate) and distancing from abuse or its memory are also valuable techniques. Such techniques may be more available to survivors with higher intelligence or healthy attachments and with communication patterns with people who will support and help them both during and after abuse.

7. While the debate over recovered memories continues, clinical practice clearly shows that memories of severe CSA can be suppressed, only to be triggered later in life by specific stimuli. Follow-up research on verified CSA survivors indicates that some do completely forget or repress details of abuse.

8. Simply remembering CSA and talking about it, writing about it, or engaging in other cathartic activities such as arts therapy with a sympathetic female therapist or survivor group can be an important step on the road to psychological recovery.

9. Symptoms of acute anxiety and post-traumatic stress may indicate repressed CSA memories. Many CSA survivors are hypervigilant, and this is associated with high levels of adult anxiety. Substance abuse and suicide attempts may be caused by massive anxiety attacks in the adult survivor. Hypervigilance and reactivity to unwanted sexual touching may also lead to low pain tolerance. Nevertheless, efforts to "diagnose" post-traumatic stress syndrome have little clinical value for survivors.

10. Paradoxically, even as adults, children can remain loyal to their abuser and hostile to the parent who did not protect them. Therapists must not blame or express disgust for the abuser when therapy begins.

11. Primary care physicians should be alerted to CSA as a possible cause of eating disorders and of treatment-resistant chronic gastrointestinal symptoms and pelvic pain. Many survivors do not link CSA and their current symptoms, and making such a link is an important step in psychological healing.

12. The therapist must understand the cognitive style of a CSA survivor. Often, an inappropriate cognitive style underlies a self-defeating way of coping with body, psyche and the external world. A survivor who believes that she is bad and responsible for the sexual, physical or emotional abuse she has suffered is likely to develop a stable, attributional style of self-blame as well as low self-esteem and feelings of inadequacy and powerlessness in human relationships. This negative attributional cognitive style leads survivors to blame themselves for external, uncontrollable negative events. Cognitive therapies can help survivors absolve themselves of blame for the abuse and develop a sense of competence in self-appraisal and social relationships. Cognitive therapy aims to eliminate irrational and negative beliefs through individual cognitive restructuring and has demonstrated effect in longitudinal evaluations.

ABUSERS: ASSESSMENT, PROCESSING AND THERAPY

Compared with the many studies on victims of CSA and on teaching children to help prevent their own victimization, the literature on men and women who abuse children is disturbingly small. Relatively little research has focused on how to prevent potential abusers from abusing children and how to treat them effectively when they are apprehended. One problem is that almost all published studies concern men already in the criminal justice system. These men are probably the most persistent, impulsive, violent or incompetent abusers, the ones most likely to be pursued by police, most likely to be caught, and most likely to be brought to trial. Only a few researchers have identified or recruited men with long histories as sexual abusers. At least two-thirds of these men were never arrested, but they admitted in confidential interviews to abusing scores or hundreds of children. Unfortunately, in most jurisdictions in North America, reporting laws designed to reduce CSA prevent current but undetected abusers from obtaining non-punitive treatment that could prevent further offending.

1. The classic study by Groth and Birnbaum (1978) identified two apparently quite separate groups of abusers: regressed offenders (typically, incestuous abusers) and fixated abusers (typically, paedophiles with a history of offending that originated in adolescence and with a personal history of CSA—such men are more likely to assault extrafamilial boys). Later research suggests a continuum rather than a dichotomy because there is also an intermediate, perhaps larger, group of incest offenders who have histories of violence and other offences, sometimes including extrafamilial CSA. Another typology has identified social competence (low or high) and degree of fixation (low or high) as defining four types of abusers. Offenders with low social competence and high fixation are most likely to be caught and prosecuted. Some paedophiles marry women with children to gain sexual access. Seductive paedophiles can be infinitely patient in selecting and grooming a child for gradual acclimatization to sexual activity. Other paedophiles lack empathy for the suffering of their victims. Empathy training could be an important part of therapy, although this has not been formally evaluated. There is clearly a need for further work on classifying abusers to refine strategies for treatment and for predicting capacity to reoffend.

2. Offenders have been described as lacking social skills, ego strength, and self-esteem; however, these traits could reflect the pain and humiliation of prosecution and incarceration. Some male CSA survivors may abuse children during fugue or dissociative states or under the influence of alcohol, and they often deny that they committed abuse or that such abuse is harmful. It is clear, however, that many paedophiles approach and seduce children at great risk to themselves. Paradoxically, seducing children requires considerable determination and is not the act of a timid man. No model that integrates these paradoxical findings has yet appeared, and separate

models of motivation may have to be constructed for various subgroups of abusers.

3. The origins of paedophilic motivation are diverse, but they usually lie in childhood. Some men bonded to an abuser and internalized his role as they escaped from emotionally and physically abusive homes. Others acquired a powerful sexual motivation through the imprinting of sexual acts with peers or adults. The sexual exploitation of children by incest offenders seems to represent a combination of lust and the expression of a fragile sense of dominance and power in men with little self-esteem or ego strength. The sexual motivation for many paedophiles is overwhelmingly strong, which is why "chemical castration" is sometimes used to treat them. This sexual motivation may be linked to temporal lobe and pituitary gland abnormalities, which are found in about 25 percent of detected offenders. Genetic factors have also been implicated, as have certain temperaments.

4. Finkelhor's (1984) four-factor model of paedophile motivations has received strong empirical support. In this model, all four of the following factors must be present for CSA to occur: (a) motivation to sexually abuse a child; (b) overcoming internal inhibitions about CSA; (c) overcoming external inhibitions or controls; and (d) overcoming the child's resistance or reluctance by some form of control, authority or quasi socialization.

5. Standardized psychological assessment has produced disappointing results. The Minnesota Multiphasic Personality Inventory profiles of abusers are often similar to those of controls. Some evidence suggests that apprehended abusers have lower IQs than controls; this might reflect either some underlying brain functions associated with paedophile motivation or simply that clever paedophiles and incest offenders are less likely to be caught. Paedophiles are often able to camouflage their psychological characteristics and sexual interests and have normal marital relations when they choose. In phallometric studies, many paedophiles are capable of normal responses to conventional erotic stimuli. Apprehended offenders may also "fake good" or "fake bad" on psychological measures, according to the setting and purpose of the testing; for example, they may "fake bad" on measures that imply a diminution of responsibility.

6. Alcoholism is an important factor in incest. Alcohol increases libido, lowers inhibition, impairs sexual function, harms social relationships and, unless addressed directly, impedes therapy. Incest abusers may also give alcohol to their victims to reduce opposition to sexual contact. Most incestuous abuse occurs in families with disordered patterns of communication, impaired attachments between children and adults, and the physical or emotional abuse of children, or both.

7. Overcoming denial of the offence and countering the offender's minimization of its impact are important first steps in treating sexual abusers of children. Many first-time offenders can be treated in the community and will not reoffend, especially if they abused only one victim and that

victim was a member of their family. However, community treatment requires a cooperative judicial system that permits probation if the offender enters therapy and participates in therapy for his victim and his family. A family systems approach based on an understanding of sexism and classism may be successful in this respect. Unfortunately, careful follow-up studies of treatment regimes for offenders are rare.

8. For incarcerated offenders, therapy to prevent reoffending is important. Without treatment in prison, the offender is likely to be released with unmodified, deviant sexual patterns and is therefore likely to reoffend. Treatment in prison costs relatively little and could be highly cost effective.

9. In addition to lack of treatment in prison, other predictors of reoffending are being a CSA survivor; having begun to abuse children during adolescence; having brief, serial sexual encounters with several extrafamilial children, usually boys; remaining unmarried; and having several previous convictions. Some men with many risk factors can be successfully treated, but others seem untreatable by available therapies. Taxonomic studies may identify subgroups requiring more specific types of treatment to prevent recidivism.

10. Combining cognitive-behavioural treatment with drug therapy to reduce testosterone or sex drive can reduce recidivism in fixated paedophiles to 10 to 30 percent, compared with a recidivism rate of about 50 percent in untreated offenders.

CASE STUDIES

The Development of Research and Policy on Child Sexual Abuse in Canada: A Case Study of Exemplary Research and Policy Development

The impetus for change in the way CSA is regarded, treated and prevented in Canada began in the late 1970s, as a result of several local initiatives (e.g., in Calgary, Vancouver and Toronto). Political responsiveness by the government of the day led to the establishment of the Committee on Sexual Offences Against Children and Youths (Canada), chaired by Dr. Robin Badgley and sponsored jointly by the Department of Justice and Health and Welfare Canada. In 1984, *Sexual Offences Against Children: Report of the Committee on Sexual Offences Against Children and Youths (Canada)* was published in two volumes (Badgley 1984). Based on four national surveys of CSA survivors and processing and treatment of victims, the Badgley Report was an intellectual and moral *tour de force*, and its 52 recommendations fueled debate and community input that led to legal and policy changes at the federal level. As a result of a proposal in the report, the government appointed a Commissioner with broad responsibility for developing and integrating action and policy in the areas of health, welfare and criminal justice. Many of the proposed legal changes were adopted in 1988 as amendments to the *Criminal Code of Canada* and the *Canada Evidence Act* (Wells 1990), and the Commissioner issued a series of consultation papers (Rogers 1990).

In 1985, the report of the Fraser Committee on Pornography and Prostitution was published (Fraser 1985). Although the Fraser Report covered both adult and juvenile prostitution, many of its proposals resembled and reinforced the Badgley Report recommendations, with one important variation. The Badgley Report recommended making juvenile prostitution a status offence so that a youth could be prosecuted as a party to a commercial sex act, just as an underage youth can be prosecuted for purchasing and consuming liquor, but the Fraser Report successfully argued against criminalizing juvenile prostitution. This debate continues, but the fact remains that police need the power to intervene when a child or an adolescent is prostituted. Remarkably few pimps controlling juveniles are prosecuted. Purchasers of the sexual services of someone under 18 are committing a criminal offence, even when they do not know the juvenile's exact age, but it is very difficult for police to enforce this law. We are unaware of any prosecutions of customers of juvenile prostitutes in the past five years.

The research, policy and law enforcement initiatives that arose from the Badgley Report are important examples of coordinated research and action and of how a policy cycle can be launched by setting a public agenda. However, in the mid-1990s, the impetus seems to have flagged. The federal office of the commissioner for intergovernmental policy review has been abolished. No new research was commissioned after the original research was reviewed and implications were drawn (Bagley and Thomlison 1991). Federal cuts have severely limited sponsorship of CSA research by national research agencies such as the Social Sciences and Humanities Research Council and the National Health Research and Development Program. The National Institute for the Prevention of Child Abuse closed in 1995 for want of funding, and other programs are now struggling in the face of severe funding cuts. The National Forum on Health could take the lead in maintaining and promoting prevention of CSA as an item on the policy agenda.

Child Sexual Abuse and Community Regeneration: Case Study of an Aboriginal Community in British Columbia

All over North America, Aboriginal nations experienced European invasion, loss of land and livelihood, and deliberate efforts to undermine traditional family, language and religious systems. These efforts included the official removal of Aboriginal children to residential schools, where many were physically, emotionally and sexually abused. Among the sequelae are high rates of unemployment, alcohol and drug abuse, and suicide (Bagley, Wood, and Khumar 1991). The exact rates of sexual abuse experienced by Aboriginal women are unknown. Rundle (1990) interviewed 203 women at health and community centres in and around Calgary and found that 97 of them had been sexually abused before the age of 17. Many had been sexually assaulted by an adolescent or adult alcoholic who was drunk at the time— clearly implying that alcohol abuse compounds the issue of sexual abuse of Aboriginal women, among many other problems.

The Alkali Lake Band in northeastern British Columbia is a remarkable example of a regenerated community that addressed problems of alcohol abuse and, consequently, sexual abuse of children. This community development took place in the 1980s and has been well documented, particularly in a series of films produced by the Canadian Broadcasting Corporation. In a 1996 telephone interview, a member of the Alkali Lake Band Council stated that at least 95 percent of the adult population maintains sobriety. Adult CSA survivors receive support in continuing group sessions. These groups also include adults (many of them CSA survivors) who became abusers themselves. The support groups have an ethos of forgiveness and sharing emotions. Other benefits have been a sharp decrease in child neglect, and outside social workers no longer need to intrude into the lives of band members.

Alkali Lake is an important model of community action that sprang from the action of a few individuals. Other factors must, however, support such action; for example, problems of economic dependency and chronic unemployment must be solved. As we found in our Alberta research, suicide rates in bands has a direct, inverse correlation with per capita income, so a community that wants to tackle alcoholism and the legacy of CSA must address other problems first. The five elements of community regeneration are (1) solution of economic problems, including settlement of land claims, so that a band can become economically self-sufficient; (2) withdrawal of external agencies unless the Band Council requests involvement; (3) community-wide recognition of the problem and participation in defining it and its solutions (e.g., whether alcohol abuse is addressed); (4) involvement by most community members in the regeneration program; and (5) taking the necessary time to implement change, because communities do not regenerate at a predictable speed (for instance, the Alkali Lake Band needed a decade to limit alcohol abuse problems to a small minority of members).

The Alkali Lake experience shows that, other things being equal, a community can, from its own resources, overcome problems of current and past sexual abuse. This success, and the wisdom developed in achieving it, can be gathered into community development models, such as those offered at the Nechi Institute of Northern Alberta in workshops for Aboriginal health care providers.

The literature on preventing CSA covers few examples of community-based programming, self-help, mutual aid, or population health promotion.

The London Family Court Clinic

A London Family Court Clinic team headed by Dr. Louise Sas has been responsible for innovations in supporting child witnesses testifying against sexual abuse offenders (Sas 1991). The clinic received major federal funding for this project. The clinic staff includes a team of scholars and researchers from the University of Western Ontario led by Dr. David Wolfe that has contributed significantly to knowledge and practice in treating and preventing child abuse.

Attending court to testify against an alleged abuser is often traumatic, and anxiety may prevent a child from giving a clear account of events. Prosecutors sometimes drop cases because court attendance and cross-examination are likely to be too traumatic for a child victim.

In a controlled study, 144 children were randomly divided into three groups: (1) children received no pretrial preparation, but the counselling ordinarily available to known victims was available; (2) in addition to normal counselling, children were given a tour of the court and an explanation of possible events, about a week before the trial; and (3) children were given a tour of the court and, on average, five individual trial preparation sessions, including role play in a simulated courtroom, relaxation exercises and, after assessment of the child's cognitive and emotional state, specialized counselling. For legal reasons, the counsellors did not discuss any aspects of the alleged abuse, although children may have met with Crown prosecutors to discuss details of testimony and questions that might be asked in cross-examination.

Eighty percent of the children in the study were girls, 37 percent had been abused by someone with authority over them, and 34 percent had been abused by someone who threatened to use force. Most of the children were between the ages of 10 and 13, and about 20 percent had "low-functioning" intellectual levels. The most common type of assault was sexual touching (74 percent); 13 percent of the children had been subjected to vaginal intercourse; and 49 percent were suffering from post-traumatic stress disorder. Many children waited a year or more for the court to adjudicate on their allegations, and some waited as long as two years. Such delay is, in itself, traumatic, since counsellors may not address the events of abuse until the case is concluded.

Comparison of measures completed before and after the trial indicated that children in the intensive-preparation group had significantly fewer court-related fears and anxieties and less general anxiety than children in the other groups. In court, Crown attorneys found that children from the intensive-preparation group gave the clearest, least troubled testimony and that the accused in these cases were found guilty more often. Sas recommends that all children who must testify in sexual abuse trials be given comprehensive preparation to alleviate their anxiety. She also noted that many boys who had been abused but were not in the intensive-preparation group reappeared in court as abusers and that many of the untreated girls ended up in abusive or exploitive relationships. Therefore, court preparation may have positive preventive benefits far outweighing reduction of court anxiety and improvement of conviction rates.

The success of witness preparation cannot be measured solely in terms of convictions; the average time from charge to trial was 322 days. Of 144 cases, 32 were abandoned by the Crown; 127 went to trial; and only 75 trials ended with a judicial conclusion. Only 37 of the 144 men charged were found guilty, despite the testimony of their child victims. Only 6 percent of the men originally charged served time in prison.

As of 1995, this program had not been extended or replicated elsewhere in Canada. However, the London Family Court Clinic issued a key report from the child witness project on how children reveal sexual abuse and the support that a Family Court clinic can give (Sas et al. 1995). In 1995, the Clinic published the first issue of *Viva Voce*, a national newsletter for prosecutors and therapists in the child abuse field. A new problem looms in 1996: one-third of Ontario's Crown prosecutors will lose their jobs as a result of government cutbacks. This means that many men charged with CSA will not come to trial because a long delay between the laying of charges and trial makes it necessary for the court to stay the charges.

The Kingston Group's Study and Treatment of Sexual Offenders against Children

The work of W. Marshall and colleagues in Kingston is recognized internationally as leading clinical research that shows what can be done in a particular field of CSA tertiary prevention given adequate funding. Marshall's group has undertaken several key studies on sex offenders in Kingston Penitentiary and has collaborated with New Zealand researchers. This work includes a study of the effects of masturbatory reconditioning for nonfamilial child molesters (Johnston et al. 1992), a group particularly difficult to treat. In this experiment, posttreatment, phallometric arousal in reaction to erotica featuring children decreased from 61 percent to 17 percent.

Marshall et al. (1991) reviewed the effects of their own and other treatment programs for paedophile offenders. With regard to pharmacological agents, the authors concluded that cyproterone acetate, which is designed to reduce sex drive, often works on paedophiles when combined with psychological treatment and with monitoring and encouragement to ensure that the paedophile takes the drug as ordered. Cognitive-behavioural programs with institutionalized offenders have several components, including cognitive reorientation (focusing on habitual beliefs and perceptions), social skill development, assertiveness training, desensitizing of deviant fantasies, aversive stimuli (electric shocks, ammonia inhalation) when presented with deviant pictures or stories, and biofeedback. The typical recidivism rate for men treated in this way, often in combination with pharmotherapy, is about 10 percent five years after release for a first offence, compared with about 35 percent in untreated men. Follow-up of offenders from Kingston Penitentiary found that 57 percent of the untreated group sexually reoffended, compared to 39 percent in the treated group, which included some multiple offenders. Therefore, the cognitive-behavioural program has been relatively successful. On the basis of these results, the authors altered and improved many aspects of the program and hope to reduce recidivism rates further. The authors recommend the development of further aspects to cognitive-behavioural programming, and for more evaluative research (Barbaree and Marshall 1991). Marshall (1994) also reported on a relatively successful program to counter denial in offenders, which is essential to further therapy. After group treatment, only 2 of 26 male participants remained in denial, and only 2 of the 9 minimizers remained unchanged.

Marshall et al. (1991) summarized their research at the Sexual Behaviour Clinic in Kingston. They showed that the reoffense rate for men who have been through their program is 25 percent less than that for untreated prisoners and pointed out that each reconvicted sex offender costs the federal and provincial governments about $200,000. Therefore, over a two-year period when 100 offenders were treated, Marshall's programs saved the government about $4 million. Such programs are highly cost effective, but, in an era of cuts, program funding has decreased.

Addressing Dilemmas Inherent in the Process of Reports of Child Sexual Abuse: The Quebec Model

A major dilemma in frontline work with allegations of CSA is the degree to which a full range of professionals should be involved in investigating and processing cases. If police and Crown prosecutors are to be involved, careful coordination with child protection and therapy teams is needed. In the United States and Canada, according to literature reviewed above, about 60 percent of CSA complaints turn out to be unfounded because of mistaken assumptions about child sexual knowledge (not because of false allegations). One solution to the difficult and often wasteful deployment of scarce resources is to leave the decision to involve police and Crown prosecutors to investigating social workers. The merit of the Quebec model is that much of the system-induced trauma that effects children and adolescents when CSA is investigated can be avoided.

The Quebec legal system is not like the common law one of Anglophone North America. The Quebec Civil Code allowed the provincial legislature to set up an entirely new youth protection procedure, in which abused children are referred to a Youth Protection Director at local Social Service

Centres. The Youth Protection Director evaluates the situation and directs everyone involved to the appropriate help.

This nonjudicial process of dealing with abuse allegations gives Youth and Family Counselling Centres the authority to treat incest cases in the way that their professional judgment indicates would best serve the child's interest. These centres distinguish between incest resulting from a marked sexual deviation (in which case the paedophile abuser is separated from a family on application to a court) and incest that can be treated with other, concurrent family problems. In this latter case, prosecution of the abuser is not usually sought.

Legislation on endangered children was codified in the Quebec *Youth Protection Act* of 1988 (Sansfacon and Presentey 1993). Police who learn of a CSA case must report it to the Youth Protection Service (YPS), but the YPS is not obligated to report CSA cases to the police, as in other Canadian provinces. The YPS has a specific mandate to avoid criminal processing of CSA cases whenever possible, particularly when CSA occurs within a family. However, Sansfacon and Presentey used case histories to show that social workers can and do use criminal prosecution for leverage in cases of incestuous abuse (e.g., requiring the male abuser to leave the family setting and desist from sexual abuse). About 25 percent of cases dealt with by Youth Protection Workers are referred to the criminal justice system when the offender's "voluntary cooperation" is doubtful. The sentence most frequently imposed in the adult courts for sexual abuse of children is probation. However, for charges of requiring a child under the age of 12 to engage in prostitution or for charges of violent rape of a child, conviction usually results in imprisonment. Quebec has several CSA assessment and treatment centres that use family-based therapy based on Giarretto's (1991) humanistic model.

This important Quebec initiative has yet to be evaluated or compared with the system in an Anglophone province. Crucial questions are (a) whether the Quebec system causes less trauma to CSA victims; and (b) whether leaving social workers to decide when to report CSA to police results in less or more recidivism (e.g., further abuse of the child or of other children in the family) and is consistent with other social policies, such as gender equity and cultural sensitivity.

The York Region Abuse Program: Community-Based Service Coordination

The population of York region increased from 252,000 in 1981 to 505,000 in 1991, and growth is expected to continue. Located just north of Metropolitan Toronto, the region comprises multicultural suburban communities (in the south) and agricultural communities (in the north).

The York Region Abuse Program (YRAP) is the only North York agency formally identified as serving sexual abuse survivors. However, the YRAP design assumes interagency cooperation and coordination between the social service, health, religious, educational, legal and government sectors, with community participation through the Board of Directors and operational committees. Twenty-six other agencies work with YRAP, which offers training for professionals and coordination of services involved with each client. The multidisciplinary nature of YRAP is revealed by the fact that it uses external case managers, who can be any health care or social service professional (e.g., physician, social worker, nurse) who works individually with the client and who will follow up after treatment. The YRAP Internship Program provides extensive training for professionals from other agencies (15 trained in 1994), who may then lead groups and train other interns.

YRAP was initially funded as a demonstration project by the Institute for Prevention of Child Abuse in the Ontario Ministry of Community and Social Services to provide group treatment and support services. (The institute has been disbanded.) YRAP is now funded by a variety of sources. The sources and the proportion of YRAP funding each contributed for 1993–94 and 1995, respectively, were as follows: Ontario Ministry of Community and Social Services, 45 and 49 percent; Ontario Ministry of Health, 14 and 14 percent; the City of North York, 7 and 5.5 percent; the United Way, 8 and 7.5 percent; and community fundraising, 26 and 20 percent. In 1995, the York Regional Board of Education contributed 2 percent and other donors contributed 2 percent. Funding was relatively stable for two years, with local contributions (United Way, the municipality and community fundraising) accounting for almost 50 percent of the operating budget. The advantages of deriving funding from a variety of sources are that the program maintains community support and can be flexible about starting new initiatives with the money raised. The disadvantages are a lack of job security for staff and an increase of stress in an already stressful occupation. (The program had an operating deficit for the first time in 1994–95.)

The group treatment program is comprehensive and free of charge. It includes male and female CSA survivors in several age groups: preschool; aged 6 to 8; aged 8 to 10; aged 10 to 12; teenage; and adult. YRAP also provides groups for male and female developmentally challenged survivors, non-offending parents, teenaged offenders, adult offenders, sexual assault survivors, and survivors who must testify in court. In 1994, 323 children and adults attended 24 types of groups. The Abuse Prevention Program, which operates through the public and separate school boards, includes (1) an information session for principals and superintendents; (2) two plays performed by high school students and designed for developmental stages (a) kindergarten through Grade 4 and (b) Grades 5 to 8; (3) three-hour workshops for teaching and non-teaching staff that include preparing students before the plays and dealing with disclosure; (4) identification and training of a resource person for each school; (5) a two-hour orientation and education session for parents before the play; (6) psychoeducational support for the student actors; (7) a one-hour evening meeting for parents of high school students; and (8) a classroom kit for each school that introduces primary and secondary prevention concepts and activities for teachers to use. In 1994, 30 schools—19,000 students, 3,500 parents and 1,350 teachers—were included.

The Reach Out and Recover (ROAR) program is one of the most unique features of YRAP. Clients who are or have been in group therapy form self-help groups, and a volunteer program provides services that increase access to YRAP: telephone support for people on program waiting lists; child care at the YRAP offices; representation of YRAP at community events; administrative support; transportation for clients; homemaking relief for parents; and fundraising. Through ROAR, YRAP moves beyond tertiary prevention for individuals to facilitation of social support, social network building, and social action (Breen 1994). The process resembles emancipatory education programs in which participants are encouraged to understand the experiences of all members or to form collective consciousness.

Several community actions oriented to primary and secondary prevention have resulted from YRAP. Parents offered mutual aid and support (tertiary prevention) and applied their skills to primary prevention. The capacity of YRAP is thereby exponentially greater than that of programs in which individuals and individual families work in isolation. The capacity of individuals and families is also increased as they learn and practise new skills and make connections.

YRAP incorporates evaluation into many of its programs and includes advocacy and research in its mission. Among the research contributions have been a study of group supervision of group therapists (Steadman and Harper 1995); an evaluation of the effectiveness of group treatment for adult female CSA survivors (Breen et al. 1994); and an evaluation of the self-help program.

End the Silence: A Program for Nonverbal Survivors of Childhood Sexual Abuse

In the past, service providers for people with disabilities lacked training in sexual abuse prevention, while service providers for victims of sexual assault lacked training in the needs of people with disabilities. In 1993, two Calgary nonprofit organizations began to discuss forming an interagency relationship to address the sexuality education needs of women with disabilities who use augmentative communication. The agencies were the Calgary Birth Control Association (CBCA), which provides information and counselling on healthy sexuality; and the Technical Resource Centre (TRC), which is committed to enhancing the lives of people with physical disabilities by providing information, education and access to advanced technology. Both agencies have executive directors, a board of directors, fewer than 10 staff and funding primarily from the United Way. TRC received special United Way funding to develop the End the Silence (ETS) info kit, which comprises a brochure, a poster and a self-teaching manual. A United Way partnership grant enabled TRC and CBCA to work together to pilot the kit. The ETS kit contains information, problem-solving strategies and suggestions for improving communication between women with disabilities (including nonverbal women) and service providers and to help service providers develop accessible, appropriate services for nonverbal women who have experienced sexual abuse. The United Way suggested establishing an advisory committee that included nonverbal women, and the coordinator agreed. The 14 advisory committee members were stakeholders from all targeted groups (nonverbal women with physical disabilities; a disability and sexual assault counsellor; caregivers; and providers of legal, educational and rehabilitation services) to contribute information, feedback and guidance.

The coordinator believed that unless all stakeholders could share their perspectives, skills and abilities, it would be impossible to achieve effective communication, understanding and problem solving around the issues. It was hoped that the committee process and its members' experiences would set an example of increased communication and understanding, coalition-building, and shared problem solving among verbal and nonverbal stakeholders. The advisory committee agreed to document and evaluate the process. A university researcher evaluated three aspects of ETS: the content of the kit; the advisory committee process; and the partnership.

The three evaluations showed that the coordinator received extensive feedback from committee members with a wide range of experience and that the committee members began to establish connections and share perspectives and expertise. The committee members also drew in professionals from the community, who contributed time and expertise to the kit project. However, the goal of effective communication was not achieved. Although the project was intended to empower nonverbal women with disabilities, meetings tended to replicate society's interaction patterns. Inadvertently, despite the best of intentions, patterns that perpetuated the silence of the women continued.

This example shows that community agencies can collaborate to meet special needs associated with CSA and other sexual abuse and that universities can provide important support. An excellent resource was developed at relatively little cost, advancing community education at the same time. The evaluation was yet another opportunity to learn and to disseminate not only the kit itself, but also the knowledge gained. This case also illustrates that the promotion of population health faces many challenges.

Misinterpretation of Research, Policy, Treatment and Prevention Activities: An Urban Example

Most major Canadian cities now have practice and policy initiatives for treating CSA survivors. In 1980, Calgary activists and professionals organized a CSA conference, which helped pressure the federal government into setting up the Badgley Commission in 1983. Judge Herb Allard of Calgary, one of the Commissioners, wrote the Badgley Report's hard-hitting chapter on juvenile prostitution, which recommended making juvenile prostitution a status offence. Since the 1985 release of the Badgley Report, Calgary has done much to get child and adolescent prostitutes off the streets. These efforts have been supported by, among others, the city's Department of Social Services, members of City Council, and the United Way. Street teams, police procedures and residential shelters have been established. In 1994, as a result of all this activity, an American tabloid featured Calgary as "the child prostitution capital of Canada." This is almost certainly not true— activists had given the problem a high profile, creating the impression that Calgary has extensive juvenile prostitution (Bagley 1995). The Calgary example is important because people tend to be uneasy about services and programs that make their communities seem more "deviant" than others.

CONCLUSIONS AND POLICY IMPERATIVES

The review of clinical and research literature indicates how complex CSA prevention and treatment issues are and how difficult it is to propose solutions that apply to all situations and all children. Therefore, although we have grouped our conclusions under several headings, the policy implications are clearly not mutually exclusive. We remind policymakers that with CSA, as with most health issues, there are no policy vacuums; failing to address CSA means overlooking the short- and long-term well-being of many children.

Research

1. Clearly, the problem deserves more research and better conceptualizations. Models are needed for programs based on theories of individual and social change. Well-designed techniques are needed for evaluating treatment and prevention strategies for children, adolescents and adults. Improving the research effort will require epidemiologic and other quantitative methods triangulated with grounded theory, phenomenology, case studies and other qualitative methods.

2. The extent of both short- and long-term harm varies. Primary prevention is the ultimate goal, but it is unlikely that CSA will be eliminated. More research into the resiliency of victims is needed so survivors' own

resources can be promoted. Clearly, the determinants of health (namely, income, education and social status, social support, coping skills and competence, and health services designed to promote health) are important in this regard.

3. Population health research and health promotion have not given enough serious attention to gender and the health concerns of women. CSA research must be gender sensitive; for example, simply controlling for gender in multivariate analysis is misleading when separate models are actually needed.

The Family in Social Context

4. The family context in which CSA occurs must be understood, as must the emotional and physical abuse and child neglect that often precede and accompany CSA.

5. The family must be viewed in the context of broader social forces. CSA prevention requires multisectoral collaboration. The institution of the family has undergone rapid change in the last two decades, and social policies on issues such as child care can affect certain families' ability to cope with external and internal stresses. At the population level, we must recognize the social isolation of families and foster the idea that seeking help is both appropriate and admirable.

6. Family support programs are needed for families with stepfathers (a major CSA risk factor) and to promote father-infant bonding (a deterrent to father-daughter incest).

7. Support programs are needed for families with severe problems such as alcoholism and parentification of children, which place them at higher risk of CSA.

8. Community support for the role of mothers in protecting their children from CSA and in supporting their children when incest is revealed is an important policy need.

Treatment and Prevention Services

9. The prevention focus must be shifted from children to adults and community institutions, who have the real power to stop CSA.

10. Treatment and prevention work must address all types of child maltreatment and neglect. Service agencies must collaborate and coordinate their efforts to avoid operating in isolation from each other and from the community. This integration of effort makes the scholarship associated with the promotion of population health important, especially the study of concomitant community development and provision of clinical services.

11. Serious long-term psychological problems appear to be caused by (a) repeated sexual abuse experienced in childhood, along with other forms

of family pathology, including disordered communication and attachment patterns, as well as emotional abuse and neglect; and (b) violent rape experienced in adolescence. Children with such experiences need the earliest possible intervention.

12. Current prevention strategies targeting children may be ineffective and might actually make children more vulnerable to CSA. Prevention education must target adolescents, who are both potential victims and potential abusers, and adults with paedophilic potential. Prevention education must be based on sound theory, research and evaluation.

13. Adult CSA survivors may have health problems that can be resolved only when the psychosocial etiology has been addressed. Fortunately, evidence suggests that many adult CSA survivors improve when the importance of CSA in their background is acknowledged by a trusted professional, although others need additional support. All health care professionals should be trained to identify and treat the long-term consequences of CSA. CSA survivors also need more mutual aid and self-help opportunities.

Legal Issues

14. The prolonged examinations and interrogations to which sexually abused children are subjected before they testify in court can be as traumatic as the abuse itself. Two alternative models to address this have been reviewed: the Ontario Family Court Clinic approach of supporting child witnesses; and the Quebec youth protection model, in which social workers decide whether to involve police in a CSA case. A combination of these models would serve children well.

15. Police can lay Criminal Code charges against customers of juvenile prostitutes, but they rarely do. Innovative policing and social support for victims are urgently needed; making juvenile prostitution a status offence might promote such interventions.

16. Treating convicted paedophiles can be successful and, therefore, cost effective in terms of both money and prevention of assaults on children. These programs are underfunded, and many paedophiles leave custody without treatment.

17. Few CSA perpetrators actually go to trial, and the legal process is frequently devastating for victims and their families. With the legal system responsible for CSA offenders, other social institutions can wash their hands of the problem. We need to revisit this public policy, which values punishment and imprisonment more than treatment and rehabiliation by community-based services.

Populations with Special Needs

18. Acting-out, disturbed and runaway adolescents are often blamed for antisocial activities related to abusive home environments. Blaming the victim is both wrong and ineffective. Most juvenile prostitutes have been abused, and their problems are urgent. More street workers and more long-stay hostels are needed.

19. Aboriginal nations have the social and psychological resources to deal with CSA, but they need material resources as well. This means, among other things, that equitable land claim settlements and policies to end racism and discrimination are needed.

20. People with disabilities are four times more likely to be sexually abused than people of the same age without disabilities. Services must be made accessible, and services for people with disabilities must be empowered to address CSA.

21. Racism, cultural sensitivity and cultural synergy should be addressed in all programs and policies.

Funding

22. The 1980s saw many excellent innovative CSA programs in Canada. However, cuts in provincial and federal funding have increased the stress on workers, reduced creativity and innovation, and made some programs less effective. The social safety net was designed, in part, to ensure equitable access to the determinants of health. When the social safety net is torn, children fall through the holes first.

SPECIFIC RECOMMENDATIONS

I.   The major granting institutions that support research should col-laborate to promote CSA research focused on theoretical weaknesses, specific gaps in knowledge, program evaluations and dissemination of knowledge. Multidisciplinary, nonsexist, culturally sensitive, community-based research emphasizing policy applications should be supported.

II. A national or international conference to report on evaluations of models of interventions should be held to disseminate interventions, permit networking, and help establish CSA as an item on the policy agendas of Canadian communities.

III. Demonstration projects of interventions should be supported, particularly in areas where little has been done, for example, with adolescent boys who have or may become offenders; with stepfathers; with paedophiles who are not incarcerated; and with mothers of abused children. Projects should focus on capacity building in individuals and communities, rather than on professionalization.

IV. College and university curricula in every pertinent discipline should be subjected to a review like Health Canada's review of family violence.

Christopher Bagley, Ph.D., *is a social psychologist working within the discipline of social work. He began a longitudinal study of sexually abused children in 1968; the adult mental health status of this cohort was reported in his 1995 book* Child sexual abuse and mental health in adolescents and adults. *He is the author of* Children, sex and social policy: Humanistic solutions for problems of child sexual abuse *(1997) and coauthor of* Understanding and preventing child sexual abuse *(1996) and* Suicidal behaviour in adolescents and adults *(1997). His doctorate is from the University of Sussex, England and he worked at the Maudsley Hospital in London before coming to Canada to take up a chair of child welfare at the University of Calgary which he held for fifteen years before returning to England to take up a chair of social work at the University of Southampton.*

Wilfreda Thurston *has a Ph.D. in epidemiology and health care research. She has worked in government, and community health and human services. She specializes in health promotion program planning and evaluation with an emphasis on the health of women and ethnocultural groups. She is an associate professor in the Department of Community Health Sciences, director of the Office of Gender and Equity Issues for the Faculty of Medicine, and chair of the University Women's Health Research Group.*

BIBLIOGRAPHY

Note: The literature reviews above are drawn from Bagley and Thurston (1996a and 1996b), to which volumes the reader is referred for a full list of citations.

BABINS-WAGNER, R. 1991. Development and evaluation of a family systems approach to the treatment of child sexual abuse. In *Child Sexual Abuse: Expanding the Research Base on Program and Treatment Outcomes*, eds. B. THOMLISON and C. BAGLEY. Calgary: University of Calgary Press. pp. 103–128.

BADGLEY, R. (chair). 1984. *Sexual Offences Against Children in Canada. Volumes I and II*. Ottawa: Minister of Supply and Services Canada.

BAGLEY, C. 1995. *Child Sexual Abuse and Mental Health in Adolescents and Adults in Canada and Britain*. Brookfield: Avebury.

BAGLEY, C., and KING, K. 1990. *Child Sexual Abuse: The Search for Healing*. London: Tavistock-Routledge.

BAGLEY, C., and RAMSAY, R. 1990. Sexual abuse in childhood: Psychological outcomes and implications for social work practice. *Journal of Social Work and Human Sexuality* 4: 33–47.

BAGLEY, C., and THOMLISON, R. 1991. *Child Sexual Abuse: Critical Perspectives on Prevention, Intervention, and Treatment*. Toronto: Wall and Emerson.

BAGLEY, C., and THURSTON, W. E. 1989. Preventing child sexual abuse: Reviews and research. *Rehabilitation and Health Monograph Series No. 18*. Faculty of Social Work, University of Calgary.

_____. 1996a. *Understanding and Preventing Child Sexual Abuse. Volume I—Children: Assessment, Social Work and Clinical Issues, and Prevention Education*. Aldershot: Arena Social Work Pubs.

_____. 1996b. *Understanding and Preventing Child Sexual Abuse. Volume II—Male Victims, Adolescents, Adult Outcomes, and Offender Treatment*. Aldershot: Arena Social Work Pubs.

BAGLEY, C., WOOD, M., and KHUMAR, H. 1991. Suicide and careless death in an Aboriginal population. *Canadian Journal of Community Mental Health* 9: 127–142.

BARBAREE, H., and MARSHALL, W. 1991. Treatment of the adult male child molester. In *Child Sexual Abuse: Critical Perspectives on Prevention, Intervention and Treatment*, eds. C. BAGLEY, and R. THOMLISON. Toronto: Wall and Emerson. pp. 217–256.

BENTOVIM, A. 1988. *Child Sexual Abuse within the Family: Assessment and Treatment*. London: Wright-Butterworth.

BRIERE, J. 1992. *Child Abuse Trauma: Theory and Treatment of the Lasting Effects*. Newbury Park: Sage.

BREEN, H. 1994. Child sexual abuse: Parent group leads to community and social action. *Canadian Journal of Public Health* 85: 381–384.

BREEN, H., HARPER, K., STALEY, S., STEADMAN, J. H., WARGEL, K., and WATSON, E. 1994. Effectiveness of group treatment for female adult survivors of child sexual abuse. Unpublished manuscript.

BUKOWSKI, W. 1992. Sexual abuse and maladjustment considered from the normal development process. In *The Sexual Abuse of Children: Theory and Research*, eds. W. O'DONAHUE and J. GEER. Hillsdale (NJ): Erlbaum. 1: 261–282.

CANADA. 1994. *Strategies for Population Health: Investing in the Health of Canadians*. Ottawa: Minister of Supply and Services Canada.

DONALDSON, L. 1995. Personal communication from Professor Donaldson, Faculty of Education, University of Calgary.

EPP, J. 1986. *Achieving Health for All: A Framework for Health Promotion*. Ottawa: Health and Welfare Canada.

FINKELHOR, D. 1984. *Child Sexual Abuse: New Theory and Research*. New York: Free Press.

_____. 1995. The victimization of children: A developmental perspective. *American Journal of Orthopsychiatry* 65: 177–189.

FRASER, P. 1985. *Pornography and Prostitution in Canada: Report of the Special Committee on Pornography and Prostitution.* Ottawa: Minister of Supply and Services Canada.

GIARRETTO, H. 1981. A comprehensive child sexual abuse treatment program. In *Sexually Abused Children and Their Families*, eds. P. BEEZLEY MRAZEK and C. H. KEMPE. Oxford: Pergamon Press. pp. 179–198.

GOLD, E. 1986. Long-term effects of sexual victimization in childhood: An attributional approach. *Journal of Consulting and Clinical Psychology* 51: 471–475.

GROTH, A.N., and BIRNBAUM, H. J. 1978. Adult sexual orientation and attraction to underage persons. *Archives of Sexual Behaviour* 7: 175–181.

HERTZMAN, C. 1994. The lifelong impact of childhood experiences: A population health perspective. *Journal of the American Academy of Arts and Science* 123: 167–180.

JEHU, D. 1988. *Beyond Sexual Abuse: Therapy with Women Who Were Child Victims.* Chichester, U.K.: John Wiley & Son.

JOHNSTON, P., HUDSON, S., and MARSHALL, W. 1992. The effects of masturbatory reconditioning with nonfamilial child molesters. *Behavioural Research and Therapy* 30: 559–61.

KILPATRICK, A. 1992. *Long-Range Effects of Child and Adolescent Sexual Experiences: Myths, Mores and Menaces.* Hillsdale (NJ): Lawrence Erlbaum.

LARSON, J., and MADDOCK, N. 1995. *Incestuous Families: An Ecological Approach to Understanding and Treatment.* New York: Norton.

MARMOR, T. R., BARER, M. L., and EVANS, R. G. 1994. The determinants of a population's health: What can be done to improve a democratic nation's health status? In *Why Are Some People Healthy and Others Not? The Determinants of Health of Population*, eds. R. G. EVANS, M. L. MORRIS, and T. R. MARMOR. New York: Aldine de Gruyter. pp. 217–230.

MARMOT, M. G. 1994. Social differentials in health within and between populations. *Journal of the American Academy of Arts and Science* 123: 197–216.

MARSHALL, W. 1994. Treatment effects on denial and minimization in incarcerated sex offenders. *Behavioural Research and Therapy* 32: 559–565.

MARSHALL, W., JONES, R., WARD, T., JOHNSTON, P., and BARBAREE, H. 1991. Treatment outcome with sex offenders. *Clinical Psychology Review* 11: 465–485.

MOELLER, T., BACHMANN, G., and MOELLER, J. 1993. The combined effects of physical, sexual and emotional abuse during childhood: Long-term health consequences for women. *Child Abuse and Neglect* 17: 623–640.

MRAZEK, and C. H. KEMPE. Eds. n.d. *Sexually Abused Children and Their Families.* Willowdale (ON): Pergamon Press. pp. 179–198.

PELLETIER, R. 1980. Advantages for children of a non-judiciary and family approach to cases of sexual abuse. In *Enfance et sexualité*, ed. J.-M. SAMSON. Montreal: Éditions Études vivantes. pp. 21–34.

PUTNAM, F. and TRICKETT, P. 1993. Child sexual abuse: A model of chronic trauma. *Psychiatry* 56: 82–95.

ROGERS, R. 1990. *Reaching for Solutions: Report of the Special Advisor to the Minister of National Health and Welfare on Child Sexual Abuse.* Ottawa: Queen's Printer.

RUNDLE, G. 1990. Child sexual abuse of Native women. Ph.D. thesis, University of Calgary, Calgary.

RUSSELL, O. E. 1986. *The Secret Trauma: Incest in the Lives of Girls and Women.* New York: Basic Books.

SANSFACON, D., and PRESENTEY, F. 1993. *Processing of Child Sexual Abuse Cases in Selected Sites in Quebec.* Ottawa: Department of Justice.

SAS, L., CUNNINGHAM, A., and HURLEY, P. 1995. *Primary and Secondary Prevention Strategies for Child Sexual Abuse: Developing a Prediction Model Based on the Facilitators and Inhibitors of Child*

Disclosures. London (ON): Family Court Clinic for Family Violence Prevention, Division of Health Canada.

SAS, L., HURLEY, P., HATCH, A., MALLA, S., and DICK, T. 1991. *Reducing the System-Induced Trauma for Child Sexual Abuse Victims through Court Preparation, Assessment and Follow-Up.* London: Family Court Clinic.

SIGURDSON, E., MARGINET, C., and ONYSKO, R. 1991. A child abuse risk index. In *Child Sexual Abuse: Critical Perspectives on Prevention, Intervention, and Treatment*, eds. C. BAGLEY and R. THOMLISON. Toronto: Wall and Emerson. pp. 49–78.

STEADMAN, J. H., and HARPER, K. 1995. Group supervision of group psychotherapy. *Canadian Journal of Psychiatry* 40: 484–488.

TUTTY, L. 1992. The ability of elementary school children to learn sexual abuse prevention concepts. *Child Abuse and Neglect* 16: 369–384.

_____. 1993. Parent's perceptions of their child's knowledge of sexual abuse prevention concepts. *Journal of Child Sexual Abuse* 2: 83–103.

_____. 1994. Development issues in young children's learning of sexual abuse prevention concepts. *Child Abuse and Neglect* 18: 176–192.

WELLS, M. 1990. *Canada's Law on Sexual Abuse.* Ottawa: Department of Justice.

WOLFE, D., SAS, L., and WEKERLE, C. 1994. Factors associated with the development of post-traumatic stress disorder among child victims of sexual abuse. *Child Abuse and Neglect* 18: 37–50.

Preventing Unintentional Injuries among Children

Barbara A. Morrongiello, Ph.D., C.Psych.

Professor of Psychology
University of Guelph

SUMMARY

In Canada, injuries account for more child deaths than the next six causes combined. Injuries are also a leading cause of children's hospitalizations and trips to emergency rooms. Many injury control measures and programs have been implemented. However, too often the efficacy of these has not been established. This paper critically reviews programs aimed at preventing injuries among children under 13 years of age.

The objectives of this paper are (1) to identify broad-based approaches and specific programs that have proven effective in promoting children's safety practices, decreasing injury risk behaviours, and reducing injuries; (2) to discuss some program evaluation issues; and (3) to discuss policy implications based on these findings.

The paper includes the following sections:
- *a brief review of epidemiology-based findings about injuries among children and discussion of the implications of these findings for injury prevention programs (i.e., what kinds of programs are needed for children at various developmental stages);*
- *a brief discussion of the merits and costs of active approaches (i.e., require some action by individuals) and passive approaches (i.e., require no action by individuals) to injury control;*
- *a discussion of program evaluation issues in the literature;*

- *a critical review of programs that aim to prevent injuries among children;*
- *conclusions and recommendations for future programs to reduce injuries among children; and*
- *a discussion of policy implications.*

The section evaluating the programs provides details on the structural characteristics, content and efficacy of programs aimed at preventing the most common types of child injuries: motor vehicle injuries to passengers; motor vehicle injuries to pedestrians; burns; spinal cord injuries and head trauma; and in-home injuries. The programs were identified through discussions with Canadian professionals who work in this field and an extensive computer-based search of internationally published literature. Programs that have been implemented but never formally evaluated were not included.

A number of conclusions are given:

1. Passive approaches are extremely cost effective and reach a large proportion of the target population, resulting in significant declines in child mortality rates. In short, these approaches are highly successful.

2. Active approaches show varying degrees of success, depending on several factors:

- *Those that emphasize education seldom result in changes to behaviour and are, therefore, largely ineffective as a means of injury control when presented in isolation.*
- *The effectiveness of these programs can be increased if they target groups at risk for particular types of injuries and are delivered in a personal, one-to-one context. To improve efficacy of programs that target children directly, the message must be delivered while involving the child in a participatory way.*

3. Interventions that aim to change behaviour (decrease risk-taking; increase safety practices) are much more effective than education programs. Behavioural programs often result in good short-term compliance and declining (but still above baseline) rates over longer intervals (6–12 months). Effectiveness is maximized if a combination of features is incorporated in the program (role playing or modelling, feedback, rewards). High compliance rates can be maintained over long periods if booster (retraining) sessions are given periodically.

4. Community-based interventions can very effectively produce behavioural and attitudinal changes. The successful programs have one goal (e.g., promoting helmet use among cyclists) and have an education component (e.g., local television advertisements) and a behavioural component (e.g., reward programs). The successful programs also communicate information through many sources simultaneously, creating interventions that are so pervasive as to make it difficult for individuals not to become informed and involved. These can be very cost-effective interventions.

Several recommendations follow from these conclusions:

1. Use passive approaches to injury control whenever possible.

2. Select active approaches based on considerations of cost-effectiveness, the target audience (e.g., high risk or not), and the behaviours to be changed. Limit the focus to the most frequent or serious type of injury, rather than targeting a broad array simultaneously. Make the programs as multifaceted as possible given the financial and personnel resources available.

- *Combine legislation with public education and enforcement strategies.*
- *Ensure that education interventions are delivered to the individual, communicated by respected individuals, target specific high-risk populations, and have a narrow focus.*
- *Follow up behavioural interventions with an occasional booster message to promote high compliance rates over time. To reduce costs, restrict access to those at particular risk for specific injuries.*
- *Design community-based interventions so that they have education and behavioural components and a bottom-up (i.e., community derived) as opposed to top-down (i.e., organizationally imposed) strategy and ensure that the intervention matches the intended audience and respects the culture of the target community.*

A number of policy implications are discussed:

1. Injury control must be established as a national priority in Canada and should be managed at a national, not provincial, level. A national agenda must be developed. There must be efforts made to raise public, private sector and governmental awareness of this national health threat.

2. A key stakeholder group should be given the mandate, power and resources to develop and to implement a national strategy to achieve injury control and eliminate duplication of efforts.

3. Although program evaluations cost money and there are challenges in deciding on appropriate outcome measures and evaluation strategies, these are necessary components of intervention and prevention programs. Face validity (i.e., the degree to which the program appears to address the injury issue in question) is not sufficient.

4. Because injury data are critical to identifying injury control issues at local and national levels and to tracking the effectiveness of prevention programs, injury surveillance must include comprehensive collection of information, be common across hospitals, and be technically current.

5. High-risk populations must become a central focus in injury prevention programs. However, research is needed to identify the key determinants of health among these populations (e.g., boys, low-income children, Aboriginal children). Implementing programs without a thorough appreciation of the factors and processes that decrease or increase injury risk among these populations is likely to lead to failure.

TABLE OF CONTENTS

If a disease were killing our children in the proportions that accidents are, people would be outraged and demand that this killer be stopped.

– C. Everett Koop, M.D. (former U.S. Surgeon General), 1991

In Canada, as in many industrialized countries, unintentional injuries are the number one cause of death for children beyond 1 year of age (CICH 1994). Child mortality is only part of the problem. Injuries are also a leading cause of children's hospitalizations and trips to emergency rooms. Thus, injuries pose a national threat to the health and well-being of Canadian children.

As mortality rates from infectious diseases and unsanitary conditions dropped over the past 20 years, attention shifted to child injury. Many measures and programs to prevent or control injuries have been implemented. However, too often their efficacy has not been established or is found lacking. This paper critically reviews programs that aim to prevent unintentional injuries (that is, excluding suicide) among children under 13 years of age.

The primary aim of this paper is to discuss success stories—programs that have been evaluated and shown to produce gains in preventing injuries among children. The paper has several sections. First, there is a review of patterns of injuries, highlighting the types of injuries that are prevalent at different developmental stages and the correlates of those injuries. Next is a general discussion of the merits and limitations of passive and active prevention strategies. Some program evaluation issues are raised, and there is a review of specific programs organized according to injury type. This is not an exhaustive selection of programs, but an attempt was made to identify and discuss programs that target populations at increased risk for childhood injuries. The programs are sampled from an international database. Finally, the paper provides recommendations for future injury prevention programs and discusses the policy implications of these findings.

PATTERNS OF INJURIES AMONG CHILDREN

The type and number of injuries among children are influenced by several factors, including the child's developmental level, gender and socioeconomic status (SES).[1] Each of these factors is discussed below.

---

1   Other influences on injury statistics (e.g., family background, geography, urban or rural context, race, temporal variation, historical influences) are reviewed, for example, by Baker et al. (1984), Rivara and Mueller (1987), Wilson et al. (1991), and CICH (1994).

Developmental Patterns

The location and types of injuries that commonly occur among children vary greatly, depending on the child's developmental level (Shanon et al. 1992). These differences have implications for the targeting of prevention programs.

Injuries among infants (prelocomotor) often occur in the home. In-home injuries include falls from heights, suffocation, choking, burns from water or food, and drownings in bathtubs. Motor vehicle injuries arise from not riding in a safety seat, riding in an improperly fitting or incorrectly facing infant car seat, or riding in a seat that is not properly secured to the vehicle. According to the Canadian Institute of Child Health (CICH 1994), the leading causes of injury-related deaths among Canadian infants are suffocation, burns, drownings, falls and motor vehicle–related incidents. Falls are the leading cause of hospitalizations. Because these injuries often result from caregivers' decisions and behaviour, prevention programs to reduce injuries among infants target caregivers.

Like infants, toddlers (having locomotor capabilities but limited communication skills; aged 12 months to 3.5 years) continue to experience primarily in-home injuries and vehicle-related injuries. However, the toddler's behaviour is more often implicated in the injury. In the home, injuries often result from the child's increasing curiosity, need to be active, and desire to explore the surroundings. Such injuries include poisonings from opened medicines and home cleaners, choking on small objects like buttons and coins, suffocation from playing with plastic bags or blind cords, drownings in large buckets and planters, cuts from sharp objects like knives or tools, burns from playing with cigarette lighters, and falls from heights or down stairs or from pulling furniture down onto themselves while trying to climb. According to the Canadian Institute of Child Health (CICH 1994), the leading causes of injury-related deaths among toddlers are motor vehicle–related incidents, drownings, burns and suffocations. Falls are the leading cause of hospitalizations.

Vehicle-related injuries start to include pedestrian injuries (e.g., from running out into the street), although these are less common than at older ages. Since many injuries to toddlers result from caregivers' poor judgment, inadequate supervision or lack of knowledge, programs to reduce injuries among toddlers also focus on caregivers.

Preschool children (3.5–6 years old) and young school age children (under 10 years old) are at increased risk for motor vehicle–related pedestrian injuries. Programs to reduce this type of injury are diverse, with some targeting caregivers and others targeting the children directly. Most child-directed programs are delivered by the schools. Many preschoolers and young school children are involved in bicycling and other sports, resulting in many injuries. Children on bicycles are often hit by vehicles or crash into them and stationary objects. Such accidents may produce fall-related injuries (cuts, broken bones, etc.) and head trauma. Bicycle safety programs usually target children directly, although some programs to increase helmet use by children focus on caregivers. As is true for infants and toddlers, falls are the leading cause of hospitalizations among Canadian school children and preschoolers (CICH 1994).

Finally, for Canadian children 10–13 years old, the leading causes of injury-related deaths are motor vehicle–related incidents, burns, suffocations and drownings. Falls continue to be the leading cause of hospitalizations (CICH 1994). Programs to reduce injuries among this group of children focus directly on the child.

Gender Patterns

For nearly every kind of injury at every age beyond 1 year, males are at higher risk than females (Baker et al. 1984; CICH 1994). This gender difference in injury rates is not specific to childhood—it persists until the seventh decade of life (Rivara and Mueller 1987). Depending on the type of injury, males have two to four times more injuries than females. This difference is particularly sizeable for injuries involving speed or the mechanical transfer of energy, such as motor vehicle–related injuries and play- and sport-related injuries (Rivara and Mueller 1987). In addition to having a greater incidence of injuries, boys also suffer more severe injuries.

The factors that lead to increased injuries among males are complex and not fully understood. Differences in injury rates are not simply due to differential risk exposure—statistical correction for participation rates still reveals, and sometimes even magnifies, the gender difference (Routledge et al. 1974; Rivara et al. 1982). Research suggests that inborn differences in impulsivity and activity level (Manheimer and Mellinger 1963; Matheny 1980, 1988), more aggressive and daring play by males than females (Smith and Daglish 1977), and greater risk taking by males than females (Ginsberg and Miller 1982) contribute to the gender differences in injury rates.

Recent research in my own laboratory reveals a strong relationship between children's attitudes and beliefs about injuries and their risk-taking behaviour. Boys 6–10 years old show more optimism (belief that one is less likely to be hurt than one's peer) than girls in the same age group; rate the perceived severity of experienced or potential injuries lower than girls do; and attribute injuries to bad luck more often than girls do (Morrongiello and Rennie, in press).

Even though there are these gender differences in injuries, a review of the prevention literature revealed no programs that target male audiences differently from female audiences.

Socioeconomic Patterns

A survey of epidemiological studies of injuries reveals that the incidence of injuries also varies with SES (Baker et al. 1984; Wilson et al. 1991; CICH 1994). Maternal education, often taken as an indirect index of SES, has been shown to be inversely associated with risk for childhood injuries (Rivara and Mueller 1987). Lower SES is associated not only with higher rates of injuries but also with more severe and often fatal injuries (Rivara and Mueller 1987). In a well-designed study in Maine, for example, poor children had a twofold greater risk of death due to injury than children who were not poor (Nersesian et al. 1985). In Canada, Aboriginal children, who are too often from low-income families, have a rate of injury four to seven times greater than the national average rate for children (CICH 1994).

The way in which SES influences injury rates among children is not well established, but it is likely that several paths of influence are operating. Areas of low SES, for example, often provide more hazardous environments and fewer satisfactory play areas (Lueller et al. 1990). Children in these areas are more likely to use the streets as their playgrounds and to play with hazardous materials instead of toys (e.g., stick instead of a baseball bat, rock instead of a baseball). Often, families in areas of low SES are noisier and more chaotic, and these characteristics are related to elevated injury risk. Parental characteristics also may contribute to increased risk. Parents in poor areas often have limited knowledge of child development and may exercise poor judgment about their children's abilities, thereby placing their children at increased risk of injury (e.g., Rivara and Howard 1982). Whatever the factors increasing the risk of injury among lower SES children, the statistics make clear that programs need to target these high-risk groups if injury control is to be achieved. Toward this aim, this paper focuses on successful prevention programs that target high-risk and low-income populations.

ACTIVE VERSUS PASSIVE APPROACHES TO INJURY PREVENTION

Injury control strategies are often categorized as active or passive (Williams 1982), although the case has been made for viewing them on a continuum (Wilson and Baker 1987).

Passive Strategies

Passive strategies are community- or population-based approaches to injury control and require limited or no action by individuals. These are sometimes called environmental or structural approaches to injury control because protection is achieved by making changes in product design or the environment. Legislated childproof caps on medicines, air bags in cars, and fire-resistant sleepwear for children are examples of passive prevention.

Wilson and Baker (1987) summarized the goals of this approach as (1) not creating new hazards, (2) eliminating or minimizing existing hazards, and (3) implementing strategies to reduce risk from unchangeable hazards. While passive approaches that meet these criteria have proven highly effective in preventing several types of childhood injuries, other passive interventions sometimes create new hazards. For example, some flame retardants in children's sleepwear proved to be carcinogenic (Blum and Ames 1977). Speed bumps, which are designed to promote slower speeds, sometimes actually increase car crashes because drivers lose control (Allen and Walsh 1975; Turturici 1975). Obviously, when deciding whether to adopt passive injury control strategies, one must evaluate and weigh possible negative effects against the gains expected.

In the injury control literature, the consensus is that passive approaches are more effective than other approaches (Williams 1982; Wilson and Baker 1987). Perhaps the most significant reason for passive approaches not being used more often is the difficulty in getting them implemented and accepted (Roberts 1987). Despite their impressive effectiveness, legislated changes take enormous amounts of time and effort before they are implemented. Lobbyists must document the scope and significance of the injury problem, demonstrate that the proposed intervention will alleviate or minimize the problem, and convince the policymakers that the effects will be significant enough to merit such an intervention. Furthermore, the more politically charged the issue (e.g., gun control), the less likely it is that consensus on taking a legislative approach will be reached.

Despite evidence of the effectiveness of regulatory approaches to injury control, struggles between advocates for individual freedom and advocates for children's safety persist and limit the use of passive approaches to injury control (Roberts and Brooks 1987; Peterson and Roberts 1992).

Active Strategies

Active strategies are individual-based approaches to injury control and require repeated action by the individual to prevent an injury from occurring. For example, car passengers must take the initiative to secure their seat belt every time they ride in the car. Since passive approaches to injury control cannot be applied to all situations, there has been considerable interest in determining ways to promote the success (individual's compliance) of active approaches to injury control.

Many successful active interventions draw on psychological principles and use behavioural techniques to modify an individual's unsafe behaviour. Such interventions include education (e.g., about passenger injury statistics), modelling safe behaviours (e.g., seat belt use), and rewarding compliance (e.g., giving children stickers for wearing seat belts on the drive to school). Periodic booster (retraining) sessions may be used to maintain high compliance levels over time (Roberts et al. 1987). Earlier active approaches relied solely on education, and these were largely ineffective (see Pless and Arsenault 1987). Incorporating psychological principles has increased the effectiveness of active approaches to injury control, making them attractive alternatives when passive measures are not feasible.

Limitations in active strategies for injury control have been discussed by several investigators (e.g., Rivara and Mueller 1987; Wilson and Baker 1987). These limitations include the following:

- Individuals may be unwilling or unable to take the required action.
- Active interventions may not be appropriate for some injuries. Thus, decisions need to be based on a thorough understanding of the circumstances of injury.
- Because individuals may feel bombarded by messages urging them to change a number of health-related behaviours (e.g., nutrition, smoking, exercise, safety), it is necessary to concentrate on changing behaviours that result in frequent and serious injuries (Etzioni 1978).
- There may be undesirable side effects, known as risk compensation. For example, drivers may actually speed up when using seat belts or driving in cars with air bags (Streff and Geller 1988; Wilde 1982).

Legislative requirements for safe behaviour by individuals (e.g., mandatory helmet use by motorcyclists) is an approach to injury control that is active in emphasis but carries consequences for individuals apart from decreasing potential injuries—failure to comply with the law may result in a fine. Although the negative consequence of a fine may not motivate all individuals enough to change their behaviour, the rates of compliance with safe behaviours are higher than without these laws. Obviously, to achieve maximum compliance, legislated interventions place demands on enforcement resources. To maximize its effectiveness, a legislated intervention needs to be embedded in a broader context that includes public education and an enforcement strategy.

In sum, in cases where passive approaches to injury control are not feasible and the potential severity of injury is great (e.g., 70–85 percent of motorcycle fatalities are due to head trauma) (NHTSA 1980), legislative active approaches have been proven effective in promoting safe behaviours (e.g., helmet use) and in curtailing injury rates (e.g., Watson et al. 1980).

EVALUATION ISSUES

In the area of program evaluation, one issue that continues to be debated is the question of what is an appropriate outcome measure. A decline in injury rates is the ideal standard for deciding whether a program is successful. However, for a variety of reasons, very few program evaluations use this measure. For example, categories of injuries that have a low probability of occurrence are a problem. Injury rates may not show statistically significant declines, but the injury may be so severe (e.g., head trauma) and result in such long-term personal and financial costs that evaluators might consider the program a success if it reduces injury rates at all. Obviously, statistical significance and practical significance do not always indicate the same level of success for a program.

For programs that incorporate behavioural techniques, some researchers argue that an increase in safety promotion behaviours (rather than a decline in injury outcomes) is an appropriate measure of program success. One difficulty with this measure, however, is that in many behavioural programs there is a difference between short-term and long-term compliance rates. Specifically, the level of success (i.e., safety behaviours) may decline over time, making it difficult to compare across programs that evaluate success at different points after the intervention.

Timing also affects the evaluation of community-based programs. Immediate gains in compliance, for example, may diminish once program rewards or incentives are discontinued or if the individual must exercise some effort to maintain compliance (e.g., replace batteries in smoke detector). On the other hand, initial low levels of compliance may increase as a result of gradual shifts in attitudes and beliefs, with a similar change in behaviours. For financial reasons, few programs incorporate both short-term and long-term measures of success. This is unfortunate because one often observes different outcomes over time.

A related issue is that many evaluations are based on self-reported behaviours rather than on actual observations. This is a particular problem in evaluations of programs to prevent spinal cord and head trauma injuries. The issue becomes more apparent if one considers the possible effects of having participated in a program to reduce spinal cord injuries: it is possible that the child has been persuaded by the intervention program to use seat belts, but it is equally plausible that the child has learned that saying he uses a seat belt is the socially desirable response or thinks that he may appear foolish to say otherwise (i.e., the child should remember from the program to endorse this response). It is difficult to know what to make of "successful" programs that have used self-reported behaviour as the outcome measure.

The reader may notice the lack of uniformity of outcome measures across injury types: sometimes success is measured by a decline in injury rates (more stringent types of program evaluations); sometimes it is measured by an increase in safety behaviours without a corresponding decline in injury rates; and sometimes it is measured in terms of self-reported behaviours instead of actual observations.

Using the incidence of events as the only outcome measure in program evaluations is also problematic, particularly for some injury categories. For example, burn prevention programs often teach people how to minimize burn severity once the skin has already been burned. As a result, interventions may not affect the general incidence of burns, but it may result in less severe burn outcomes because people are more knowledgeable and take action more quickly.

Several other program evaluation issues are evident in the literature. For example, one issue that is seldom addressed in evaluations of injury prevention programs concerns confounding sources of prevention information. Prevention programs are often a response to elevated injury statistics. With media focus on both the statistics and factors leading to these injury outcomes, it is impossible to speak with certainty about the "pure" effects of the injury prevention program. A related issue is that many programs are multifaceted in scope. Although this promotes a program's success (see below), evaluators are often unable to discern which component is responsible for that success. This limits one's ability to make informed decisions about essential components if a scaled-down version of the program is sought.

It also deserves mention that most evaluation components of programs apply the most rudimentary of statistical approaches. For example, there is often no consideration of using statistical control for possible seasonal effects on outcome measures (in winter, one might see only the most avid cyclists, and these individuals are probably most likely to use helmets anyway, thereby limiting evaluation accuracy for helmet promotion campaigns). Often, there are no baseline measures taken in control communities that are to be compared with target communities to evaluate the success of a program. Rather, comparison communities are selected on the basis of demographic variables alone. This approach makes it difficult to interpret differences in outcome rates after the intervention has been implemented in the target community.

Given these caveats, the following section reviews program successes in greater detail. Where appropriate, it also provides a discussion of program failures and the factors that differentiate successes and failures.

PROGRAMS TO PROMOTE INJURY CONTROL: THE "SUCCESS STORIES"

Motor Vehicle Injury to Passengers

Programs to Promote the Use of Safety Seats

Motor vehicle collisions are the leading single cause of childhood death and injury (Roberts et al. 1987). Health professionals have estimated that as many as 70 percent of these could be eliminated if children were properly secured in car seats (infants), booster seats (toddlers, preschoolers), or seat belts (larger preschoolers, school-age children).

Early programs focused on educating caregivers and relied on lay persons (e.g., teachers, volunteers), physicians and other public health professionals to promote the use of car seats. Generally, any effects that were realized were more positive when physicians communicated the messages than when lay persons or other health care professionals did. That is, *who* the communicator is matters: the more a person is deemed an expert in the area, the more powerful is the effect of his message on caregivers' behaviours (Bass 1993).

Similarly, to the extent that prenatal messages had any impact at all, they had more impact on caregivers' decisions to use infant safety seats than postnatal messages did. That is, *when* the information is communicated matters: it is best to convince caregivers of the importance of use before they develop a false sense of security (Allen and Bergman 1976; Kanthor 1976).

Although limited, there also is evidence suggesting that educational messages that focus on positive inducements for car seat use (e.g., discussion of benefits) have more impact on caregivers' behaviours than educational messages that focus on negative ones (e.g., appeals to fear). That is, the *nature* of the communication matters (Treiber 1986).

Overall, however, positive effects of these education-only approaches, if any, are short lived (see Pless and Arsenault 1987 for a review). For example, one program considered the effect of discussion, pamphlets, formal prescriptions for car seats, and a demonstration by a paediatrician on the correct use of restraints (Reisinger et al. 1981). A 72 percent difference between target and nontarget groups' use of car seats was found 2 months after the program, but this difference decreased to only 9 percent by 4 months (see also Geddis and Pettengell 1982). Thus, education-only approaches are not especially effective for promoting long-term use of safety seats by caregivers.

Alternative approaches have included legislated requirements for child restraint, loaner programs to make safety seats widely available, and the incorporation of behavioural techniques in caregiver training on the use of safety seats.

Legislated requirements are in place throughout North America. Generally, observational studies reveal no more than a 50 percent compliance rate with the law (American Academy of Pediatrics 1984; Decker et al. 1984; Reagan 1984; Ziegler 1989). Even though this is a less than ideal outcome, the increase in safety seat use has been sufficient to produce a significant decline in child passenger deaths (Decker et al. 1984). Not surprisingly, the stronger the enforcement program is, the greater the rate of compliance. For example, in a locally funded study at two sites in Philadelphia, the initiation of a strong enforcement program resulted in increasing use of toddler safety seats from a baseline of 71.8 and 60.9 percent to 76.8 and 71.4 percent, respectively; correct usage increased from 67 and 57.5 percent to 72.8 and 69.3 percent, respectively (Decina et al. 1994). Obviously, when enforcement is increased and this is publicized (along with educational information about the merits of child restraint), caregivers respond by increasing their use of safety seats for their children. Thus, to be effective, legislated mandates must be accompanied by a strong program of enforcement and public education about injury control.

Loaner programs (e.g., administered by hospitals, Lions' Club, Rotary Club) seek to overcome the cost barrier to safety seat use by providing seats for free or at very low cost (the benefits of promoting caregiver safety practices by providing free or low-cost safety devices will also be discussed later). These programs have yielded mixed results (e.g., Reisinger and Williams 1978; Greensher 1984), which illustrates that making safety devices available does not ensure their use. Nonetheless, loaner programs can be quite successful (e.g., Colletti 1984 reported rates of infant seat use exceeding 70 percent at the time of hospital discharge, in contrast to 16 percent before the program) if certain features are incorporated into the program. Christophersen et al. (1985), for example, documented the importance of a comprehensive program that includes not only education material about the benefits of infant safety seats and availability of the seats, but also demonstrations of their use, written material reviewing this demonstration, and the opportunity for caregivers to practise using the car seats and receive feedback.

Incorporation of behavioural techniques in caregiver training significantly increases caregivers' use of safety seats. This is not surprising, given the success of behavioural methods to promote the use of seat belts by adults (e.g., Geller et al. 1982). Drawing on learning theory, these approaches seek to evoke behavioural changes through the judicious use of rewards. The basic premise is that behaviours that result in positive consequences are likely to increase in frequency. Thus, with positive incentives, parents are likely to alter their behaviour and use safety seats for their children. The findings support this assumption.

Christophersen and Gulay (1989), for example, sought to increase parents' use of child restraints by advocating the positive effects for parents of their doing so (e.g., children would be better behaved and less distractive or intrusive if they were properly secured). The authors found some positive effects of having health care professionals provide a written protocol for parents highlighting the fact that children are better behaved when restrained in vehicles and also providing guidelines for getting children to remain in safety seats. Five of eight mothers began using child restraint devices after the intervention; at 6 months there were still five parents complying, although this dropped to three at the 1-year follow-up.

Behavioural programs that provide tangible rewards to parents for using safety seats produce even greater levels of compliance. Roberts and Turner (1986), for example, used this approach with parents participating in two private daycare settings. If children were secured in car safety seats when they arrived at daycare, their parents were rewarded with tokens, some of which were redeemable for prizes. Local businesses donated pizza, hamburger, chicken, taco, or fish dinners, movie passes, ice-cream cones, and cookies—an estimated $500 in prizes. Businesses were acknowledged in letters to parents and in local advertising about the program. Every day that the parents arrived with their child in a car seat, trained observers gave the parent a token, some of which said "You win" and others of which said "Try again." The odds of winning were high initially and then declined as compliance rates increased. Results indicated that rewards increased car seat use from 49 percent to 80 percent after 2 weeks at one daycare facility (upper- and middle-class families) and from 11 percent to 64 percent at the other (lower- and middle-class families). Typically, with behavioural interventions, the high compliance rates drop off once rewards are discontinued. Nonetheless, the rates remain substantially above baseline levels. Thus, behavioural approaches to injury control are typically quite effective.

Success in reducing the incidence of child passenger deaths is limited not only by the moderate compliance rates in caregivers' use of safety seats, but also by improper use of safety seats. For example, a Transport Canada (1992) observational and telephone survey of child restraint practices sampled 21,844 children and found that 21 percent of infant safety seats, 19 percent of car seats, and 5 percent of booster seats were used incorrectly. These findings suggest the following: (1) Indices of compliance may suggest a more favourable situation than actually exists, since improper use compromises safety. This is difficult to determine by simple observation as a car drives by. Passenger injury rates are therefore likely to provide a more sensitive index of program effectiveness than observations alone. (2) More emphasis on education in proper use of safety seats is warranted to achieve greater injury control.

A key barrier to promoting proper use of safety seats is the abundance of models on the market, each with different features and closing mechanisms. This variety precludes making any public statements about what constitutes proper use in general terms (aside from the tether strap feature, which is common across front-facing infant seats). The instruction manuals are often difficult to follow and are usually in English only, which compounds the problem of achieving proper use among non-English-speaking segments of the population.

The problem of improper use could be addressed by car designs that incorporate child safety seats as part of the car (not just top-of-the-line models, but all cars; for example, top-of-the-line Volvos have this feature, eliminating the need for separate toddler safety seats). Similarly, car dealers could expand their service domain to include inspection of customers' installation of safety seats in their vehicles and provide feedback. A common motivator for purchasing a new car is the expected growth in family membership; thus, this service feature could be an appealing one. Another possibility is to have safety seat manufacturers provide videotapes about correct installation of different types of safety seats. These videotapes could be rented at local video stores, with money refunded upon their return (the use of videotaped instruction has proven quite successful in promoting do-it-yourself projects in the home). Similarly, detailed instruction manuals showing correct installation—for example, "Before You Turn the Key," a resource guide produced by the Infant and Toddler Safety Association in Kitchener (Lee 1995)—could be made available through local libraries. Holding free safety seat inspections and providing feedback to correct problems (e.g., Esso has sponsored such community-based programs through Safe Kids Canada in Ontario) also have proven useful.

Probably one very effective way to motivate caregivers to learn about proper use of safety seats is to take a passive-strategy approach and make proper use a stipulation of the child restraint laws. An approach recently being developed in Alberta is based on this premise, although the legislation has not yet been enacted (Anna Lovasik, Injury Prevention Centre, Alberta, personal communication). In this program, a "zero-tolerance" approach is advocated, and the emphasis in education about safety seats is on correct use. Toward this aim, drivers may receive a fine if a child is improperly restrained. They can avoid payment by, for example, attending a 45-minute session on proper use of safety seats. Although the program is still being implemented and has not yet been evaluated, this approach speaks directly to what is emerging as a key issue in child restraint in Canada and elsewhere—improper use of safety seats by caregivers.

Programs to Promote Children's Use of Seat Belts

Two types of programs are commonly used: education and behavioural programs.

Education programs directed toward children are generally not very effective. However, they are fairly inexpensive to implement and can reach large numbers of children (e.g., through the school system). Thus, schools persist in delivering these programs, using props such as Elmer the Elephant colouring books. Recent evidence suggests that effectiveness can be enhanced if education includes a participatory or interactive component. For example, Lehman and Geller (1990a) demonstrated that having kindergarten and young school-age children practise (2 weeks of rehearsal, including practising seat belt use in the classroom) and present a 15-minute safety belt skit increased the seat belt use of those children who were initially inconsistent users (increased from 47 percent to 82 percent) and also increased use among parents who watched the skit (increased from 36 percent to 56 percent). These positive gains were still evident 3 months later.

Another education program, also noteworthy for its success, actively involved children (4–9 years old) in several ways. This program (Morrow 1989) was delivered by familiar teachers as a 1-month intensive curriculum intervention (May Is Buckle Up Month). Children read books, saw movies, and were involved in a number of activities (e.g., making posters) to create seat belt promotion messages. The curriculum (reading, math, art) was revised to present seat belt use in a positive way (no appeals to fear) that involved the children and promoted a sense of mastery of their environment.

The program also incorporated "Flash for Life" (see Geller et al. 1985), a participatory component that had the children request other people to use a seat belt. Specifically, as the children rode in a vehicle, they displayed a postcard to unbelted passengers and drivers in nearby cars that read "Buckle Up—I Love You" and flipped the card to say "Thank You" once the person put on the seat belt. Although not singled out by the program developers, this feature of the program may have been critical to the success of the program for several reasons. First, research indicates that this feature alone results in significant increases in seat belt use among adults (Geller et al. 1985). Second, the card could have served to remind children to use their own seat belts. Third, to participate in this way the children would have had to be modelling seat belt use themselves. Fourth, this feature may have provided intrinsic rewards for the children (promotion of self-esteem and a sense of mastery and control over the environment, including over adults' behaviours).

The program improved the rate of seat belt use by children as well as that of their parents, although parents were not directly targeted. Children's use increased from 46 percent to 66 percent, and the parents' use increased from 47 percent to 61 percent. These improvements persisted for 3 weeks following the program.

Behavioural programs, in contrast to education programs, are extremely effective but are relatively costly to implement and are therefore, typically, limited in scope to small numbers of children. Some of the most innovative work in this area has been done by Roberts and Turner (1986), Roberts and Layfield (1987), and Roberts et al. (1988). They showed that applying behavioural principles (e.g., rewards) leads to a significant increase in seat belt use among children, and this is true whether the target audience is the parent (on behalf of the child) or the child directly (see Roberts and Fanurik 1986). It is noteworthy too that programs aimed at the child often result in an accompanying increase in seat belt use by parents (Roberts and Layfield 1987) and even younger siblings (Roberts et al. 1988), which suggests that children can evoke behavioural change among other family members by requesting or modelling such changes themselves (e.g., Morrow 1989). These generalization effects improve cost-effectiveness and suggest that targeting either children or their parents may be sufficient to reduce passenger injuries among both populations.

One behavioural program stands out as a noteworthy exception to the problem that these programs are typically directed to only a small number of children. The program involved 27 schools (low- to middle-income levels) and more than 10,000 children (5–11 years old) in public and private school systems (Roberts et al. 1990). Incentive rewards (certificates for free pizza) were given to promote seat belt use. The program cost $13,600 to implement, and a local pizza company absorbed the costs in return for promotion of its name.

The program lasted 4 weeks, with a different focus each week. In week 1, there were public information announcements, and all children received program materials. Media coverage was extensive throughout the program, and the month was publicly designated as "Buckle Up, We Care Month." Children received Flash for Life notebooks, including information on how to use the notebook to encourage others to use seat belts. They were encouraged to "flash" to at least one person each day. They also received a bumper sticker for parents to place on the rear bumper of their vehicle, indicating they were participating in the buckle-up program ("Please Buckle Up, I Care" was printed on the sticker, along with the logo from the pizza sponsor). Parents and children received information about the program and were told of the role of the police force (when a car was observed with the bumper sticker and with all occupants buckled up, the officer gave a gift certificate for a pizza dinner). The names of each day's winners (five per day) were announced on the evening weather forecast of the local television station.

During week 2, the reward program was implemented in all schools. Volunteers gave coloured stickers to school children who were wearing seat belts on arrival at school; if anyone in the car was not buckled up, the child did not receive a sticker. The sticker said "Buckle Up, I Care" and showed the logo of the pizza store. During week 3, the volunteers randomly selected 2 days of the 5 on which to give stickers. This dropped to 1 day during the fourth week of the intervention.

This reward-based program was effective in increasing seat belt use. For example, in one school, rates changed from a baseline level of 23.5 percent to 31 percent during week 1, to 42 percent during week 2, to 34 percent during week 3, to 44 percent during week 4, and to 42 percent in the 2 weeks after the program. It is noteworthy too that in this project children obtained reward stickers only when everyone in the vehicle was properly restrained. This requirement produced an indirect benefit: seat belt use rates increased for parents and siblings too.

Obviously, behavioural principles can be applied on a large scale, and successfully so. What are required, however, are enough volunteers to distribute rewards, observers to record incidence of safe behaviours, and funding to supply rewards and support materials to families. Other ways that communities have become involved in behavioural interventions include obtaining assistance from local businesses (such as donation of billboard space) and recruiting sponsorship for purchase of billboard space or advertising space in local newspapers. Public endorsement campaigns are run by local groups (law enforcement units, pediatricians, universities, medical auxiliaries, etc.), to promote community awareness and support of the intervention program (e.g., Roberts et al. 1988). Obviously, the more pervasive and multifaceted the community intervention is, the greater the degree of success, even in the case of behavioural programs that typically already enjoy high levels of success.

One issue that has been raised in the literature on behavioural interventions is whether rewards are essential for success. Since the reward feature of these programs often results in prohibitive costs, this speaks directly to the issue of cost-effectiveness. Lehman and Geller (1990b) recently argued that rewards are not essential for motivating children to use seat belts if group interaction is incorporated in the education program. Intrinsic rewards may somehow be built into the intervention process in interactive-based education programs (teacher support for compliance may be rewarding, a sense of mastery of the material may be rewarding, etc.). However, further research is needed to establish the validity of this claim. In any case, the likelihood of success in behavioural programs is greater if rewards for compliance are provided.

Motor Vehicle Injury to Pedestrians

Children between the ages of 5 and 9 are at particular risk for pedestrian injuries. These injuries typically occur in residential areas close to home, frequently during play. Among children, the most frequent type of accident observed is the midblock dart out from between parked cars (Malek et al. 1990).

The majority of programs aimed at teaching pedestrian safety to children are school-based ones. Most programs provide a conceptual framework, with some strategies or rules that are applicable across several situations (Ampofo-Boateng and Thomson 1990). Classroom teaching usually involves talks from police officers or crossing guards, possibly supplemented by written material or visual aids (posters and videos). Unfortunately, the success of such programs is not inspiring: there are often increases in knowledge of road safety, but little generalization to behaviour in the traffic environment (Numenmaa and Syvanen 1974; Ryhammer and Berglund 1980). Reductions in injuries seldom exceed 10 percent (e.g., Howarth and Repetto-Wright 1978).

Probably the most significant criticism of classroom instruction is that it bears little relationship to the real task facing children when they are pedestrians in the street. Much less widely used, but a closer approximation to reality, is simulation or practical training, which involves behavioural rehearsal by the child. Rothengatter (1984) developed such a program. He taught kindergarten mothers and teachers how to instruct children about safe crossing, and these adults then taught 5- and 6-year-old children in real traffic situations. Even after a 4-month delay, there was improvement in the children's crossing skills. Other programs have been modelled on this demonstration project, but evaluations have not yet been published. Recently, a program called Kidestrians was launched in southwestern

Ontario. This program holds great promise, since it seeks to teach children how to cross safely at midblock locations and from between parked cars. Traditional education approaches rejected these goals, even though most injuries to child pedestrians happen under exactly these circumstances.

Recent intervention efforts have also taken a more systematic approach to determine exactly what skills are needed for children to cross streets without incident (e.g., Ampofo-Boateng and Thomson 1990; Thomson 1991) and to relate skill levels to injury outcomes (e.g., Pless et al. 1989, 1995; DeJoy 1992). Similarly, an analysis of common characteristics of sites of child pedestrian injuries (Ampofo-Boateng 1987) led to some innovative experimental-based approaches that have shown encouraging results in road safety education. For example, a training study has shown that children at 5 years of age can acquire the necessary skills to find safe routes along which to cross a road (Ampofo-Boateng et al. 1993). One feature common to this training study and Kidestrians-type programs is that the children are taught in actual traffic situations, thereby providing opportunities for modelling, rehearsal and feedback (including rewards, such as praise), which are features of behavioural programs that have succeeded in achieving injury control.

The Safe Kids/Healthy Neighborhoods Coalition

One success story I have chosen to review in depth is a program that was initiated in Harlem, New York, in response to elevated injury rates (Davidson et al. 1994). This program targeted a high–injury risk, inner-city population in which poverty was prevalent.

Description – The study spanned 9 years and represented an intensive and coordinated community-based effort to promote safety. The basic premise was twofold: to reduce outdoor injuries, children need safe places to play and supervision of their play activities.

Reasons for the initiative – Parents and educators in Central Harlem requested a program in playground safety from health professionals. The playgrounds were sites for drug dealing and were in poor condition. The lack of safe play areas and supervised play activities was assumed to contribute to high rates of outdoor injuries among children.

A review of the injury statistics for the area by the Northern Manhattan Injury Surveillance System revealed that (1) the incidence of severe injuries (requiring hospitalization or resulting in death) was twice as high in Central Harlem as in nearby Washington Heights (since the communities were similar in many other ways, Washington Heights became the control site); (2) the incidence was increasing among 5–16-year-old children and adolescents and decreasing among children under 4 years old; and (3) the leading causes of injuries were falls and motor vehicle with pedestrian collisions.

At the end of 1988, the Harlem Hospital Injury Prevention Program, in conjunction with community groups and city agencies, initiated the Safe Kids/Healthy Neighborhoods Coalition, the goal of which was to reduce outdoor injuries among children and adolescents 5–16 years old. Specifically, the Coalition worked to (1) renovate playgrounds; (2) involve children and adolescents in safe, supervised activities that would also teach them useful skills (dance, sports, horticulture, carpentry); (3) provide education on injury and violence prevention; and (4) provide bicycle helmets at reasonable costs.

Actors – Over the first 3 years (1988–1991), 26 city agencies, voluntary organizations and citizen groups participated in the intervention. For example, the Department of Parks repaired all playgrounds and involved children in mural painting, and the Department of Transportation initiated an intensive pedestrian safety education program in the schools, reaching all children in Grade 3. The Harlem Hospital Injury Prevention Program initiated a dance program, an art studio, a Little League program, a winter baseball clinic, and a soccer league. More than 1,000 children participated in these programs, and more than 500 bicycle helmets were made available to the community.

Results – To evaluate the effectiveness of the program, the control site and test site were compared. Sophisticated statistical analyses were applied to the data, and adjustments were made for seasonal and annual trends that were independent of the intervention. Initially, severe injuries were two times higher in Central Harlem than in Washington Heights. By the end of the 3-year intervention, there had been a significant decline in the injury rates in Central Harlem, with a 26 percent reduction in the overall injury rate in the targeted age group of children and adolescents 5–16 years old. No such reduction was observed in the nontargeted younger age group. Within the targeted-injury category, motor vehicle–related and assault injuries decreased significantly, although outdoor injuries did not (possibly because the sports programs increased children's exposure to the risk of outdoor falls).

Replicability – Relatively few community-based programs have used changes in injury rates as outcome measures; many use increases in safety promotion behaviours instead. Nonetheless, in two similar large-scale projects in which injury rates for control and test sites were compared, there were some positive gains demonstrated. The Massachusetts Statewide Childhood Injury Prevention Program (SCIPP) found a reduction in one of the targeted areas (motor vehicle injuries to passengers) (Guyer et al. 1989). In Sweden, a 4-year grassroots project resulted in a 28 percent reduction in motor vehicle–related injuries, as well as a 27 percent reduction in in-home injuries (Shelp 1987, 1988). These results suggest that community-based intervention can be quite effective in reducing injuries among children (further elaboration of these ideas is given in the section on in-home injuries).

Funding – The project was supported in part by grants from the Centers for Disease Control, Health of the Public, Mellon Foundation, and Robert Wood Johnson Foundation.

Evaluation – This intervention, targeting a specific low-income, high-injury risk urban population, significantly reduced pedestrian-related injuries among children and adolescents 5–16 years old. Rarely are injury prevention interventions as rigorously evaluated as in this program. Indeed, this program could serve as a model for what evaluations should be like. The success of this program derived primarily from creating safe alternatives (playgrounds) to children playing near streets and from offering attractive supervised activities at these play locations. Both features effectively removed the potential hazard (proximity to cars). It is likely that the school-based programs on safe pedestrian practices increased knowledge and sensitized children to the hazards of cars. However, results from earlier research suggest that this type of program probably has little impact on safe crossing skills (see above review). In fact, there was no measure of safe crossing skills before or after the intervention.

This program demonstrates that large-scale programs that target prevention of specific types of injuries can be effective. It is noteworthy that the program was not effective, however, in reducing outdoor injuries. This probably resulted, in part, from the lack of specificity in programming (e.g., falls were not targeted in any particular way). It is clear in the injury prevention literature (see, for example, the section on spinal cord injuries and head trauma) that the more behaviourally specific the intervention is, the greater the likelihood of successfully decreasing injury risk behaviours and increasing safety promotion practices. As suggested above, the incidence of serious falls may not have declined during the intervention period because the sports activities that were advocated as a substitute for playing on the streets increased the exposure to the risk of outdoor injuries. Possibly, this was an intervention that was successful in reducing one type of injury (pedestrian injuries) but actually increased the likelihood of another type of injury (falls), resulting in no change in the rate of injuries due to falls.

To summarize, effective strategies to reduce pedestrian injuries among children are those that provide street-crossing training in a real-life or simulation context (e.g., Kidestrians program) or minimize exposure to the hazard by redirecting children to other activities and by creating safe outdoor play areas. Classroom instruction increases awareness of the hazard but does not produce significant changes in street-crossing behaviours; therefore, it is not very cost effective. Ideally, an emphasis on pedestrian education should occur during the preschool and early school years, when children are at increased risk for these injuries and are just acquiring these skills.

Burns

Several approaches have been taken to prevent fire-related injuries to children. Some interventions focus on modifying the environment (e.g., by installing smoke detectors, using flame-retardant fabrics for children's clothes, turning down the temperature of the water heater). Others attempt to teach children, using behavioural approaches, to minimize the injury risk in potentially hazardous situations. Because burn prevention programs have generally yielded only modest levels of success, there is no single success story to be discussed. Rather, a general overview is provided of the types of programs that aim to reduce burns among infants and children.

The realization that 70 percent of all burns to infants were related to their clothing catching fire led to the passage of legislation throughout Canada and the United States requiring children's sleepwear to be flame retardant. Like most other passive interventions, this one was quite successful, resulting in a significant drop in both in the number and the severity of burns from sleepwear ignition (McLoughlin et al. 1977).

Similarly, although very few places have adopted fireworks legislation (I could locate only one study on this topic), it is noteworthy that this approach to burn control has been shown to be extremely effective in the United States: the rate of injuries related to fireworks is significantly greater in those states that do not restrict access to the product (Berger, Kalishman, and Rivara 1985; Smith and Falk 1987). Thus, legislated strategies to restrict access to dangerous products work to control burn-related injuries.

Smoke detector programs were initiated in response to two key statistics on house fires: (1) 75 percent of fires in homes occur between 9 p.m. and 7 a.m., when members are likely to be asleep (National Fire Protection Association 1982); and (2) 26 percent of fire victims die from burns, and the remaining 74 percent die from smoke-related injuries because they do not escape in time (Levin and Radford 1977). In fact, if a smoke detector is not installed, individuals are 2.5 times more likely to be killed if there is a fire (Federal Emergency Management Agency 1983). For example, in a large study in Ontario that involved 79,000 homes over a 4-year period, smoke detectors gave early warning in 85 percent of house fires, thereby preventing serious injury and death (Ontario Ministry of Housing 1978).

Although loaner approaches to controlling in-home injuries and passenger vehicle injuries have produced mixed results (see those sections for review), giveaway programs are generally successful in recruiting families to use smoke detectors (Miller, Reisinger, and Blatler 1982). For example, in a Baltimore study involving a low-income urban area at high risk for house fires, a survey of 231 randomly selected households that had requested and received smoke alarms 8–10 months earlier (3,720 were distributed) revealed that 92 percent had installed the alarms and 88 percent of these were operational (Gorman et al. 1985). The success of this program is noteworthy because it required active initiative by consumers. Those who could afford to buy the alarms were able to purchase them at cost, but they had to go to firehalls to do so. Those who could not afford to buy the alarms had to request them from the fire department directly, either in person or by phone, or by placing a sign in their window that could be seen by firefighters riding along the city streets; the alarms were then delivered to their door.

Another approach to modifying the environment is taken by burn prevention programs aimed at having caregivers reduce the temperature of their tap water (e.g., to 55 °C). Approximately 10 percent of all paediatric admissions for burns are due to tap water scalds (Green et al. 1984), and these often involve greater total body surface and a higher mortality rate than other scalds (Smith and O'Neill 1984). Thus, hot water is a significant source of injury among children, particularly those under 3 years of age (Raine and Azmy 1983; Green et al. 1984; Smith and O'Neill 1984).

Several approaches have been used to try to convince caregivers to reduce tap water temperature. Most approaches involve education (pamphlets, counselling) to inform caregivers of the risks and teach them how to adjust water heater thermostats to safer settings; a thermometer may also be provided so that they can measure their water temperature. Like most other programs that emphasize education about injury risks, these programs are not especially effective. Furthermore, they can be quite costly because of the need to provide thermometers as part of the education package. For example, in a community-wide, multimedia study that was impressive in scope, Katcher (1987) encouraged people in a population of 2.1 million to request information (pamphlet, thermometer) at no cost. More than 140,000 requested information. A follow-up telephone survey revealed 61.5 percent actually used the thermometer; and of these, 43 percent reported unsafe water temperatures. Of those reporting unsafe temperatures, however, only 52 percent lowered their thermostat to safer levels. Thus, this program, which cost $200,000, resulted in only 20,000 or so families lowering the temperature of their water heater to safer levels.

In other studies, as in Katcher's (1987) study (which obtained only 52 percent compliance), there is evidence that convincing people to change their behaviour after they are familiar with the issues is a key barrier to success (e.g., Webne et al. 1989). The design of water heaters may be partially to blame. Many manufacturers label the setting "hot" when the water temperature is 70 °C (i.e., scalding) and "warm" when the water temperature is 50 °C. Relabelling these settings "scalding" and "safe" may lead more consumers to adjust the temperature downward (Webne et al. 1989). Caregivers may also have developed a false sense of security from having bathed their children without burn incidents in the past. This makes it difficult to convince caregivers of the hazard of their current water temperatures.

In addition to structural interventions, such as relabelling settings, a passive legislative approach requiring manufacturers to pre-set heaters at lower temperatures would go a long way toward solving this problem. Although the net gains in reducing hot water–related burns would likely take years (most residential water heaters need replacing only every 10 years or so), legislative intervention will produce the required effects over time. Indeed, a review of U.S. data from areas with laws controlling water heater temperature indicate that a convincing case can be made for a passive intervention to address this injury risk. For example, Seattle, Washington, burn admissions dropped from 5.5 to 2.4 per year after legislation was enacted that required water heaters to be pre-set at 49°C (Erdmann et al. 1991).

Finally, several programs have sought both to reduce children's fear of fire and minimize their risk of burn injuries if they do encounter one. Because fear can hamper response in emergencies (e.g., Janis and Mann 1968; Jones and Ollendick 1986), fear reduction is often a component of emergency training programs targeting children. Most successful programs teaching fire safety skills have used behavioural approaches incorporating simulation conditions. The use of simulations that approximate real-life situations is likely essential for success in teaching specific safety skills. These programs indicate that children who are exposed to models demonstrating the safe behaviours, rehearse these behaviours in simulations, and receive feedback and rewards (e.g., praise) for doing so acquire proper fire safety behaviours (Jones et al. 1981, 1989).

Spinal Cord Injuries and Head Trauma

In infants and young children, falls from heights are a common source of head injury and spinal cord damage. Few programs, however, have focused on eliminating falls at these young ages. One exception was the Children Can't Fly Campaign that was launched in 1971 by New York City Health Department to combat the specific problem of children falling from windows. Such falls accounted for 12 percent of all deaths in New York City between January 1965 and September 1969. The success of this small-scale program, which reduced falls from windows by 50 percent within 2 years of implementation, led to the adoption of legislation throughout North America requiring owners of multiple dwellings to provide window guards for apartments in which children 10 years old and younger reside.

In school-age children, common sources of spinal cord injuries and head trauma include bicycling without a helmet, diving in too-shallow waters, and risk behaviours resulting in falls (e.g., climbing up trees, rollerblading without a helmet) (Stover and Fine 1986). Adolescents and young adults (15–24 years old) account for fully one-third of all spinal cord injuries, and almost half of these result from not wearing a seat belt in motor vehicle accidents (Kraus et al. 1984). It has been estimated that the lifetime cost of one spinal cord injury is U.S.$1.2 million (National Spinal Cord Injury Association 1987). Because of the high personal and financial costs of such injuries, a number of interventions have been tried to prevent these injuries.

Most interventions have several objectives: to promote the use of seat belts and helmets; to reduce injury risk behaviours; to educate children about their bodies and the impact of these injuries on their functioning; and to increase children's awareness of their vulnerability to spinal cord injuries and head trauma. The majority of the programs target junior and high school students. Fewer than 10 percent of the programs are aimed at young school-age children (Richards et al. 1991), which is surprising, given that increasing young children's awareness of the risk-taking behaviours that can lead to such injuries and the effects of such injuries, would likely foster their assimilation of attitudes and behaviours that would help them avoid these injuries as they grow up.

A review of this literature reveals that many programs have not been evaluated at all, and those that have been evaluated have yielded equivocal results. A University of Missouri program, for example, resulted in improvements in knowledge, attitudes and some behaviours 1 week after the program was presented (Lechman and Bornwich 1981). However, in other studies no such positive effects have been realized (Robertson et al. 1974; Neuwelt et al. 1989; Ng 1991). A program presented to elementary school children (kindergarten through Grade 6) resulted in improved knowledge of injury effects and preventive strategies at each grade; however, there was no impact on seat belt use (Richards et al. 1991). A preliminary study by Frank et al. (1992) examined the long-term impact of a five-component program aimed at preventing spinal cord injuries among adolescents. These researchers found more reported seat belt use and lower likelihood of riding with friends who had been drinking among those who had experienced the program 3 years earlier. However, the psychometric properties of the measures were weak, and the key behavioural data were all self-reported; possibly, exposure to the program resulted in more social desirability biases in reporting about safe behaviours. Finally, an extensive evaluation of THINK FIRST, the national program to prevent head and spinal cord injuries founded by the American Association for Neurological Surgeons and the Congress of Neurological Surgeons, reveals findings similar to those in much of this injury prevention literature: the program effectively increases knowledge and awareness but results in few behavioural changes that would promote safety and minimize risk (Englander et al. 1993).

In summary, I was unable to identify any program to prevent spinal cord and head trauma injuries that has consistently proved successful in reducing injury risk behaviours, although many programs increased awareness and knowledge. Perhaps the most striking conclusion is that we know that one-shot programs are not likely to be sufficient to alter the likelihood of injury risk behaviours that can result in spinal cord injuries or head trauma. Although one would think that a comprehensive approach (e.g., THINK FIRST) would produce the greatest results, the behavioural-intervention literature suggests that the problem with these approaches is a lack of behavioural specificity. In other words, they seek to cover too much at once. Consistent with this explanation are programs that have failed to produce positive results in areas in which other research has shown the approach to be effective when it is narrow in focus and behaviourally specific (eg., McLoughlin et al. 1982). Possibly, programs would be more effective if they sought to target only the most critical injury risk behaviour at an age, with repeated application but a different behavioural focus across age (e.g., seat belt use for 15–24 year olds; helmet use for 8–14 year olds; awareness of fall-related injury risks among 5–7 year olds). Finally, the failure of THINK FIRST to produce behavioural changes suggests that the Canadian program HEROES, which is closely modelled after THINK FIRST, may not be effective in altering risk behaviour. Given the expense of implementing programs, formal program evaluations are necessary to determine what positive effects are realized by a program like HEROES. Certainly, the injury statistics strongly suggest that increasing knowledge about head trauma risks is not sufficient to reduce injury risk behaviours. This result mirrors the common finding in health psychology literature that knowledge does not often lead to behaviour change.

Programs to Promote the Use of Bicycle Helmets

Head trauma prevention programs that are specific and focus on the use of helmets have enjoyed greater success than more general programs to prevent spinal cord injuries and head trauma. Among school-age children, bicycle accidents are the most common injuries requiring treatment in an emergency room (Rivara 1982) and the leading cause of head injury (Canadian Bike Helmet Coalition 1995). Particularly high death rates due to bicycle injuries are found among children aged 8–14: by these ages, they are likely allowed to bicycle without adult supervision. Epidemiological research indicates that 76 percent of fatalities from bicycle crashes are due to head traumas (Consumer Product Safety Commission 1983; Thornson 1984). Recent research indicates that helmets reduce head injury in cyclists by as much as 85 percent (Thompson 1989). Helmets also reduce the severity of head traumas: injured cyclists not wearing helmets are seven times more likely to suffer permanent brain damage than those with helmets (Canadian Bike Helmet Coalition 1995). Thus, a major focus in programs aimed at reducing head trauma injuries among children is to increase helmet use among cyclists.

To promote helmet use among children, a variety of intervention strategies have been used: school-based education programs, community-wide media campaigns, distribution of education materials to medical patients, and the adoption of laws requiring bicycle helmets. Each intervention has achieved some degree of success (Wood and Milne 1988; Bergman et al. 1990). Not surprisingly, programs that incorporate multiple intervention strategies are the most effective, but they are also the most costly. These findings suggest that any serious commitment to lowering the incidence of bicycle-related head injuries by increasing helmet use on a national scale in Canada will require a large financial commitment. Given the costs of head trauma, however, national strategies to achieve injury control are warranted and would certainly prove cost effective very quickly.

Legislative interventions have been shown to be effective in increasing use, although the mandatory use of helmets is a recent phenomenon and the effects are still being realized (i.e., the compliance rates may show a cumulative pattern, taking years to achieve their full impact, as did compliance rates after seat belt laws were passed). Helmet use in a Maryland suburb increased 43 percent (from 4 percent to 47 percent) following an education program and the implementation of the first law of its kind in the United States (Cote et al. 1992), compared with an increase of only 4 percent (from 7 percent to 11 percent) following an education program alone (Dannenberg et al. 1993). Similarly, after years of a concerted education campaign to increase helmet use in Victoria, Australia, helmet use was made mandatory, resulting in a dramatic increase—to more than 80 percent—in cyclist compliance and a dramatic decrease in bicycle-associated head injuries (Wood and Milne 1988; Ozanne-Smith and Sherry 1990). Thus, legislative interventions effectively increase helmet use by children and thereby achieve greater injury control.

The Seattle Children's Bicycle Helmet Campaign

Probably the most written-about active intervention to promote helmet use was a program initiated in Seattle, Washington, in response to injury statistics. This community-wide intervention resulted in modest increases in helmet use immediately and a steady increase the next year. This success story incorporates some unique features and illustrates a community-wide approach to intervention that could be applied to other types of injuries as well.

Description – This community-wide campaign was implemented from 1986–1989, initially in Seattle and then in the whole state.

Reasons for the initiative – The program grew out of a research project by the Harborview Injury Prevention and Research Center (one of five centres funded by the U.S. Centers for Disease Control) that evaluated barriers preventing children from wearing helmets. Taking into account these findings, the objectives of the community-wide intervention were (1) to convince parents that riding without a helmet is hazardous, (2) to lower the price of helmets to affordable levels, and (3) to overcome the reluctance of children to wear helmets.

Actors – Leadership and coordination of the 16-member coalition were provided by the Harborview Injury Prevention and Research Center. Participants in the coalition included members from the organized bicycle community, a helmet manufacturer, and a Public Health representative. To be a member, an organization had to provide some tangible contribution of money, services or goods. The program drew heavily on the expertise of a public relations specialist and a health education coordinator. In addition, physicians, hospitals, and County Health Department clinic personnel played significant roles in distributing educational materials.

Campaign spokespersons included physicians and surgeons who treated trauma victims and worked in rehabilitation, which added to the credibility of the program. To dispel any stigma associated with helmets, prominent local sports figures were recruited to advertise their use. Youth groups that were popular and visible in the community (e.g., Boy Scouts) helped with promotion by adding helmet use to their merit badge programs and requiring helmet use in bicycle-related activities.

The endorsement by prominent sports figures (i.e., heroes in the eyes of children) and the authoritative messages from individuals in the medical community (i.e., spokespersons likely to influence parents' views) were likely both key to the program's success.

Results – The initial results revealed that helmet use increased from 5 percent to 16 percent over a 2-year period, which is very disappointing given the scope of the program. However, use was up to 25 percent (Rivara et al. 1990) and then to 38 percent in the following year (Young 1991).

Replicability – I am not aware of the application of this program to other settings.

Funding – A program of this magnitude required considerable funds. However, most support came in the form of goods and services instead of direct contributions of money. For example, the Washington Medical Association solicited funds for printing educational materials and distributing materials to physicians, and the association even had its advertising agency help promote events. The Children's Hospital printed and distributed coupons to parents for discounts on the price of helmets and provided volunteers to monitor their redemption. The County Health Department published a pamphlet and organized a number of bicycle rodeos. The local television station sponsored several large events and provided free advertising and material, and a professional production company produced commercials at cost. Newspapers and television stations routinely ran stories on children suffering from head trauma after bicycling accidents; these stories were presented on behalf of the helmet campaign. This was the only program I located that incorporated public sharing of personal injury stories as a component of the media campaign. Because appeals to fear have not typically produced as much success in injury control as positive inducements, it would be useful to know if the strategy of publicizing personal injury stories produces any changes in attitudes or behaviours.

A key issue to be addressed was the prohibitive cost of the helmets themselves (initially U.S.$40–60). To reduce costs, a promotions manager of a helmet manufacturer was recruited to be part of the coalition. The company mass-produced helmets under another name at half the cost (U.S.$20). When a larger company took over the operation, it donated U.S.$5,000 toward the cost of advertising helmet use, with the stipulation that the posters and educational materials show a child wearing the company's helmet. In addition, discount coupons were distributed through doctors' offices, schools and youth groups, and at community events to promote the purchase of children's helmets for U.S.$25 at any of more than 59 bicycle shops throughout the state.

Evaluation – Given the low incidence of deaths (12 percent a year), it will be many years before the full impact of this intervention can be ascertained. Nonetheless, the statistics to date are encouraging.

Education and mass media campaigns, both components of this multifaceted program, have not proven very effective in isolation (e.g., Robertson et al. 1974). However, in combination with financial incentives and effective spokespersons, they constituted a comprehensive program that prompted more children to use their helmets when cycling. Reading about the intervention gives one the impression that the program permeated the community, making it impossible for children and parents to be unaware of the program. In addition, the specificity of focus differentiated this program from most earlier, less successful interventions that had a more general focus on bicycling behaviour (Halperin et al. 1983). The behavioural interventions certainly add credence to the notion that success is more likely when the intervention has a narrow and specific focus.

In-Home Injuries

Programs to Prevent Injuries among Infants and Preschoolers

The protection of infants and preschoolers from injury depends on the actions of caregivers. Consequently, a number of approaches have been taken to increase caregivers' knowledge and practice of in-home safety. The American Academy of Pediatrics and the Canadian Medical Association recommend counselling on home safety practices as part of the well-child care agenda—for example, The Injury Prevention Program (TIPP), is available to help physicians in this counselling process—although the effectiveness of such limited approaches has been questioned repeatedly in evaluation research (e.g., Berger 1981; Morrongiello, Hillier and Bass 1995).

Surprisingly, many interventions that target in-home safety have proceeded without a solid, empirically based understanding of parents' attitudes, beliefs and practices regarding child injuries and child safety (Wortel et al. 1994). Not surprisingly, many of these interventions are more effective in increasing knowledge than in producing changes in caregivers' behaviours. This had led to campaigns for passive interventions to protect children from injury (e.g., Eichelberger et al. 1990).

Health Canada recently sponsored a national survey (Morrongiello and Polak 1995) of parental attitudes toward childhood injuries. The survey revealed that parents were unaware of the scope of the childhood injury problem in Canada. The respondents did not strongly indicate a belief that many injuries to children were preventable. Similarly, in a national survey of parental attitudes and knowledge of child safety in the United States (part of the national SAFEKIDS campaign sponsored by Johnson & Johnson Products and the National Safety Council in Chicago), investigators found that parents, particularly lower SES ones, knew little about the prevention of bicycle injuries, burns and drownings. Many parents mentioned the need to "be careful," but they were unable to explain what this would mean, specifically, in terms of their own behaviour (Eichelberger et al. 1990). Parents in this survey also believed that children were more likely to listen to other authority figures (e.g, physicians, police) for advice about safety than to parents themselves (parents ranked themselves last), and many parents thought that safety was boring. The blend of indifference and ignorance certainly highlights the difficulties faced by programs that target changes in parents' behaviours as a means of reducing risk of injury among young children. The significance of this challenge is magnified by the finding that parents often overestimate their children's knowledge of risks and their children's ability to handle emergency situations (Yarmey and Rosenstein 1988). Overestimations of children's abilities may lead to fewer parental efforts to teach children about home safety practices and risk avoidance.

Recent research (Morrongiello and Dayler, in press) and common findings in the health psychology literature indicate that parental compliance rates are strongly correlated with the parents' perceptions of their child's vulnerability for the injury targeted (i.e., perceived threat) and with their attitudes and beliefs about child injuries (e.g., preventability, seriousness, responsibility for the injury). Evidence showing that parents' attitudes and beliefs direct their safety behaviours comes from research on child injury occurrences: only 39 percent of parents of a preschooler who suffered an injury requiring medical intervention changed their safety behaviours to reduce the likelihood of a recurrence (Langley and Silva 1982). The other parents obviously did not believe their behaviours contributed to their child's injury.

In summary, developing programs that target caregivers and aim to reduce in-home injuries requires foundation research to identify parental attitudes and beliefs that predispose children toward injuries and serve as barriers to parents' adopting safety practices and teaching their children about them (Greaves et al. 1994). Such research may provide insights into why boys experience a greater number of, and more severe, injuries than girls. Perhaps parents supervise sons and daughters differently or socialize them differently with respect to risk taking. Obviously, the gaps in our knowledge limit our ability to devise successful programs to prevent in-home injuries and to reduce the incidence of injuries among boys. Certainly, what is known is that increasing parents' knowledge of child safety issues is not enough to prompt changes in their home safety behaviours (Paul et al. 1994).

Some programs cited in the home safety literature aim to promote the use of in-home safety devices by parents. A recent survey revealed that outlet covers were used in only 40 percent of homes with young children (Kelly et al. 1987). A review of these programs reveals that whether parents use free home safety devices depends partly on how easy they are to use. For example, in a study of well-educated, affluent parents (Dershewitz 1979), the experimental and control groups both showed an increased use of easy-to-install devices (e.g., outlet covers) but not difficult-to-install devices (e.g., cabinet locks) when both of these were provided at no cost. The education session (20-minute individual instruction on child safety, home safety booklet, follow-up phone call to provide reinforcement and encouragement) produced a significantly greater increase in compliance in the experimental group 2 months after the intervention. Across several injury categories, the results suggest that making devices (e.g., smoke detectors, infant car seats, home safety devices, window guards) available for free or at low cost as part of a broader intervention program may promote use of these devices by caregivers, but the barriers to their use exist, and need to be addressed in future research.

Many community-based, comprehensive programs promoting in-home safety have been implemented, with various degrees of success. Safe Start, a Canadian program affiliated with British Columbia's Children's Hospital and sponsored by the Royal Bank ($500,000 over 5 years), targets families with preschoolers having a higher than average risk of injuries. The Safe Start resource materials (video, booklet, growth chart), which have been produced in six languages, are distributed through public health units, pregnancy outreach agencies, and a variety of programs serving the multicultural population. The Safe Start Mobile House is a teaching tool that provides fire prevention instruction in communities across British Columbia. Preliminary data collected by those who deliver the program reveals a great deal of satisfaction with the materials and the program as a whole (CS/RESORS Consulting Limited 1995). An outcome-oriented evaluation is expected in the next few years.

The Home Injury Prevention Program (HIPP), a unique program that was designed to reduce in-home injuries among low-income families living in substandard housing, is an example of a community-wide program that successfully achieved injury control among a high-risk urban population. HIPP, which was implemented in Massachusetts in the 1980s (Gallagher et al. 1985), took a comprehensive and multifaceted approach that combined an educational strategy (counselling parents on potential in-home hazards), a regulatory strategy (identifying violations of existing housing codes and resolving the issue), and a technological strategy (distributing and installing inexpensive safety devices at no cost to the family) to reduce injuries among children under 6 years living in substandard housing. The goal was to reduce household hazards related to burns, poisonings, falls, choking, and consumer products.

Since local health staff were required to enforce housing codes, additional duties were added to their regular assessment procedures. As well as inspecting homes, they counselled parents on specific home hazards and corrective measures, and they distributed and installed safety devices. Return visits to ensure housing code compliance gave staff an opportunity to reinforce educational messages.

Follow-up evaluation visits to 29 percent of the previously inspected dwellings were conducted about 45 days later. Household hazards were significantly reduced from 13 to 7, with most reductions occurring in the kitchen and child's room. Although all three strategies resulted in success (i.e., reducing hazards), educational counselling, which required the most effort by parents, produced the least number of changes. Consistent with general trends in the injury prevention literature, the regulatory and technological interventions were more effective than the education strategy.

The success of HIPP was probably due to several factors: (1) The counselling occurred in the homes, making the message focused and relevant to the parents. The message included the identification of both hazards and the solutions that would eliminate them. The follow-up visit allowed staff to repeat and reinforce the educational messages. The educational counselling was delivered by an authority figure, the local health agent, which probably increased its effectiveness. (2) Most safety devices were installed by the inspector, thus limiting the effort required by parents. In fact, the few devices that were left for parents to install were seldom in evidence during the follow-up inspections. (3) Failure to comply with the code had legal implications, and this was probably a motivation for compliance. (4) The multifaceted nature of the intervention, with several strategies targeting a high-risk population for which the information was directly relevant, probably promoted its success as well (e.g., Spiegel and Lindaman 1977).

In the report on this program (Gallagher et al. 1985), there is considerable discussion of the need to provide training, encouragement and support to local health inspectors to overcome their resistance to including advocacy for injury prevention in their duties. The program was cost effective because it made optimum use of the people who were already visiting these high-risk homes regularly for other reasons. Obviously, the compliance and support of local officials and community organizations are prerequisites for the success of this approach. Nonetheless, it is also apparent that such compliance and support are obtainable and can quickly produce significant decreases in home hazards in high-risk populations.

In a similar community-wide intervention that reduced in-home injuries by nearly 30 percent in a Swedish city, the participating organizations incorporated all aspects of the program into the routine activities funded by their normal budget (Shelp 1987, 1988).

The Safe Block Project

In the success story discussed below, an innovative approach to injury prevention was used: local residents were recruited to do in-home assessments in their own community.

Description – The Safe Block Project was an urban home safety program implemented in an injury risk area in Philadelphia (Schwarz et al. 1993). The project was developed by the Philadelphia Injury Prevention Program, a cooperative effort of the Philadelphia Department of Public Health, the University of Pennsylvania School of Medicine, the Children's Hospital of Philadelphia, and the Philadelphia Citizens Advisory Board for Injury Prevention. The project targeted a high-risk population that was predominantly African American and poor.

The intervention consisted of three parts: (1) home inspection to inform residents about hazards and ways to eliminate them; (2) simple modifications and repairs to eliminate hazards; and (3) education about injury prevention practices. Education programs were conducted in homes and at block and community meetings.

Reasons for the initiative – Motivated by local injury statistics, the program was undertaken to reduce the incidence of falls, fires, scald burns, poisoning and homicide in a high-injury area of Philadelphia. The goals were to (1) improve injury prevention knowledge and reduce hazards in homes; and (2) reduce the rates of injuries in homes. The target and control sites were selected on the basis of demographic information and injury statistics.

Actors – Thirteen team members (3 safety liaison people and 10 safety inspectors) were hired from the community. The team was supervised by personnel from the Injury Control Section of the Philadelphia Department of Public Health.

The liaison people recruited a volunteer from each block to act as a representative to identify local resources, make contact with block residents, and reinforce safety messages through monthly block meetings. Each month, the liaison people worked with the block representatives on a new safety topic, organizing the block meeting and identifying and providing educational materials for households on the block.

After obtaining consent, the safety inspectors carried out their mandate: inspecting the homes, helping with modifications, and educating the residents about hazards. Materials provided for each home cost U.S.$10.34 and included a smoke detector, a water thermometer (to prevent scalds in baths), a night light (to prevent falls), syrup of Ipecac (to induce vomiting if child has swallowed poison), a telephone sticker for emergency numbers, and a magnetic fridge poster listing information about preventing burns, poisonings, fall and domestic-violence injuries. The inspectors taught residents how to remove hazards (providing simple instructions for repairs); turned down the temperature of the hot-water heater; installed the safety devices provided; and checked for fall hazards (loose rugs, etc.), poison hazards (medicines, peeling paint), and electrical hazards (e.g., frayed cords). They taught caregivers how to use syrup of Ipecac and the bath thermometer and gave them information on community resources related to child restraint devices, weapon storage and domestic-violence issues.

Neighbours were asked to encourage other neighbours to participate. Households were only considered nonparticipating after three contacts had been made to enlist participation (on different days and at different times of day). The program achieved a 51 percent participation rate for households within the targeted area.

Results – Approximately 12 months after the intervention, the program team visited a random sample of target homes (72 percent) and control homes (72 percent) to assess hazards (to check whether hazards had been eliminated as recommended and whether safety devices were still intact) and injury prevention knowledge.

Compared with control homes, the target homes had more safety devices present and had fewer of the hazards that require minimal to moderate effort to alleviate (minimal: night light, syrup of Ipecac, functioning smoke detector, etc.; moderate: medications out of reach, fire escape plans formulated, tripping hazards removed, etc.). These target residents also showed a greater knowledge of safety. Among households there was no difference for hazards requiring a lot of effort to correct (unsafe kitchen flooring, peeling paint, etc.), although it is worth noting that these repairs depended not only on effort but also on the availability of money for materials for the repairs. The distribution of hazards indicated too that the areas of the house that had received the greatest attention during the safety inspection had the fewest hazards at the time of the follow-up assessment. Finally, an analysis of the types of hazards present indicated significantly fewer poisoning and burn hazards in the targeted households than in the control households. Thus, since there was specificity in the effects of the intervention, the positive effects can likely be attributed to the intervention per se.

Replicability – There are no other published reports of community-based interventions involving block-level education programs and home-based interventions with populations at high risk for injuries. HIPP (the Massachusetts intervention) also included home inspectors and took a comprehensive approach (educational, regulatory and technological strategies) and observed good success rates (see above). Finally, a community-wide program in a rural area of Sweden that incorporated home visits as a strategy reported a 10 percent decrease in injury rates following the program, although that intervention was not particularly a grassroots operation (i.e., neighbours educating neighbours) like the Safe Block Project was.

Funding – The program was funded from U.S. Centers for Disease Control and the Henry J. Kaiser Family Foundation.

Evaluation – In comparing this program with others that were much less effective (e.g., SCIPP; Guyer et al. 1989), we can see that a community-wide intervention to reduce in-home injuries among children is most likely to be effective if (1) it reflects a bottom-up, or grassroots, process (i.e., the intervention evolves from within the community, is motivated by local statistics, and derives its solutions from local resources); it involves one-to-one communication (e.g., trained neighbours talking to neighbours, respected authority figures talking to residents); (3) it provides home inspections (education and in-home counselling about specific safety hazards and how to eliminate them); (4) it offers free safety devices requiring minimal efforts to install (i.e., installation by inspectors); (5) it incorporates repeated or follow-up contacts to reinforce safety practices and eliminate hazards; and (6) it has lots of media coverage to increase awareness of the issues and promote compliance. The success of the Safe Block Project is particularly noteworthy because it was a grassroots project targeting an extremely poor, inner-city neighbourhood and included residents with little formal education as key players in the intervention.

Programs to Teach Home Safety Practices to Latchkey Children

Latchkey children are children who are left unsupervised for some period of the day, usually after school, until a caregiver returns home from work. These children have come to be referred to as latchkey children because most of them carry a house key (e.g., pinned to their shirt). A number of programs have been implemented to teach home safety practices to latchkey children. These programs draw on behavioural training techniques and require trained administrators, rewards for participants, and many training sessions involving modelling, rehearsal and feedback.

Attempts to make these programs less costly to run have generally resulted in poorer outcomes. For example, after demonstrating their success in teaching 8-year-old children home safety practices (e.g., dealing with emergencies), Peterson and colleagues sought to make the program more cost effective by reducing the instruction and training time to 10 hours (with occasional retraining sessions) and by using volunteers (e.g., parents) in place of professional teachers (Peterson 1984a, 1984b; Peterson and Mori 1985; Peterson et al. 1988). The parents of five of the children in the program received training, supervision and feedback from the investigators every week; thus, time saved by reducing the training for children was offset somewhat by time required to train the volunteer administrators of the program. These five children mastered the safety skills and performed well at a 6-month follow-up. However, another 16 children whose parents had not received professional supervision in administering the program and had been recruited for the program by the children (rather than volunteering for themselves) performed much more poorly. These findings suggest that "one gets what one pays for" in children's safety programs. Obviously, mass delivery of behavioural programs through reduced professional supervision is not likely to be successful.

Peterson and colleagues also tried to determine if one could substitute short-term group instruction for on-going, one-to-one training. Six 15-minute sessions role playing were conducted with groups of children; different safety issues were discussed during each session. Pre- and post-tests revealed improvement in safety knowledge for each topic (e.g., dealing with fire, cuts, stranger at door), but not a single child scored as well as any of the children receiving the one-to-one, intensive, home-based training program.

In summary, although there are safety programs that have been shown to increase safety skills and knowledge among latchkey children, in general, these are very costly. Attempts to trim the program to increase cost-effectiveness have not been successful.

Poisoning

The most effective interventions to prevent poisonings among children have been passive measures. Laws requiring childproof caps on medicine bottles and restricting the number of baby aspirins in a jar to 36 virtually halved the number of poisonings for children under 5 years of age (Clarke and Walton 1979). Similarly, the establishment of poison control information centres that can be reached by telephone has also helped manage the problem (Dershewitz and Christophersen 1984).

Programs such as Mr. Yuk have not proven effective in reducing poisonings because someone has to place the danger stickers on every appropriate container in the house (Fergusson et al. 1982). Interventions that target in-home injuries more generally have often incorporated poison control measures, with various degrees of success (see above).

Drowning

Strategies to prevent drownings among children include improving their swimming abilities and erecting barriers to prevent access to water hazards (e.g., pools).

There are many Water Babies programs available for infants and young children, but there is no evidence that these programs significantly decrease the number of drownings among children at these ages (Quan 1982). However, a recent training program with this goal in mind has shown encouraging results (Asher et al. 1995; Barass 1995; Smith 1995). In an effort to promote swimming skills and water safety knowledge among children, the Canadian Red Cross Society has recently expanded and revised its program, adopting a national standard for delivery, course content, prerequisites, and certification requirements. The new water safety program is being delivered at a number of pilot sites across Canada. The media attention on the new program has increased the number of participants, which fulfils one of the aims of the program (i.e., reaching more children). Only long-term evaluation, however, will determine if the program results in fewer drownings among children.

Millner et al. (1982) studied the effectiveness of fencing regulations in Mulgrave Shire, Australia, and estimated that strict enforcement of these regulations would reduce drownings by 80 percent among children under 14 years old. Over the 10-year study, no child had drowned in a fenced pool. Obviously, legislative interventions to reduce the likelihood of children contacting the hazard can be very successful in reducing injuries among young children. Since swimming pools are a common site of toddler drownings (Canadian Red Cross Society 1994), many Canadian municipalities have adopted fencing bylaws. In Canada, however, standards for pool safety do not yet exist, which makes it virtually impossible to enforce these municipal bylaws.

Suffocation

In Canada, suffocation is the leading cause of injury and death to children under the age of one (CICH 1994). Suffocation can result from several causes: entrapment in cribs (especially cribs made before the new safety standards went into effect), strangulation by ropes such as blind or phone cords, a foreign body in the airway, plastic bags or pillows that restrict the flow of oxygen, etc. Surprisingly, there have been few legislated initiatives to prevent suffocation. For example, warnings on plastic bags that say these bags pose a hazard to young children are voluntary. I could find no prevention programs that specifically target this type of injury. Rather, this injury category is usually included in programs to control in-home injuries.

Falls

Although fall-related injuries are the number one cause of hospitalizations among Canadian children 2–14 years old, there are no programs specifically aimed at reducing falls. Rather, the need to reduce this type of injury may be mentioned in home safety programs, playground safety discussions, programs to control spinal cord injuries and head trauma, etc., but often receives only secondary attention.

Playground safety, in particular, is a growing concern, owing to the number of injuries related to falls. For example, a study in Montreal revealed that falls accounted for 74 percent of all playground injuries (Lesage et al. 1993). Similarly, Ontario Trauma Registry (1995) data indicate that nearly 20 percent of children's hospital admissions due to falls resulted from falls on playgrounds. To address this problem, the Canadian Standards Association is collaborating with professionals in the United States to revise standards for playground safety and adopt one set of North American standards. This is a beginning, but other issues must be addressed, such as who will assume responsibility for the costs of upgrading and maintenance. Increasingly, as a result of limited budgets, playgrounds are being removed instead of being upgraded or maintained. This increases the likelihood that children will play in more hazardous situations, such as on the street and on hard concrete surfaces like the sidewalk. Obviously, more attention is needed to determine ways to reduce falls among children and to manage the problem of playground safety.

CONCLUSIONS AND RECOMMENDATIONS

As this review of the injury prevention literature shows, different strategies are used to address various types of injuries common to children. The findings support the following conclusions and recommendations.

Passive Strategies

Whenever possible, passive intervention (i.e., those that require no action by individuals) should be adopted. Since these are population-wide interventions, passive approaches are very cost effective and significantly reduce injury rates in a reasonable time frame. To ensure strong support, passive interventions should generally be accompanied by public education on the issues, but there will always be those who will argue against any restrictions on personal freedoms and choices. Nonetheless, passive interventions produce results and should be the intervention of choice for reducing childhood injuries. To my knowledge, there has never been a passive injury control intervention that did not produce significant declines in child mortality from injuries (for further review see Lovasik 1995).

Active Strategies

Active interventions require an individual's compliance and therefore show various degrees of success.

Legislated Prevention Strategies

Legislated interventions for injury control are generally effective in getting people to comply with safety practices. However, to maximize success, these should be embedded in a broader context that includes public education and an enforcement strategy. This comprehensive approach will likely require cooperation, coordination, and communication across a number of stakeholders, but it is essential that these conditions be met to realize the full effectiveness of a legislated prevention strategy.

Education Programs

Education programs often produce increases in knowledge but seldom produce changes in behaviour. Such programs may seem cost effective— they can reach large numbers of people at one time (e.g., television advertising, school-based safety programs)—but when these programs are delivered in isolation, they are largely ineffective.

The success of education programs is increased if they (1) target a specific group at elevated risk for particular type of injury; (2) are limited in scope (e.g., aimed at changing only one particular behaviour); (3) are delivered in a personal, one-to-one context by an authority figure (e.g., physician); and (4) incorporate individual prompts or naturally occurring rewards. For programs directed at children, success also depends on having the educational messages delivered in an interactive participatory way. Nevertheless, even if all these criteria are met, education programs are less successful in reducing rates of injury than other intervention approaches.

Behavioural Programs

Behavioural interventions have typically sought to increase safety practices (as opposed to decreasing injury risks). Most interventions have proven effective, whether they aim to change children's behaviours or caregivers' behaviours. These programs often result in good short-term compliance rates and declining (but still above baseline) rates over longer intervals (e.g., 6–12 months).

Success is maximized if these programs incorporate a combination of features: (1) narrow behavioural objectives; (2) role playing, role modelling and rehearsals; and (3) feedback and rewards. High compliance rates can be maintained over time if retraining or booster sessions are given periodically.

Despite their effectiveness, behavioural interventions have some limitations. These individualized programs require repeated training sessions led by skilled personnel, and participants need tangible rewards; thus, the cost makes it prohibitive to offer these programs to more than a limited number of participants. Behavioural programs are not a very cost effective way to achieve a significant reduction in the incidence of injuries among a large number of children. Restricting access to children who are at high risk for a particular injury may make this type of intervention more cost effective, particularly if the safety behaviour is also adopted by nonparticipating family members (e.g., programs to increase the use of seat belts often generalize to all family members).

Community-Based Interventions

Community-based interventions show great promise and should be the *primary* focus of future efforts because of their cost-effectiveness, their relatively high success rates, and the likelihood of changing attitudes as well as behaviours. Generally, these interventions reach large numbers of people and successfully draw on community resources, thereby keeping overhead costs low.

The most successful programs (1) have a narrow focus (i.e., have one key goal or target one key behaviour for change); (2) target more than one level (e.g., the individual, the setting or environment, the community); and (3) are multifaceted. Components typically include education at several levels (personal contacts as well as media-based messages); opportunities for modelling, rehearsal and feedback (i.e., some of the key aspects of behavioural interventions); and environment modification (e.g., availability of safety devices). Successful programs typically communicate information through many sources simultaneously, creating interventions that are so pervasive as to make it difficult for individuals to not become informed and involved.

The greatest challenge to community-based intervention is often the coordination of information delivery and program components. Generally, programs enjoy the most success and the most cooperation from community members when decisions are made at the grassroots level: this promotes a sense of community ownership of the program and accommodates local injury control need. To promote success, these interventions must match the intended audience and emerge from a knowledge of and respect for the culture of the target community. Injury surveillance at the local level is an essential first step in developing relevant community-wide injury prevention programs.

POLICY IMPLICATIONS

This paper has suggested several approaches to reducing the incidence of injuries among children. What is perhaps most compelling in the literature reviewed is that no one injury control strategy can be singled out and uniformly applied across all injury categories. Also apparent in the literature is that success is more likely with multifaceted interventions (i.e., programs that incorporate several injury control strategies). At present, we have a great deal of knowledge about preventing some types of childhood injuries (e.g., passenger injuries) but relatively little about preventing other types (e.g., falls). One might be tempted to use this literature review as a basis for suggesting to policymakers that they focus on reducing childhood injuries that are especially prevalent, severe and costly (e.g., in Canada, falls are the number one cause of injury-related hospitalizations among children 2–14 years old), but a broader perspective on the issue of injury control is needed to manage this national health threat. With this premise in mind, I bring the following needs to the attention of policymakers.

The Need to Establish Injury Control as a National Priority

Injuries are the number one cause of death among children and a leading cause of childhood hospitalizations, but far too few people in this country know this. We spend billions of dollars each year to treat children because of this country's failure to achieve injury control. For example, a review of 10,528 child admissions to hospitals in Ontario in 1993 revealed that 15 percent of these were injury related; the average stay in hospital was 3 days (Ontario Trauma Registry 1995). Even spending the equivalent of one-third of the treatment money on preventive programs would likely significantly reduce childhood injuries, saving much more money in the long term. For example, the measles vaccination program over an 8-year period saved $1.3 billion in long- and short-term costs (Witte and Axnixk 1975). In light of these statistics and the costs of injuries, it seems obvious that there would be a substantial return on investment in injury prevention in Canada if a commitment were made to achieve greater control over childhood injuries. A cost analysis study in the United States, for example, estimated that 22,000 child fatalities amounts to nearly U.S.$8.3 billion in future lost productivity (Rice et al. 1990).

The need to make injury control a national priority is apparent. For this to happen, however, injury control must achieve national priority status, not just among stakeholders, but also among the public. What is needed, therefore, is a national strategy for achieving injury control in Canada and for raising public awareness of the issue. Frank (1966) discussed "moral indignation" as a catalyst for evoking change in the social issues that shape our lives. Apparently, Canadians have not yet reached the level of indignation necessary to commit to national activism for injury control. Policymakers must act to help achieve this goal.

The lack of a national strategy to bring this problem under control is perhaps best indicated by the diversity in the priority assigned to the problem by the provinces and in the resources they allocate to address it. A "piecemeal approach" is perhaps a fitting description of the current approach to injury control in Canada. Working from the premise that a national strategy is needed, I offer the following suggestions to promote the development of a national strategy to reduce childhood injuries and to establish injury control as a national priority in the minds of Canadians.

1. Injury prevention strategies should be coordinated at the national level, not the provincial level. A national focus would lead to uniformity in establishing priorities, choosing interventions, and evaluating success. Such an approach would foster the emergence of injury prevention as a national health concern and lead to a coordinated national effort to reduce injuries. Redundancy would be reduced, and the development and implementation of strategies would become a national collaborative effort. In the context of the national focus, the provinces would still have an opportunity to select a particular geographic area or population to target in response to local injury statistics.

2. As part of getting injury prevention on the national agenda, we must raise public awareness of the scope of the childhood injury problem. An aware public would create demand for resources and innovative programs for injury control, thereby prompting government initiatives and increasing the likelihood of recruiting corporate sponsors to play a role as well.

A national, multimedia campaign is needed to increase awareness and promote prevention-oriented attitudes. Corporate sponsors could be sought for the campaign, but the direction and scope of the campaign should be determined by the lead agency (see next section). An appeal to fear should not be used, as this is not as effective as positive appeals (e.g., Treiber 1986) and may suggest that only severe or atypical injuries are the problem. Drawing on the health psychology and childhood injury literature, the media campaign should communicate the following:

- Injuries are the number one cause of death and a leading cause of hospitalizations among children.
- Injuries can happen to anyone (most people have an optimism bias belief—"Injuries happen to others, not to me or my children").
- Most childhood injuries are not "accidents" (i.e., chance events) but are preventable.
- Although injuries are common, and can happen to anyone, they are *not* normative (i.e., to be expected and accepted during childhood).
- Issues of inconvenience and caregivers' stress levels can lead to decisions that compromise the safety of children even when caregivers "know better" (see Morrongiello and Dayler, in press). "Safe risk" must guide caregivers' and older children's decision making (even though this principle is hard to follow at all times). The SMARTRISK Foundation in Toronto may help in defining and communicating the concept of safe risk to the public.

These messages must be communicated in such a way that they are not construed as "blaming the victim." Instead, they should promote the idea that mastery of the problem is possible, and they should appear proactive (injury control as the focus) rather than reactive (driven predominantly by injury statistics).

3. Physicians, nurses, and public health professionals—key stakeholders who have the potential to raise public awareness—should receive training in preventive medicine that includes an injury control component and stresses the importance of anticipatory guidance to promote safety among caregivers. (In a survey of physicians in London, Ontario, for example, many felt that their training had not prepared them adequately to appreciate the scope of the problem and the importance of anticipatory guidance; see Morrongiello et al. 1995.) Changes to the training curriculum and public health mandate are needed to ensure that injury control receives the attention and resources it needs to make it a priority among these key professionals.

The Need to Identify Key Stakeholders to Direct the Solution

A major barrier to achieving injury control in Canada is not that we don't understand *what* the solution should encompass (indeed, this review highlights how much we already know about what strategies lead to success), but that there is no key group or stakeholder *who* is responsible for directing the solution. The power to make decisions about injury control is distributed across many actors and agencies, each having their own agenda, issues, ideal solutions, and ideas. This distribution of power limits the progress that can be made, promotes duplication of efforts, and is even counterproductive when players are at odds on identifying priority issues. With this premise in mind, I offer the following recommendation:

1. Responsibility for establishing priorities and directing the solution has to be given to one key group of stakeholders. The most logical choice is health care providers. These stakeholders are a national group; they have the respect of most people, thereby enhancing the perceived credibility of their messages; they deal with the failures to achieve injury control; and, historically, they have publicized many injury control issues (e.g, safety seats, baby walkers, bicycle helmets) and have helped develop measures to address these issues (e.g., public advertising, fighting for legislative interventions), albeit with varying degrees of success.

   If responsibility is not given to one key group of stakeholders, then lead public health agencies should be established to coordinate efforts across the many sectors of government and to disseminate findings from injury control interventions to stakeholders (private, professional, government).

The Need to Make Program Evaluation a Requirement

Many intervention programs in Canada have been evaluated inadequately, if at all, making it difficult to identify success stories, let alone discern key characteristics for success. In times of fiscal restraint, it may be tempting to omit the evaluation component from prevention programs. However, those who are funding and developing programs must resist this temptation. Face validity, or the degree to which the program appears to address the injury issue in question, is not a sufficient measure for evaluating programs—the failure of THINK FIRST to achieve its desired goals (discussed in the section on spinal cord injuries and head trauma) is an excellent illustration of this point. Evaluation and documentation of efficacy are essential for garnering political and corporate financial support and media coverage of the magnitude of the problem of injury control. For a variety of reasons, then, outcome evaluation is a necessary component of programs that aim to reduce child mortality due to unintentional injuries. With this premise in mind, the following recommendations are offered.

1. An evaluation plan should be a requirement for receiving funding for injury prevention programs. (Alberta recently adopted this strategy in funding prevention programs—this is the kind of strong tactic that is needed to convince program developers of the necessity and role of evaluation in developing successful programs.)

2. The evaluation plan should be developed at the beginning so that the prevention program can be planned with evaluation in mind and appropriate data can be collected before, during, and following program implementation.

3. The plan should provide for both short-term and long-term evaluations, since efficacy may increase over time (many community-wide interventions show accumulating positive effects) or decline over time (behavioural programs often show a decline once rewards are discontinued). There is no standard length for a long-term evaluation, but probably a 1- or 2-year follow-up would suffice.

4. The evaluation should focus on outcome indicators (e.g., incidence of injuries or of safety practices, knowledge of injury control practices), rather than on only program specifics (e.g., materials) or process specifics (e.g., implementation).

5. To maintain integrity of the results, the evaluation plan should be managed by people who are not closely affiliated with the prevention program.

6. People implementing the prevention program must be responsive to the results of the program evaluation. The easiest way to achieve this is by making continued program support contingent on an evaluation indicating the program is achieving its goals (whether they be directly related goals, such as reduction of injury incidence, or indirectly related

goals, such as injury control education) or holds promise for doing so with some minor modifications.

7. An infrastructure is needed to make key players (e.g., public health personnel) aware of program evaluation and help them develop program evaluation skills so that they can understand the evaluation process, propose evaluation strategies, and interpret evaluation results. Some possibilities for the form this infrastructure might take are the following:

   – workshops, possibly sponsored by public health or medical associations, with the option of continuing education credits;

   – a resource list of professionals skilled in program evaluation (e.g., members of the Canadian Evaluation Society) and willing to share their expertise, possibly on a project-by-project basis and in exchange for the right to coauthor a publication about the program; or

   – a correspondence course developed by a university that offers a graduate course in program evaluation (e.g., University of Guelph, Psychology Department).

The Need to Improve Injury Surveillance

Evaluation also calls attention to the need for a system of surveillance that collects comprehensive injury process information (what the child was doing at the time, the place where the injury occurred, etc.); is common across locations (i.e., the same system is used across provinces and at local as well as regional hospitals); and is technically current, to support future developments. A search of the injury prevention literature reveals the paucity of Canadian data suitable for monitoring trends in injuries at a national level. This problem does not allow Canada to manage injury control at a national level; instead, it is managed primarily at a provincial level. Surveillance is necessary for planning our national prevention strategies and evaluating their effectiveness.

A common surveillance system would foster communication and collaboration at the national level and help track trends in injuries across the country. At the same time, community-based prevention programs need local statistics to identify injury control problem areas and track the effects of programs that aim to reduce specific injuries. Thus, surveillance, programming, and evaluation are all linked conceptually and must be addressed concurrently; otherwise, our lack of surveillance data will limit the information available for identifying prevention needs and for serving as possible outcome measures in planning evaluation strategies. With these thoughts in mind, I offer the following recommendations:

1. Funding for emergency health services could be made contingent on recording and reporting reliable injury statistics. (The State of Victoria, Australia, recently adopted this approach, so policymakers in Canada now have a source to turn to for information on implementing such a strategy.)

2. A national standard for using E-codes to report different types of injuries should be applied. (Injuries in Canada are classified according to the International Classification of Disease E-codes. The problem is that the use of the E-codes to categorize injuries varies greatly across Canada.) A 1-800 number could be set up during the first year of applying this national standard (or in developing the standard) to identify and correct problems of classification and definitions. The Canadian Children's Safety Network (sponsored by Health Canada) on-line computer system could provide stakeholders with any national reports on any modifications or implementation questions related to the standard.

3. An overview report that draws on national surveillance data to discuss injury trends in Canada should be published. An update of this report every 2–3 years would identify national shifts in injury trends and indicate the effectiveness of national initiatives targeting specific injury categories. (At present, injury data are segmented across several agencies and government departments, making it difficult to discern the "big picture." Regulatory-impact analysis statements are routinely prepared by government, but these are not widely distributed, which limits their usefulness)

The Need to Undertake Research on Factors and Processes That Lead to Injuries among High-Risk Populations

High-risk populations must become a central focus in injury prevention programs, but first we must understand more about the factors and processes that lead to injuries. Why are certain populations of children—boys, low-SES children, and Aboriginal children—at increased risk for injuries? In particular, why is the incidence of injuries among Aboriginal children four to seven times that of the national Canadian average for children? We need further research on the determinants of health. Which factors serve to increase injury liability among these groups of children? Which factors, if any, have a protective function?

Developing a program in response to injury statistics without a thorough understanding of how those results occur is premature and should be resisted. The goal in injury control should not be simply to prevent a certain type of injury that poses a risk to children because they are in a particular age group or environment. Rather, the goal should be more general: to prevent that type of injury *and* reduce the likelihood of risk taking in the future. The program must foster an injury awareness so that the children internalize a prevention orientation, which is then reflected in their attitudes toward and beliefs about safety and risk. Focusing on changing their behaviour without attention to their attitudes and beliefs is not likely to alter their general orientation to safety. With these thoughts in mind, I offer the following recommendations:

1. Researchers should investigate why boys have more injuries than girls. (My own research has revealed the multifaceted scope of the problem: boys and girls differ in a number of injury-relevant attitudes and beliefs, as well as in risk-taking behaviour; see Morrongiello 1997). Further research is needed to establish the bases for differences in attitudes toward and beliefs about injuries; to determine what other factors differentiate boys from girls; and to explain their differences in injury risk.

2. Researchers should examine the processes that influence injury outcomes among low-income, high-risk populations. Poverty confers a higher risk of injury, but fighting to reduce poverty is not the same as fighting to reduce injuries; poverty conditions are not uniform across all high-risk populations. While creating safer environments is an obvious way to reduce injury liability among low-income populations, the unique attitudes and beliefs that foster greater injury risk among low-SES children need to be addressed separately. A research-based approach to injury control is needed to develop programs that target critical factors in injury processes among low-income children.

3. Researchers should examine injury processes among Aboriginal children. I was unable to find a single program that has documented success in reducing injuries among Aboriginal children in Canada (see also Frankish et al. 1993). Research that documents the settings, situations and behaviours, as well as the beliefs and attitudes motivating those behaviours, is essential. The key factors identified through this research should be targeted by interventions to reduce injuries among Aboriginal children.

High-risk populations require innovative approaches to injury control because of the challenges posed by diversity in culture (e.g., attitudes, customs, values), SES status (e.g., lack of financial resources), and communication (e.g., native language spoken). Before we proceed to programming, however, we must conduct foundation research so that the implications of ethnic and economic diversity among high-risk populations is thoroughly understood and reflected in the planning, implementation, and evaluation of injury control programs. These challenges must be overcome if we are to achieve success in injury control among those children at greatest risk in Canada.

Barbara A. Morrongiello, Ph.D., C.Pschy., *is a professor in the Psychology Department at the University of Guelph. She has extensive research experience in the area of childhood injury and injury prevention. Her work has led to insights into factors that result in boys experiencing more injuries than girls, parental attitudes towards children's risk taking and injuries, and sibling and peer influences on children's decisions to take risks that could lead to injury outcomes. Her work has also led to the development of an effective injury prevention program among children.*

Acknowledgments

The author extends her thanks to Linda Dayler of the Trauma Prevention Council in Southwestern Ontario; Caroline Gagnon of First Aid Services at the Canadian Red Cross Society; Anna Lovasik of the Injury Prevention Centre in Alberta; Dr. Barry Pless of Montreal Children's Hospital; Judith Radford of the SMARTRISK Foundation in Toronto; Malak Sidky of Safe Kids Canada in Toronto; Jack Smith of the Canadian Safety Council in Ottawa; Jenny Tipper of the Canadian Institute of Child Health in Ottawa; Ann Williams of the Safe Start Program in British Columbia; Bev Woods of the Ontario Injury Prevention Resource Centre; members of the Family and Child Health Unit of Health Canada, particularly Lorie Root and Sally Lockhart, for suggesting and sharing specific sources of materials; and Tess Dawber, Hish Husein and Lorna McCleary for locating and copying materials. The author also thanks the many people across Canada who took time from their day to discuss programs with her and send materials pertinent to this report. Finally, a very special thanks goes to Robert Conn, Anna Lovasik, Barry Pless and Judith Radford for their discussion of policy implications, although the author alone accepts responsibility for those expressed herein.

BIBLIOGRAPHY

ALLEN, D., and BERGMAN, A. 1976. Social learning approaches to health education utilization of infant auto restraint devices. *Pediatrics* 58: 323–328.

ALLEN, C., and WALSH, L. 1975. Bumpy road ahead? *Traffic Engineering* 45: 11–14.

AMERICAN ACADEMY OF PEDIATRICS. 1984. Committee on accident and poison prevention: Automobile passenger protection systems. *Pediatrics* 74: 146–147.

AMPOFO-BOATENG, K. 1987. Children's perceptions of safety and danger on the road. Ph.D. dissertation, University of Stratheclyde, Glasgow, Scotland.

AMPOFO-BOATENG, K., and THOMSON, J. 1990. Child pedestrian accidents: A case for preventive medicine. *Health Education: Research, Theory and Practice* 5: 265–274.

AMPOFO-BOATENG, K., THOMSON, J., GRIEVE, R., PITCAIRN, T., LEE, D., and DEMETRE, J. 1993. A developmental and training study of children's ability to find safe routes to cross the road. *British Journal of Developmental Psychology* 11: 31–45.

ASHER, K., RIVARA, F., FELIX, D., VANCE, L., and DUNNE, R. 1995. Water safety training as a potential means of reducing risk of young children's drowning. *Injury Prevention* 1: 223–227.

BAKER, S., O'NEILL, B., and KARPF, R. 1984. *The Injury Fact Book.* Lexington (MA): Lexington Books.

BARASS, P. 1995. Cautionary notes on teaching water safety skill. *Injury Prevention* 1: 218.

BASS, J. 1993. Childhood injury prevention counselling in primary care settings: A critical review of the literature. *Pediatrics* 92:544–550.

BERGER, L. 1981. Childhood injuries: Recognition and prevention. *Current Problems in Pediatrics* 12: 6–59.

BERGER, L., KALISHMAN, S., and RIVARA, F. 1985. Injuries from fireworks. *Pediatrics* 75: 877–882.

BERGMAN, A., RIVARA, F., RICHARDS, D., and ROGERS, L. 1990. The Seattle Children's Bicycle Helmet Campaign. *American Journal of Diseases of Children* 144: 727–731.

BLUM, A., and AMES, B. 1977. Flame retardant additives as possible cancer hazards: The main flame retardant in children's pyjamas is a mutagen and should not be used. *Science* 195: 17–22.

CANADIAN BIKE HELMET ASSOCIATION PAMPHLET, 1995. "How to Organize a Community Project." Available from the Canadian Institute of Child Health Ottawa, Ontario. Cited on p. 202–203.

CHRISTOPHERSEN, E., and GULAY, J. 1989. Parental compliance with car seat usage: A positive approach with long-term follow-up. *Journal of Pediatric Psychology* 6: 301–312.

CHRISTOPHERSEN, E., SOSLAND-EDELMAN, D., and LECLAIRE, S. 1985. Evaluation of two comprehensive infant car seat loaner programs with 1-year follow-up. *Pediatrics* 76: 36–42.

CICH (CANADIAN INSTITUTE OF CHILD HEALTH). 1994. *The Health of Canada's Children.* 2nd ed. Ottawa (ON): CICH.

CLARKE, A., and WALTON, W. 1979. Effect of safety packaging on aspirin ingestion by children. *Pediatrics* 63: 687–693.

COLLETTI, R. 1984. A statewide hospital-based program to improve child passenger safety. *Health Education Quarterly* 11: 207–213.

CONSUMER PRODUCT SAFETY COMMISSION. 1983. *Hazard Analysis Related to Bicycles.* Washington (DC): U.S. Consumer Product Safety Commission, Bureau of Epidemiology.

COTE, T., SACKS, J., LAMBERT-HUBER, D., DANNENBERG, A., KRESNOW, M., LIPSITZ, C., and SCHMIDT, E. 1992. Bicycle helmet use among Maryland children: Effect of legislation and education. *Pediatrics* 89: 1216–1220.

CS/RESORS CONSULTING LIMITED. 1995. An Evaluation of "Give Your Child a Safe Start Injury Prevention Resources". Vancouver (BC).

DANNENBERG, A., GIELEN, A., WILSON, M., and JOFFE, A. 1993. Bicycle helmet laws and educational campaigns: An evaluation of strategies to increase children's helmet use. *American Journal of Public Health* 83: 667–674.

DAVIDSON, L., DURKIN, M., KUHN, L., O'CONNOR, P., BARLOW, B., and HEAGARTY, M. 1994. The impact of the Safe Kids/Healthy Neighborhoods Injury Prevention Program in Harlem, 1988 through 1991. *American Journal of Public Health* 84: 580–586.

DECINA, L., TEMPLE, M., and DORER, H. 1994. Increasing child safety seat use and proper use among toddlers. *Accident Analysis and Prevention* 26: 667–673.

DECKER, M., DEWEY, M., HUTCHESON, R., and SCHAFFNER, W. 1984. The use and efficacy of child restraint devices: The Tennessee experience, 1982 and 1983. *Journal of the American Medical Association* 252: 2571–2575.

DEJOY, D. 1992. An examination of gender differences in traffic accident risk perception. *Accident Analysis and Prevention* 24: 237–246.

DERSHEWITZ, R. 1979. Will mothers use free household safety devices? *American Journal of Diseases of Children* 133: 61–64.

DERSHEWITZ, R., and CHRISTOPHERSEN, E. 1984. Childhood household safety. *American Journal of Diseases of Children* 138: 85–88.

EICHELBERGER, M., GOTSCHALL, C., FREELY, H., HARSTAD, P., and BOWMAN, L. 1990. Parental attitudes and knowledge of child safety. *American Journal of Diseases of Children* 144: 714–720.

ENGLANDER, J., CLEARY, S., O'HARE, P., HALL, K., and LEHMKUHL, L. 1993. Implementing and evaluating injury prevention programs in the traumatic brain injury model systems of care. *Journal of Head Trauma Rehabilitation* 8: 101–113.

ERDMANN, T., FELDMAN, K., RIVARA, F., HEIMBACH, D., and WALL, H. 1991. Tap-water burn prevention: The effect of legislation. *Pediatrics* 88: 572–577.

ETZIONI, A. 1978. Caution: Too many health warnings could be counterproductive. *Psychology Today* Dec., pp. 20–22.

FEDERAL EMERGENCY MANAGEMENT AGENCY. 1983. *Fire in the United States.* 4th ed. Washington (DC): FEMA. pp. 1–5, 25, 26.

FERGUSSON, D., HORWOOD, L., and BEAUTRAIS, A. 1982. A controlled field trial of a poisoning prevention method. *Pediatrics* 69: 515–520.

FRANK, J. 1966. Galloping technology, a new social disease. *Journal of Social Issues* 22: 1–14.

FRANK, R., BOUMAN, D., CAIN, K., and WATTS, C. 1992. A preliminary study of a traumatic injury prevention program. *Psychology and Health* 6: 129–140.

FRANKISH, C. J. 1993. Injury prevention projects with Native populations: A review and critique of the literature. *Final report prepared for Health and Welfare Canada.* Alberta (BC): University of British Columbia, Institute of Health Promotion Research.

GALLAGHER, S., HUNTER, P., and GUYER, B. 1985. A home injury prevention program for children. *Paediatric Clinics of North America* 32: 95–112.

GEDDIS, D., and PETTENGELL, R. 1982. Parent education: Its effect on the way children are transported in cars. *New Zealand Medical Journal* 95: 314–316.

GELLER, E., BRUFF, C., and NIMMER, J. 1985. "Flash for Life": Community-based prompting for safety belt promotion. *Journal of Applied Behavior Analysis* 18: 309–314.

GELLER, E., JOHNSON, R., and PELTON, S. 1982. Community-based interventions for encouraging seat belt use. *American Journal of Community Psychology* 10: 183–195.

GINSBURG, H., and MILLER, S. 1982. Sex differences in children's risk-taking behavior. *Child Development* 53: 426–428.

GORMON, R., CHARNEY, E., HOLTZMAN, N., and ROBERTS, K. 1985. A successful city-wide smoke detector giveaway program. *Pediatrics* 75: 14–18.

GREAVES, P., GLIK, D., KROENFELD, J., and JACKSON, K. 1994. Determinants of controllable in-home child safety hazards. *Health Education Quarterly* 9: 307–315.

GREEN, R., FAIRCLOUGH, J., and SYKES, P. 1984. Epidemiology of burns in childhood. *Burns Including Thermal Injuries* 11: 368–371.

GREENSHER, J. 1984. How anticipatory guidance can improve control of childhood "accidents." *Paediatric Consulting* 3: 1–8.

GUYER, B., GALLAGHER, S., CHANG, B., AZZARA, C., CUPPLES, L., and COLTON, T. 1989. Prevention of childhood injuries: Evaluation of the Statewide Childhood Injury Prevention Program (SCIPP). *American Journal of Public Health* 79: 1521–1527.

HALPERIN, S., BASS, J., MEHTA, K., and BETTS, K. 1983. Unintentional injuries among adolescents and young adults: A review and analysis. *Journal of Adolescent Health Care* 4: 275–281.

HOWARTH, C., and REPETTO-WRIGHT, R. 1978. Measurement of risk and attribution of responsibility for child pedestrian accidents. *Safety Education* 144: 10–13.

JANIS, I., and MANN, L. 1968. A conflict theory approach to attitude change and decision making. In *Psychological Foundations of Attitudes*, eds. A. GREENWALD, T. BROCK, and T. OSTRUM. New York (NY): Academic Press.

JONES, R., and OLLENDICK, T. 1986. Fire emergency skills in children: The impact of fear and anxiety. Paper presented to the South Eastern Psychological Association, Orlando (FL). April.

JONES, R., KAZDIN, A., and HANEY, J. 1981. Social validation and training of emergency fire safety skills for potential injury prevention and life saving. *Journal of Applied Behavior Analysis* 14: 249–260.

JONES, R., OLLENDICK, T., MCLAUGHLIN, K., and WILLIAMS, C. 1989. Elaborative and behavioral rehearsal in the acquisition of fire emergency skills and the reduction of fear of fire. *Behavior Therapy* 20: 93–101.

KANTHOR, H. 1976. Car safety for infants: Effectiveness of parent counselling. *Pediatrics* 58: 320–328.

KATCHER, M. 1987. Prevention of tap-water scald burns: Evaluation of a multimedia injury control program. *American Journal of Public Health* 77: 1195–1197.

KELLY, B., SEIN, C., and MCCARTHY, P. 1987. Safety education in a paediatric primary care setting. *Pediatrics* 79: 818–824.

KOOP, C. E., 1991. *Healthy People 2000: National Health Promotion and Disease Prevention Objectives.* Washington (DC): Public Health Service, U.S. Department of Health and Human Services.

KRAUS, J., BLACK, M., HESSOL, N., LEY, P., ROKAW, W., SULLIVAN, C., BOWERS, S., KNOWLTON, S., and MARSHALL, L. 1984. The incidence of acute brain injury and serious impairment in a defined population. *American Journal of Epidemiology* 119: 186–201.

LANGLEY, J., and SILVA, P. 1982. Childhood accidents: Parents' attitudes to prevention. *Australian Paediatric Journal* 18: 247–249.

LECHMAN, B., and BONWICH, E. 1981. Evaluation of an education program for spinal cord injury prevention: Some preliminary findings. *Spinal Cord Injury Digest* 3: 27–34.

LEE, V. 1995. Before you turn the key. *A Resource Guide Produced by the Infant and Toddler Safety Association*, Kitchener (ON).

LEHMAN, G, and GELLER, E. S. 1990a. Participative education for children: An effective approach to increase safety belt use. *Journal of Applied Behavior Analysis* 23: 219–225.

———. 1990b. Educational strategies to increase children's use of safety belts: Are extrinsic rewards necessary? *Health Education Research* 5: 187–196.

LESAGE, D., ROBITAILLE, Y., DORVAL, D., and BEAULNE, G. 1993. *Study of the Conformity of Children's Playspaces and Equipment to Voluntary Canadian Standard CSZ Z614-M90.* Montreal (QC): Public Health Unit, General Hospital.

LEVIN, M., and RADFORD, E. 1977. Fire victims: Medical outcome and demographic characteristics. *American Journal of Public Health* 67: 1077.

LOVASIK, A. 1995. Building toward breakthroughs in injury control: A legislative perspective. Report prepared for Health Canada. Alberta (BC).

MALEK, M., GUYER, B., and LESCOHIER, I. 1990. The epidemiology and prevention of child pedestrian injury. *Accident Analysis and Prevention* 22: 301–313.

MANHEIMER, D., and MELLINGER, G. 1967. Personality characteristics of the child accident repeater. *Child Development* 9: 87–101.

MATHENY, A. 1980. Visual perceptual exploration and accident liability in children. *Journal of Paediatric Psychology* 5: 343–351.

———. 1988. Accidental injuries. In *Handbook of Paediatric Psychology*, ed. D. ROUTH. New York (NY): Guilford.

MCLOUGHLIN, E., CLARK, N., STAHL, K., and CRAWFORD, J. 1977. One paediatric burn unit's experience with sleepwear-related injuries. *Pediatrics* 60: 405–409.

MCLOUGHLIN, E., VINCE, C., LEE, A., and CRAWFORD, J. 1982. Project burn prevention: Outcome and implications. *American Journal of Public Health* 72: 241–247.

MILLER, R., REISINGER, K., and BLATLER, M. 1982. Paediatric counselling and subsequent use of smoke detectors. *American Journal of Public Health* 72: 492.

MILLNER, N., PEARN, J., and GUARD, R. 1982. Will fenced pools save lives? A 10-year study from Mulgrave Shire, Queensland. *Medical Journal of Australia* 2: 510–511.

MORRONGIELLO, B. 1997. Children's perspectives on injury and close-call experiences: Sex differences in injury-outcome processes. *Journal of Pediatric Psychology* 22: 499–512.

MORRONGIELLO, B., and DAYLER, L. In press. A community-based study of parents' attitudes and beliefs relevant to childhood injury prevention. *Canadian Journal of Public Health Assocation.*

MORRONGIELLO, B., and POLAK, A. 1995. *Parental Attitudes toward Unintentional Childhood Injuries.* Results of a national survey. Presented to Health Canada, Family and Children Branch, Ottawa (ON). May.

MORRONGIELLO, B., HILLIER, L., and BASS, M. 1995. "What I Said" versus "What You Heard": A comparison of physicians' and parents' reporting of anticipatory guidance on child safety issues. *Injury Prevention* 1: 223–227.

MORROW, R. 1989. A school-based program to increase seat belt use. *Journal of Family Practice* 29: 517–520.

NATIONAL FIRE PROTECTION ASSOCIATION. 1982. *Home Fires, Time of Occurrence.* Fire Record no. FR56–2, Boston (MA).

NERSESIAN, W., PETIT, M., and SHAPER, R. 1985. Childhood death and poverty: A study of all childhood deaths in Maine 1976 to 1980. *Pediatrics* 75: 41–50.

NEUWELT, E. et al. 1989. Oregon head and spinal cord injury prevention program and evaluation. *Neurosurgery* 24: 453–458.

NHTSA (NATIONAL HIGHWAY TRAFFIC SAFETY ADMINISTRATION). 1980. *A Report to Congress on the Effect of Motorcycle Helmet Use Repeal—A Case Report for Helmet Use.* Washington (DC): NHTSA, U.S. Department of Transportation. HF-805-312.

NUMENMAA, T., and SYVANEN, M. 1974. Teaching road safety to children in the age range 5–7 years. *Paedagogica Europea* 9: 151–161.

NG, M. 1991. SHIP (Spinal Cord and Head Injury Prevention Project) Evaluation. Honolulu (HI): Rehabilitation Hospital of the Pacific.

ONTARIO MINISTRY OF HOUSING. 1978. *Smoke Detectors in Ontario Housing Corporation Dwellings.* OMH, Toronto (ON).

ONTARIO TRAUMA REGISTRY INFOPAGE JULY 1995. Pediatric injury in Ontario. 2: 1–4.

OZANNE-SMITH, J., and SHERRY, K. 1990. Bicycle-related injuries: Head injuries since legislation. *Hazard* 6: 1–8.

PAUL, C., SANSON-FISHER, R., REDMAN, S., and CARTER, S. 1994. Preventing accidental injury to young children in the home using volunteers. *Health Promotion International* 9: 241–249.

PETERSON, L. 1984a. The "Safe at Home" game: Training comprehensive safety skills in latchkey children. *Behavior Modification* 8: 474–494.

_____.1984b. Teaching home safety and survival skills in latchkey children: A comparison of two manuals and two methods. *Journal of Applied Behavioral Analysis* 17: 279–293.

PETERSON, L., and MORI, L. 1985. Prevention of child injury: An overview of targets, methods and tactics for psychologists. *Journal of Consulting and Clinical Psychology* 53: 586–595.

PETERSON, L., and ROBERTS, M. 1992. Complacency, misdirection, and effective prevention of children's injuries. *American Psychologist* 47: 1040–1044.

PETERSON, L., MORI, L., SELBY, V., and ROSEN, B. 1988. Community interventions in children's injury prevention: Differing costs and differing benefits. *Journal of Community Psychology* 16: 188–204.

PLESS, I. B., and ARSENAULT, L. 1987. The role of health education in the prevention of injuries to children. *Journal of Social Issues* 43: 87–104.

PLESS, I. B., TAYLOR, H., and ARSENAULT, L. 1995. The relationship between vigilance deficits and traffic injuries involving children. *Pediatrics* 95: 219–224.

PLESS, I. B., VERREAULT, R., and TENINA, S. 1989. A case-control study of pedestrian and bicyclist injuries in childhood. *American Journal of Public Health* 79: 995–998.

QUAN, L. 1982. Prevention of drowning. In *Preventing Childhood Injuries*, ed. A. BERGMAN. Report of the 12th Ross Roundtable on Critical Approaches to Common Paediatric Problems. Columbus (OH): Ross Laboratories. pp. 54–57.

RAINE, P., and AZMY, A. 1983. A review of thermal injury in young children. *Journal of Paediatric Surgery* 18: 21–26.

REAGAN, R. 1984. National child passenger safety awareness day, 1984: Proclamation 5210 of June 18, 1984. *Federal Register* 49: 25217–25218.

REISENGER, K., and WILLIAMS, A. 1978. Evaluation of programs designed to increase protection of infants in cars. *Pediatrics* 62: 280–287.

REISENGER, K., WILLIAMS, A., WELLS, J., ROBERTS, T., and PODGAINY, H. 1981. Effects of paediatricians' counselling on infant restraint use. *Pediatrics* 67: 201–206.

RICE, D. 1990. *The Cost of Injury in the United States: Report to Congress.* Washington (DC).

RICHARDS, J., HENDRICKS, C., and ROBERTS, M. 1991. Prevention of spinal cord injury: An elementary education approach. *Journal of Paediatric Psychology* 16: 595–609.

RIVARA, F. 1982. Epidemiology of childhood injuries. In *Preventing Childhood Injuries*, ed. A. BERGMAN. Report of the 12th Ross Roundtable on Critical Approaches to Common Paediatric Problems. Columbus (OH): Ross Laboratories. pp. 13–18.

RIVARA, F., and HOWARD, D. 1982. Parental knowledge of child development and injury risks. *Journal of Developmental and Behavioral Pediatrics* 3: 103–105.

RIVARA, F., and MUELLER, B. 1987. The epidemiology and causes of childhood injuries. *Journal of Social Issues* 43: 13–31.

RIVARA, F., DiGUISEPPI, C., and KOEPSELL, T. 1990. Reply. *Journal of the American Medical Association* 263: 1915.

ROBERTS, M. 1987. Public health and health psychology: Two cats of Kilkenny? *Professional Psychology* 18: 157–162.

ROBERTS, M., and BROOKS, P. 1987. Children's injuries: Issues in prevention and public policy. *Journal of Social Issues* 43: 105–118.

ROBERTS, M., and FANURIK, D. 1986. Rewarding elementary school children for their use of safety belts. *Health Psychology* 5: 185–196.

ROBERTS, M., and LAYFIELD, D. 1987. Promoting child passenger safety: A comparison of two positive methods. *Journal of Paediatric Psychology* 12: 257–271.

ROBERTS, M., and TURNER, D. 1986. Rewarding parents for their children's use of safety seats. *Journal of Paediatric Psychology* 11: 25–36.

ROBERTS, M., ALEXANDER, K., and KNAPP, L. 1990. Motivating children to use safety belts: A program combining rewards and "Flash for Life." *Journal of Community Psychology* 18: 110–119.

ROBERTS, M., FANURIK, D., and LAYFIELD, D. 1987. Behavioral approaches to prevention of childhood injuries. *Journal of Social Issues* 43: 105–118.

ROBERTS, M., FANURIK, D., and WILSON, D. 1988. A community program to reward children's use of seat belts. *American Journal of Community Psychology* 16: 395–407.

ROBERTSON, L., KELLY, A., O'NEILL, B., WIXOM, C. EISWORTH, R., and HADDON, W. 1974. A controlled study of the effect of television message on safety belt use. *American Journal of Public Health* 64: 1071–1080.

ROTHENGATTER, T., 1984. A behavioral approach to improving traffic behavior of young children. *Ergonomics* 27: 147–160.

ROUTLEDGE, D., REPETTO-WRIGHT, R., and HOWARTH, C. 1974. The exposure of young children to accident risk as pedestrians. *Ergonomics* 17: 457–480.

RYHAMMER, L., and BERGLUND, G. 1980. *Children and Instruction in Road Safety.* Sweden: University of Uppsala, Uppsala Reports on Education, no. 8.

SCHWARZ, D., GRISSO, J., MILES, C., HOLMES, J., and SUTTON, R. 1993. An injury prevention program in an urban African American community. *American Journal of Public Health* 83: 675–680.

SHANON, A., BASHAW, B., LEWIS, J., and FELDMAN, W. 1992. Nonfatal childhood injuries: A survey at the Children's Hospital of Eastern Ontario. *Canadian Medical Association Journal* 146: 361–365.

SHELP, L. 1987. Community intervention and changes in accident pattern in a rural swedish municipality. *Health Promotion* 2: 109–124.

_____. 1988. The role of organizations in community participation: Prevention of accidental injuries in a rural Swedish municipality. *Social Sciences Medicine* 26: 1987–1093.

SMITH, G. 1995. Drowning prevention in children. *Injury Prevention* 1: 216.

SMITH, G., and FALK, H., 1987. Unintentional injuries. In *Closing the Gap: The Burden of Unnecessary Illness*, eds. R. AMBLE and N. DOLD. New York: Oxford University Press. pp. 143–163.

SMITH, P., and DAGLISH, L. 1977. Sex differences in parent and infant behavior in the home. *Child Development* 48: 1250–1254.

SMITH, R., and O'NEILL, T. 1984. An analysis into childhood burns. *Burns Including Thermal Injuries* 11: 117–124.

SPIEGEL, C., and LINDAMAN, F. 1977. Children Can't Fly: A program to prevent child mortality and morbidity from window falls. *American Journal of Public Health* 67: 1143–1146.

STOVER, S., and FINE, P. Ed. 1986. *Spinal Cord Injuries: The Facts and the Figures.* Birmingham (AL): National Spinal Cord Injury Statistical Center, University of Alabama at Birmingham.

STREFF, F., and GELLER, E. 1988. An experimental test of risk compensation: Between-subjects versus within-subjects analyses. *Accident Analysis and Prevention* 20: 277–287.

THOMPSON, R. 1989. A case-control study of the effectiveness of bicycle safety helmets. *New England Journal of Medicine* 320: 1361–1367.

THOMSON, J. 1991. *The Facts about Child Pedestrian Accidents.* London, U.K.: Cassell.

THORNSON, J. 1984. Pedal cycle accidents. *Scandinavian Journal of Social Medicine* 2: 121–128.

TRANSPORT CANADA. 1992. Report on "Drivers' use of safety seat restraints for children". Toronto.

TREIBER, F. 1986. A comparison of the positive and negative consequences approaches upon car restraint use. *Journal of Paediatric Psychology* 11: 15–25.

TURTURICI, A. 1975. An evaluation of speed-curtailing bumps. *Public Works* 106: 73–76.

WATSON, G., ZADOR, P., and WILKS, A. 1980. The repeal of helmet use laws and increased motorcycle mortality in the United States. *American Journal of Public Health* 70: 579–585.

WEBNE, S., KAPLAN, B., and SHAW, M. 1989. Paediatric burn prevention: An evaluation of the efficacy of a strategy to reduce tap-water temperature in a population at risk for scalds. *Developmental and Behavioral Pediatrics* 10: 187–191.

WILDE, G. 1982. The theory of risk homeostasis: Implications for safety and health. *Risk Analysis* 2: 209–225.

WILLIAMS, A. 1982. Passive and active measures for controlling disease and injury. *Health Psychology* 1: 399–409.

WILLIAMS, A., and WELLS, J. 1981. The Tennessee child restraint law in its third year. *American Journal of Public Health* 71: 163–165.

WILSON, M., and BAKER, S. 1987. Structural approach to injury control. *Journal of Social Issues* 43: 73–86.

WILSON, M., BAKER, S., TERET, S., SHOCK, S., and GARBARINO, J. 1991. *Saving Children: A Guide to Injury Prevention.* New York (NY): Oxford University Press.

WITTE, J., and AXNIXK, N., 1975. The benefits from ten years of measles immunization in the United States. *Public Health Reports* 90: 205–207.

WOOD, T., and MILNE, P. 1988. Head injuries to pedal cyclists and the promotion of helmet use in Victoria, Australia. *Accident Analysis and Prevention* 20: 177–185.

WORTEL, E., DEGEUS, G., KOK, G., and VAN WOERKUM, C. 1994. Injury control in preschool children: A review of parental safety measures and the behavioral determinants. *Health Education Research* 9: 201–213.

YARMEY, D., and ROSENSTEIN, S. 1988. Parental predictions of their child's knowledge about dangerous situations. *Child Abuse and Neglect* 12: 355–361.

YOUNG, A. 1991. A community-based head injury prevention program. *Family and Community Health* 14: 75–78.

ZIEGLER, P. 1989. *The Use of Child Safety Seats.* Washington (DC).

Youth

Strategies to Promote the Optimal Development of Canada's Youth

BENJAMIN H. GOTTLIEB, PH.D.

Professor of Psychology
University of Guelph

SUMMARY

Strategies to Promote the Optimal Development of Canada's Youth

Adolescence is fraught with risks and challenges. It is a developmental transition involving rapid growth and change for both the individual and his external environment. It is a time of heightened self-consciousness, preoccupation with appearance and social acceptability, and emerging independence and responsibility. Because it is also a period when decisions and choices shape later life prospects, concerted efforts must be made to provide the counsel, support and skills that are needed to place youth on a safe and productive life course.

Increasing evidence reveals that adolescents who show resilience when faced with adversity have three kinds of protective factors: a cohesive and stable family, sources of external support, and particular coping skills and resources. Some of these elements change more easily than others and are, therefore, targeted by programs and policies to promote the mental health, social competence and future life prospects of adolescents.

This position paper critically reviews a range of initiatives that have been effective or show promise in promoting adolescent personal and social development. It also offers guidelines for successfully implementing such programs, for avoiding pitfalls and for embedding such programs in the community and its institutions. Finally, it notes implications for policy by making suggestions to guide the actions of governments, educational authorities and other youth-serving organizations.

The paper begins with a brief definition of adolescent mental health and a concise description of the "state of the adolescent" in Canada. It then addresses the specific protective factors that have been identified (Garmezy 1983; Rutter 1983) in the literature on the subject of resilience, highlighting factors that can be changed through planned intervention.

The model programs or "success stories" highlight three program strategies: (1) behavioural training in problem-solving and social competence skills; (2) participation in community-based youth development organizations, particularly those that offer opportunities for service to others; and (3) the mobilization of social support, including initiatives involving support groups, opportunities to mentor and be mentored, and environmental restructuring. Some attention is devoted to youth who are at special risk due to economic disadvantage, stressful life events or membership in an ethnic or minority group, but these strategies emphasize universal rather than targeted recruitment of youth.

The paper offers detailed descriptions of the structure and content, and evaluates three specific examples of successful social competence training: (1) the Social Decision Making and Problem Solving (SDM-PS) program, developed by Elias and Clabby (1989) and widely implemented in, among others, the New Jersey school systems; (2) The Social Competence Promotion Program for Young Adolescents (SCPP-YA), developed by Weissberg and colleagues (Weissberg, Jackson and Shriver 1993), and implemented in public schools throughout New Haven, Connecticut and selectively in 25 other states and 4 countries; and (3) Positive Adolescent Choices Training (PACT), developed by Yung and Hammond (1995) which also promotes social skills and competence but focuses on preventing violence, particularly among African American youth.

Although some youth development programs are national in scope, most are grassroots initiatives that express the local culture and the needs and wants of local youth. Because these initiatives tend to be modestly funded and serve relatively small numbers of youth in their home communities, they are generally not evaluated. The paper briefly reviews several local Canadian initiatives, including: (1) MAD (Make a Difference) for Youth, a self-help youth development program in Antigonish, Nova Scotia; (2) Quebec's 180 Maisons de jeunes (Youth Houses) where youth aged 12 to 18 can devote part of their leisure time to learning about one another and community life; (3) the creation, of a storefront youth services bureau in a Toronto-area shopping mall offering culturally sensitive counselling, community support and referral services, and alternative educational programs to youth aged 12 to 24; and (4) in Saskatchewan, the Rancho Ehrlo Society's recreation, support, social and cultural activities for Aboriginal youth, and its youth-focused community development work with several Saskatchewan bands.

Two additional programs, for which evaluation data are available, are described in more detail: (5) a program that trains and assigns teenage volunteers to befriend children with severe handicaps and provides opportunities for the children to participate in community activities (Cooley, Singer, and Irvin 1989);

and (6) PALS (Participate and Learn Skills), an Ottawa, Ontario, community-based skill development initiative for the children aged 5 to 15 in a public housing project (Jones and Offord 1989).

The third set of programs is based on strong, consistent evidence pointing to the role of family or an adult attachment figure in building resilience for youth, and in buffering them from the adverse effect of life events and chronically stressful transitions and environments. The paper describes several individual interventions (e.g., mentoring arrangements) and group interventions (e.g., groups for children whose parents have separated or divorced) designed to introduce support early in the stress process and, thereby, maintain adaptive functioning. The paper introduces evaluation data and guidelines for successful practice.

The final section of the paper discusses the characteristics of mental health promotion programs that are successful at the community implementation level and attract youth. Policy implications are addressed with recommendations to school officials and government policymakers.

TABLE OF CONTENTS

INTRODUCTION AND OVERVIEW

Four centuries ago, William Shakespeare, one of the keenest social observers of the day, had this to say about adolescence:

> I would there were no age between ten and three and twenty, or that youth would sleep out the rest; for there is nothing in the between but getting wenches with child, wronging the ancientry, stealing, [and] fighting.

It is important to remember that, timeless as it is, Shakespeare's statement reflects the dismal health, economic and social conditions that characterized the lives of urban youth in sixteenth-century England. Today, a commitment to enhancing the life prospects of adolescents should not only prevent the development of an underclass of young people cut off from the mainstream, but should also optimally foster adolescents' talents and mental health, as well as their potential to become productive adults.

This paper takes the position that a comprehensive strategy designed to achieve these goals must embrace initiatives that promote adolescents' social competence, involve them in meaningful community activities, particularly in human service roles, and marshal support for them.

Adolescence is fraught with risks and challenges. It is a transition period of accelerated growth and change, not only in the individual, but also in his or her external environment. It is a time of heightened self-consciousness, preoccupation with appearance and social acceptability, and emerging independence and responsibility. Early adolescence is particularly challenging because of its vast physiological changes, its academic and social demands, and the emergence of sexuality. Because the decisions and choices of this period shape life prospects, concerted efforts must be made to provide the counsel, support and skills that are needed to place youth on a safe, productive life course.

AIMS AND ORGANIZATION

This position paper critically reviews a range of initiatives that have demonstrated effectiveness or show great promise in promoting adolescent mental health and social competence. In addition, it offers guidelines for successfully implementing such programs, for avoiding pitfalls, and for embedding such programs in the fabric of the community and its institutions. A third objective is to draw out the implications for policy by articulating a set of principles that may guide the actions of governments, education authorities, and other youth-serving organizations.

The paper begins by addressing the specific protective factors identified in the literature on resilience, highlighting factors that are amenable to change through planned interventions. The literature concludes that:

although no single developmental path optimizes mental health and success in the transition to adulthood and full citizenship, intervention strategies that foster strong interpersonal relationships, effective problem-solving and decision-making skills, and involvement in personally meaningful activities show the greatest promise in fashioning constructive, satisfying lives for adolescents.

The next section of the paper offers a definition of adolescent mental health, and a concise description of the "state of the adolescent" in Canada, especially in youth mental health.

The bulk of the paper then spotlights model programs or "success stories", concentrating on three programmatic strategies: (1) behavioural training in problem-solving and social competence skills, with special attention to measures that reduce the likelihood of violence among youth; (2) participation in community-based youth development organizations, particularly those that offer opportunities for service to others and for the assumption of leadership roles; and (3) the mobilization of social support through the creation of support groups, mentoring relationships, and environmental restructuring. For each of these three intervention strategies, although some attention is devoted to youth who are at special risk due to economic disadvantage, the occurrence of stressful life events, or ethnic/ minority group membership, universal rather than targeted recruitment of youth is emphasized.

The paper focuses on primary prevention strategies supported by empirical data or showing promise because they attract youth or represent strategic partnerships. The paper does not address strategies to prevent specific mental health-linked problems among high-risk youth identified as targets for intervention.

KEY CONCLUSIONS FROM THE LITERATURE REGARDING THE DETERMINANTS OF HEALTH

Sources of Resilience among Youth: Psychosocial Determinants of Health and Competence

There is a growing body of evidence revealing that adolescents who overcome adversity, manifesting resilience despite the odds against them, have access to three kinds of protective factors: a cohesive and stable family, sources of external support, and certain personal resources that protect them (Garmezy 1983).

With respect to the family environment, research shows that parents who adopt an "authoritative-democratic" style characterized by warmth, firm control and limit setting, and attention to the development of the child's social and cognitive skills tend to foster self-confidence, self-control and effective coping skills in their children. By contrast, authoritarian-autocratic or *laissez-faire* parents, especially severely critical, protective or anxious parents, tend to undermine their children's sense of self-worth and self-efficacy, impairing psychological development and mental health (Baumrind 1971).

With respect to external support, evidence indicates strongly that children in chronically stressful circumstances, such as poverty, and children who experience painful life events, such as the death of a parent or sibling, withstand these hardships more effectively when they have at least one significant, positive adult attachment. Access to a caring, concerned confidant who offers guidance and security sharply reduces the probability of adverse developmental outcomes (Garmezy 1983).

Finally, the personal characteristics that distinguish children who remain stable when stressed include personality assets, such as self-esteem and autonomy; intellectual skills, such as problem-solving abilities; social skills, such as cooperation, social engagement and responsiveness; a sense of self-efficacy; and an easygoing temperament (Garmezy 1983; Rutter 1983).

Certain elements of this triad of protective factors are more amenable to change than others, and therefore constitute the focus for programs and policies aimed to promote the mental health, social competence, and future life prospects of adolescents. However, before reviewing these initiatives, it is important to present a rationale and framework for promoting the positive development of adolescents, and to catalogue some of the risks and circumstances that Canadian adolescents face.

Defining Adolescent Mental Health

Defining the criteria for adolescent mental health is daunting because of the many perspectives on how youth function and the many values underlying concept of positive mental health. Indeed, some believe that the mental health of adolescents cannot be separated from their physical and spiritual health, and that health promotion programs must, therefore, be comprehensive, embracing diet, exercise, social skills and self-perception, and working through all the primary socialization settings, including school, family, peer groups, and youth-serving institutions in the community. This is why leaders in the field of adolescent health call for "multi-component, multi-year, theoretically guided risk-reduction and protection-enhancing models incorporating both skills training and environmental change" (Consortium on the School-Based Promotion of Social Competence 1994). Interventions that are short-term, focused on only one dependent variable (e.g., self-esteem or diet), based on knowledge rather than skills and segregated from the social network and primary socialization contexts of the client base are comparatively unsuccessful, not only in recruiting and retaining participants, but also in effecting desired, lasting change. Because multiple risk factors have been shown to predict adolescent health and behavioural problems, nothing short of coordinated, systematic intervention is likely to succeed.

This paper uses Compas' (1993) definition of mental health:

> A process characterized by development toward optimal current and future functioning in the capacity and motivation to cope with stress and to involve the self in personally meaningful instrumental activities and/or interpersonal relationships (p. 166).

Recognizing that social, ethnic, racial and cultural expectations and norms differ, Compas adds that "Optimal functioning is relative and depends on the goals and values of the interested parties, appropriate developmental norms, and one's sociocultural group" (p. 166).

The conceptual framework for primary preventive initiatives must account for two main factors: (1) the central developmental challenges and transitions of adolescence; and (2) the central life arenas of functioning in which adolescents participate. The developmental challenges adolescents face involve issues of relatedness, competence and autonomy, whereas the transitions are biological, developmental and environmental, involving sexual maturation, school changes, employment, and the gradual assumption of adult responsibilities. As for the central life arenas in which adolescents participate, the family, school and peer group offer youth the opportunity to assume valued social roles. For many teenagers, community organizations and paid employment also foster the development of values, commitments and identity.

This framework suggests that preventive interventions must foster competence, autonomy and reciprocal relationships through coordinated strategies at home, at school, in peer groups and in community organizations. Although no single developmental path optimizes mental health and success in the transition to adulthood and full citizenship, intervention strategies that foster strong interpersonal relationships, effective problem-solving and decision-making skills, and involvement in personally meaningful activities show the greatest promise in fostering constructive, satisfying lives for adolescents.

CHARACTERISTICS AND CONDITIONS OF CANADIAN ADOLESCENTS

According to the 1991 census, more than 1.8 million youth aged 15 to 19 were living in Canada, making up 7 percent of the total population. The most recent report of the Canadian Institute of Child Health (1994) revealed that this segment of the population was at increased risk of death and injury due to motor vehicle collisions, suicide, unwanted pregnancy and sexually transmitted diseases. Suicide is the second leading cause of death for both sexes, the rate for teenage men (23 per 100 000 in 1991 according to Statistics Canada) being six times that for teenage women (Statistics Canada 1994). Interestingly, the rate of hospitalization for attempted suicide among women is twice that of men, revealing that they too suffer from feelings of desperation but tend not to use lethal means as often as men do.

The emotional well-being of Canada's teens is also flagging; less than 50 percent of those surveyed about self-perceptions strongly agreed that they felt good about themselves (45 percent of males and 30 percent of females), that they have several good qualities (43 percent of males and 35 percent of females), and that they are self-confident (33 percent of males and 22 percent of females). More young women than young men consistently perceive their lives as stressful; 37 percent of males reported that life was "somewhat" or "very" stressful compared with 63 percent of young women. Feelings of loneliness and depressed moods are prevalent among Canadian youth, especially among young women. According to several surveys cited by the Canadian Institute of Child Health, between 10 and 25 percent of youth state that they are often lonely (23 percent of women; 17 percent of men), depressed (28 percent of women, 22 percent of men), and that they suffer from emotional distress (16 percent of women, 11 percent of men).

Because of high fertility rates and low life expectancy, Canada's Aboriginal population has a much larger proportion of young people than in the Canadian non-Aboriginal population. Specifically, 58 percent of Canadian Aboriginal people are under 24 years of age, compared with 39 percent of the Canadian population (Assembly of First Nations 1988). About 40 percent of Canadian Aboriginal people are below age 15. Unemployment is especially acute among Aboriginal adolescents, as is suicide. Only 24 percent of Aboriginal youth aged 16 to 24 are employed, and their annual income is half that of non-Aboriginal youth and well below Statistics Canada's poverty line. The education system does not seem to meet the needs of Aboriginal students, as dropout rates are two to four times higher than for non-Aboriginal youth (Warry 1991).

The rate of suicide among Aboriginal youth is truly shocking. Aboriginal adolescents aged 10 to 14 commit suicide at a rate that is almost 9 times the national average and, among 15- to 24-year-olds it is 5 to 7 times the national average. Violence and accidental death related to substance abuse are also exceptionally high. It is estimated that 70 percent of suicides, 80 percent of homicides, 52 percent of motor vehicle accidents and 54 percent of other accidents are alcohol-related.

According to Warry (1991), the long-term needs of Aboriginal youth can be met only through the development of culturally sensitive education and the provision of meaningful job opportunities. At the same time, the immediate needs of Aboriginal youth must be addressed by programs that enhance their life skills, prevent suicide and substance abuse, and improve educational and leisure activities. Above all, Warry (1991) maintains that programs and services must be planned in a community-based, participatory way to reflect the values, goals and priorities of Aboriginal youth and to combat powerlessness and futility. One such example is the work of the Rancho Ehrlo Society, described in the section on community-based youth development organizations.

STRATEGIES FOR PROMOTING ADOLESCENT MENTAL HEALTH: THE SUCCESS STORIES

School-Based Problem-Solving, Social Competence and Life Skills Programs

According to the Consortium on the School-Based Promotion of Social Competence (1994), social competence is:

> The capacity to integrate cognition, affect, and behaviours to achieve specified social tasks and positive developmental outcomes. Social competence consists of a set of core skills, attitudes, abilities and feelings given functional meaning by the contexts of culture, neighbourhood, and situation (p. 275).

Social competence can be seen as a set of culturally relevant life skills for handling diverse instrumental and socioemotional tasks in varied settings.

Although programs differ in their relative emphases, researchers agree that a core set of cognitive and affective factors underlie social competence in contrasting situations and settings. These factors include: attending to and accurately interpreting relevant social cues, generating effective solutions to interpersonal problems, realistically assessing alternative solutions, translating social decisions into effective behaviours, and expressing self-efficacy.

In general, social competence promotion programs seek to enhance personal and interpersonal effectiveness by teaching developmentally appropriate skills, and fostering prosocial, health-protective values (Caplan et al. 1992). From the risk perspective, these programs were developed to help prevent antisocial and aggressive behaviour), unwanted pregnancy, drug use and dropping out of school. However, from the health promotion perspective, they equip youth with resources for resisting stress and learning adaptive behaviours.

The three programs described below teach adolescents goal-setting, decision-making and problem-solving skills through structured, school-based curricula. Although each program has a different emphasis, duration and technology, all three associate the behavioural practice of skills with social competence. Evaluation data also reveals that these programs are truly success stories because their participants have comparatively favourable social and psychological outcomes. Finally, all three programs have been designed by academically based, applied researchers, and have been widely implemented at community level. The original models were funded by a combination of federal, state and local grants, as well as from foundation money. For example, the designers of the third social competence program, which focuses on preventing youth violence, received initial funding from the U.S. Department of Health and Human Services, the Ohio Commission on Minority Health, the Ohio Governor's Office of Criminal Justice Services, and the Mathile Family Foundation.

The Social Decision Making and Problem Solving (SDM-PS) program is an extended and refined established primary prevention program that was first delivered to very young children to develop their social problem-solving skills. In the present version, teachers deliver a structured curriculum with three developmental phases. The Readiness phase involves two eight-lesson modules, in which eight core problem-solving skills are taught. In the first Readiness module, students learn self-control skills like listening, concentrating, following directions, remembering, resisting provocation by others, resisting the urge to provoke others, and self-calming. In the second Readiness module, participants learn group and social awareness skills, such as giving and receiving help and praise, showing caring, selecting friends, and playing roles.

Following this priming, the core problem-solving skills are presented in the Instructional phase, in 20 lessons. The first two lessons set the ground rules for group discussion and motivate decision making about routine social problems. The next 16 sessions focus on the eight core problem-solving skills, including:
 − looking for signs that feelings have changed,
 − self-talk about what the problem is,
 − identifying goals,
 − generating multiple alternative solutions,
 − anticipating the consequences of each solution,
 − selecting the best solution,
 − planning its execution, and
 − implementing the solution and monitoring its effects.
The final two lessons focus on integrating the eight steps for specific problem situations.

The third and final phase of the SDM-PS program emphasizes applying the skills to everyday life. Teachers prompt students to implement the skills when interpersonal problems occur naturally, and integrate the skills into classroom routine through specific techniques such as recording episodes on a class problem-solving chart and discussing them later in groups. Children also use personal diaries to record how they applied the skills and which skills they found most useful. Such behavioural techniques promote generalization and transfer of skills to everyday school and home situations.

Empirical evidence reveals that, relative to a control group, the children who received the SDM-PS curriculum improved their social decision-making and problem-solving skills, and used them both inside and outside the classroom. The curriculum also fostered prosocial skills, such as helping, sharing and empathy, both immediately after the program terminated and on entrance to high school. Program participants showed less antisocial, self-destructive or socially incompetent behaviour than the control group (Elias and Clabby 1992).

The SDM-PS program has been widely implemented throughout the New Jersey school system, in several other states and in England. Hence implementation settings and funding arrangements vary. Ideally, school authorities will find permanent funding for the SDM-PS curriculum. To implement and manage the program, the program designers recommend formation of a Social Decision Making and Problem Solving Committee to ensure that all stakeholders are fully informed about the program, to guide project implementation, to consult with teachers, and to evaluate the implementation of the project and its effect on teachers, administrators and students. A one-day training session has been designed for the planning committee, including instruction on ways to expand and institutionalize the program.

Having introduced the program in various community contexts, Elias and Clabby (1992) spell out some of the most important issues to consider in the implementation process:

- *Values*. Does introduction of the program hinder or enhance the organization's basic mission?
- *Information*. How will schools share program information to resolve problems and maximize success?
- *Circumstances*. What formal and informal politics influence the successful program development?
- *Timing*. Are there any factors which will affect the introduction of the program, such as upcoming staffing changes?
- *Obligation*. Will the host community make the necessary changes to accommodate the program?
- *Resistance*. Is there resistance to the new program? If so, how much and where is it coming from?
- *Yield*. What are the program's benefits?

The second program, the Social Competence Promotion Program for Young Adolescents (SCPP-YA), was developed by Weissberg and colleagues, who refined a generic social problem-solving approach by adding a generalized thinking strategy. This program is a success because it has been implemented in middle schools throughout the New Haven, Connecticut, school system, and has spread to 25 other states and 4 countries. In 1992, the SCPP-YA program received the Lela Rowland Prevention Award from the National Mental Health Association in recognition of excellence in mental health promotion initiatives.

The SCPP-YA program concentrates on skills for emotional and behavioural self-control, stress management, problem solving, decision making and communication. The long-term goal is prevention of adolescent pregnancy, conduct disorders, aggressiveness and juvenile delinquency.

Although variations exist, the basic program design involves a 27-lesson social problem-solving module that features an intriguing "stoplight" technique. The step, "red light," means "stop, calm down and think before acting." The "yellow light" means "think about the problem" which includes thinking about and expressing feelings, setting a positive goal, generating alternative solutions and anticipating the consequences of the various solutions. The "green light" means "implement the best solution." These core lessons are followed by two nine-lesson modules that apply the core skills to preventing substance abuse and high-risk sexual behaviour.

Teachers deliver the program by means of didactic instruction, class discussion, role playing, daily diaries, videotapes, worksheets and homework assignments. Additional school and community activities are introduced to reinforce classroom teaching, and parents are enlisted as advocates and agents of reinforcement. Support for teachers includes extensive (five-day) pre-delivery training, on-site coaching during classroom instruction, a carefully structured curriculum guide featuring scripted class lessons that clarify key concepts, and attractive lesson materials, including worksheets.

Successful implementation of the program depends on teacher training and support, and the development of material that makes the teacher's job easier. Nevertheless, there is evidence that some teachers implement the program more effectively than others, and are more faithful to the program blueprint. Not surprisingly, teachers with good classroom management skills, who relate well to young adolescents and are highly motivated tend to master both the methods and the content of the program. Because the program is detailed and long, motivation is critical and teachers require continuous support.

Evaluation reveals that, relative to a control group, the 421 urban youth who received the program improved their problem-solving skills, developed more positive attitudes toward conflict resolution, were rated better on impulse control and sociability by teachers and reported fewer conflicts with the law. In an extension and replication of the program, Caplan and colleagues (1992) reported broad improvements in participants' social adjustment (constructive conflict resolution, impulse control and cognitive coping skills), and reduced use of intoxicating substances. As well, relative to a control group, both an African American inner-city youth sample and a suburban sample of youth of European descent showed the positive effects of the program.

Positive Adolescent Choices Training (PACT) also teaches young adolescents social competence and communication skills, but it has a sharper focus on preventing violence, particularly among African American youth. The cognitive and behavioural group training was designed to be sensitive to the cultural and linguistic patterns of African American teenagers, and to equip them to handle interpersonal conflict safely and constructively. For example, the participants can identify with the dress, speech and situation of the youth and adults featured in video materials.

This school-based group program serves youth aged 12 to 15 identified by teachers as being at higher risk of perpetrating or suffering interpersonal violence. Target social skills include: giving positive feedback (thanking or complimenting); learning to receive negative feedback by listening, understanding and reacting appropriately; resisting peer pressure by saying no, giving personal reasons and suggesting alternative actions; and learning to compromise, negotiate and engage in a general problem-solving cycle. Because the program targets children at risk (an indicated intervention), it was particularly important to give it the most positive title possible, and to make it welcoming and accepting to participants.

The program is implemented by trained leaders who are skilled in group interactions, knowledgeable about adolescent development, and experienced in working with minority and disadvantaged youth. Groups of no more than 10 engage in role playing, behavioural practice and observation of peer models, with many target skills introduced in video vignettes. Videos are also used to shape and refine the newly learned skills. An interesting innovation is the development of a companion parent-training module that concentrates on anger management and provocation and is used in a group format. However, the program designers say that it is very difficult to enlist parents, who tend to suspect mainstream institutions as agents of social control.

Evaluation of a pilot program, comparing 15 youth who completed training with 13 who did not, but who were also referred by teachers on the basis of aggression or a history of victimization, shows not only that the target skills are learned correctly (formative evaluation), but also that the participants who completed training had fewer incidents of violence than those who did not (Hammond and Yung 1991). An analysis of in-school and out-of-school suspensions and expulsions showed that none of the participants who completed the program were suspended or expelled from school because of violence, whereas two of the 13 participants who did not complete the program were expelled and seven were suspended. Of these, six received in-school suspensions and one an out-of-school suspension.

In a larger outcome study, Hammond and Yung (1993) randomly assigned 169 middle-school students to treatment or control groups, the former receiving 20 weekly one-hour PACT sessions over the course of a semester. Data collected for a three-year period following training showed that only 17.6 percent of the PACT-trained youth were referred to juvenile court; compared with 48.7 percent of the control group youth. Moreover, the control group youth were more likely to have been charged with violent offenses than the PACT-trained youth.

Working from their consulting and training experience, Yung and Hammond (1995) recently developed a Program Guide for PACT that includes ideas and advice about strategic implementation issues. They suggest establishing an advisory group comprising all relevant stakeholders to secure support from influential figures, serve as a problem-solving forum, provide access to needed resources and market the program. Second, although they maintain that the programs should be implemented in schools, which offer access to youth, adults to reinforce and support program gains, and opportunities to measure school-related behavioural outcomes, Yung and Hammond advise caution in inserting the programs into schools. Specifically, they advise careful explanation of how the program relates to education, selection of appropriate personnel to lead the groups (e.g., guidance personnel, often associated with school discipline, may not be desirable), and caution in identifying and forcing unwilling candidates to attend PACT sessions.

A universal, rather than targeted, recruitment strategy appears to reduce barriers to youth participation, as does the program's positive title. Program advertising should be equally upbeat, emphasizing skills to be learned rather than problems to be prevented, and brochures should describe social and recreational activities and additional incentives such as academic credit, store coupons and recognition certificates. Program graduates offering personal testimony and demonstrating new skills are effective recruiters. The appeal of the program to ethnic or minority youth can also be enhanced by special emphasis on cultural fit, achieved by choosing program leaders from relevant backgrounds who are familiar with the language, culture and activities of the program participants. It is especially important to learn the language of conflict and physical violence, such as "You're gettin' in my face," "Don't diss' me," or "He's punkin' you." In the PACT program, African American role models appear in the videos, popular media figures are discussed, and current events of interest to this group are addressed.

Group leaders are not selected for their academic qualifications but for their personal characteristics. Group leaders must understand adolescents, consciously set a good example, be capable of team building and clarifying values, and be experienced in group dynamics. They should be committed, enthusiastic, confident, assertive, persuasive, reinforcing and observant. They must also be aware of their own values and beliefs about violence (especially beliefs about the inevitability of its occurrence in certain contexts), and of negative stereotypes about African American youth they may have. Finally, group leaders must understand and believe in the program materials, rationales and role-playing techniques.

Parents can get involved in ways that range from learning about the program to leading a PACT group. Options include serving as volunteers or as paid program aides, participating in the training with their children to learn the skills and learn how to reinforce them at home, or becoming adjunct, at-home trainers offering regular practice sessions like those practised in the peer training group. Yung and Hammond acknowledge how difficult it is to enlist parents, and suggest that a program representative "pitch" the program at a parent-teacher meeting. The pitch should emphasize that parental participation is voluntary and that, whatever decision a parent makes, children will have free access to the program. Parents should also be guaranteed child care assistance and transportation to the program.

In an extensive review and critique of the practice literature, the Consortium on the School-Based Promotion of Social Competence (1994) identified the key features of successful social competence promotion programs.

Participation in Community-Based Youth Development Organizations

Community-based youth programs are perhaps the most overlooked resource for promoting youth development. They offer opportunities for youth to form secure, stable relationships with peers and adults, to develop leadership and life skills, to gain a sense of belonging and involvement in the community, and to acquire a sense of competence and usefulness to others. There are many community organizations that serve elementary and pre-school children but, although youth increasingly need enjoyable, valuable after-school activities and are often able to develop and lead them, there are not nearly enough community programs for adolescents. Hence, more creativity is needed in planning and implementing programs cooperatively with youth. A range of programs must be created, including but not limited to sports and music, to appeal to a culturally diverse youth market, cultivate their skills, and prepare them in practical ways for adulthood.

Research documents the amount of time adolescents spend unsupervised after school. The *National Education Longitudinal Study* reported that in 1988, about 27 percent of U.S. eighth graders spent two or more hours at home alone after school, and youth from the lowest socioeconomic group are most likely to be home alone for more than three hours (U.S. Department of Education 1990). During this unsupervised time, they are at greatest risk of engaging in sexual intercourse and substance abuse. Richardson and colleagues (1989) reported that, for eighth graders unsupervised for more than 11 hours a week, the risk of substance abuse was twice as high as those who had some form of adult supervision.

However, extracurricular after-school activities are designed neither to keep youngsters out of trouble, nor to provide adult supervision. Adolescents are unlikely to participate in after-school and weekend programs if they have no control over how they spend their time if they feel stigmatized by participation, or if the activities are unchallenging or inappropriate for their age group. In short, programs must be designed to be lively and enjoyable, and to give expression to youths' creativity, develop their skills, and provide opportunities for them to gain recognition, support and a sense of being useful.

Several diverse examples of thoughtfully planned, grassroots initiatives are described below. Despite a lack of formal evaluation data, these programs can be considered successful because they attract youth, they give youth a sense of belonging and reliable alliance with peers and particular adults, they provide youth with constructive alternatives to hazardous activities and they teach the leadership, teamwork and organizational skills that a successful transition to adulthood requires.

The first example is a program featured in a 1995 compendium that resulted from the National Symposium on Community Action for Children, which was jointly sponsored by the Canadian Institute for Advanced Research and the Centre for Studies of Children at Risk. This program, called MAD [Making a Difference] for Youth: Adolescent Health Project, was launched by three mothers in Antigonish, Nova Scotia. They had been aware of difficulties facing teens in the community, but were catapulted into action by three teen suicides. They created an advisory committee of 12 to 16 youth aged 14 to 19 who came from diverse backgrounds. The advisory committee surveyed 400 teens and helped to design and carry out an assessment of adolescent health needs. The products of this assessment were a report and a video called *The Voice of Teens*.

The report identified three priority areas: use and abuse of intoxicants, mental wellness, and relationship issues. To address these topics, the youth committee worked with agencies and parent volunteers on several activities, including health promotion events, community forums, workshops, media presentations, a peer health education program and several cooperative projects, such as a drug awareness committee.

Recently, MAD for Youth opened a storefront on Main Street in Antigonish for youth interested in promoting the well-being of youth in the community. Plans are underway to open a cafe and a health centre for youth, and to launch a youth newspaper. MAD has also developed partnerships with community service organizations, school officials, health and mental health agencies, law enforcement agencies and political figures, and is reaching out to local businesses and town and county councils.

MAD encountered opposition and hostility from parents who claim that the organization refers youth for abortions. MAD hopes to gain greater access to Antigonish municipal council to refute these accusations and persuade Council to acknowledge youth in their decision-making process.

At the time of writing, no data on the numbers and characteristics of MAD participants were available. There are no data on how MAD participation affected youths' decisions about sexual, drug-related or academic conduct, or on mental health or family and school relations. Nevertheless, the program stands out as a sustained, grassroots effort to involve youth in self-advocacy and leadership. Moreover, MAD has engaged in a useful cycle of research and partnership building that offers a model for other communities wishing to foster youth development through creative, participatory problem solving.

A second example, also from the Maritime provinces, is the Summerside Boys and Girls Club in Prince Edward Island. It provides recreational, educational and leadership activities for children and youth aged 6 to 18. Within this organization, the Keystone Club, involves youth aged 14 and up in volunteer service and leadership development. Recently, Keystone Club members have helped the local health agency implement some of the recommendations for province-wide youth development, contained in a provincial planning document. Youth who are sentenced to community service sometimes perform it through the club.

Recognizing the significance of settings designed and reserved for adolescents, the province of Quebec has created approximately 180 *Maisons de jeunes* (Youth Houses) where teens aged 12 to 18 can devote part of their leisure time to learning about one another and the community. The setting allows youth to develop independence, leadership and a sense of responsibility by organizing activities based on common interests and local needs. Each *Maison* is governed by a youth-dominated board of directors, and youth run committees and operate a canteen. One *Maison* recently reviewed a draft of the provincial Department of Justice document that sets out the rights and laws affecting Quebec youth, to ensure that the language and organization were user friendly.

The Ontario Coalition for Children and Youth is a youth-led group that includes individual youth, youth-serving organizations and youth coalitions. The Coalition sponsored a conference and report, and is now holding focus groups and community forums across the province to help build a youth constituency to meet the needs of young people in Ontario.

In one unusual initiative, the management of a Toronto shopping mall has addressed gang and drug-dealing problems by adapting its physical environment to discourage large groups from congregating and by employing youth workers to handle problems so it is not necessary to call police. The management created a youth services bureau in the mall by combining youth, parents, police authorities, local schools and youth-serving agencies such as Parks and Recreation and social welfare. From its storefront, the bureau offers culturally sensitive counselling, community support and referral services, as well as alternative educational programs for youth aged 12 to 24. The result has been a 16 percent reduction in arrests and convictions of youth in the mall, renewed patronage of the mall by the public (especially elderly residents) and new store leases by better-quality retailers.

In Saskatchewan, the Rancho Ehrlo Society offers recreation, support, social, and cultural activities to Aboriginal youth, and conducts youth-focused community development work with several Saskatchewan bands. For example, a northeastern Saskatchewan band that was alarmed by solvent use among their youth received the Society's assistance in surveying youth needs. On this basis, the band created a summer camp that was attended by 150 youth in 1994. Youth who gathered the original survey data were hired as counsellors, while a Rancho Ehrlo staff member directed the camp with the assistance of several other adults. The camp reopened the following summer without the Rancho Ehrlo director, and again proved highly successful. The band is currently planning to set up a year-round recreation program for its seven communities.

A second Society project that received considerable media exposure recruited Aboriginal youth to collect and distribute used hockey equipment to other Aboriginal youth in Regina's inner city. More than 100 hockey outfits and 300 pairs of skates were gathered and distributed from an Aboriginal drop-in centre. The next year, the Society formed a hockey league, drawing large numbers of Aboriginal youth and their parents to three inner-city rinks located in parks that were once considered dangerous, but are now busy social centres properly maintained by the city. Although there are no data on the social, psychological or skill-related effects of the Society's projects, the sheer number of Aboriginal youth and families that have become involved attests to the socially integrative value of the project.

A final example comes from the United States, and is featured because it represents a highly effective public/private partnership. In Los Angeles, California, UNOCAL Petroleum Corporation has joined with the local 4-H club, the Los Angeles City Council, Volunteers in Service to America (VISTA), the University of California, the housing authority and the school system to create an after school program that serves 7- to 13-year-olds in five public housing projects. The participants receive homework assistance, complete 4-H projects in gardening, computers, cooking, photography, and arts and crafts, and are involved in sports and cultural activities (Carnegie Council on Adolescent Development 1992).

The private sector may be particularly responsive to funding community-based youth programs because of the programs' relatively low cost, and employees' concerns about their children's safety and well-being after school. When employees cannot concentrate on work because of preoccupation with their children's whereabouts and activities after school, productivity decreases and absenteeism increases. Business enterprises also wish to be seen as responsible corporate citizens that enhance the community's quality of life and recruit talented youth for their labour force.

Businesses provide release time or flextime arrangements for employees who wish to volunteer their time to youth organizations, extend technical assistance to youth-serving agencies in management, budgeting or strategic planning, offer internships and mentor local youth.

Although evaluation data are sketchy, there is nevertheless strong support for participation in youth-serving community organizations. For example, a 1987 survey of alumni of youth groups such as 4-H reported that participation gave them pride in their accomplishments, the ability to set goals and cooperate with others, self-confidence, and employment and leadership skills. Similarly, four annual evaluations of the Association of Junior Leagues' Teen Outreach program, a school-based life skills and community service program for middle and high school students, revealed that participants were less likely than peer nonparticipants to become pregnant, drop out or be suspended from school.

A final success story deserves attention because it is a very promising and well-evaluated community-based skill development initiative that was extended to all children aged 5 to 15 in a public housing project in Ottawa, Ontario (Jones and Offord 1989). In 1980, PALS (Participate and Learn Skills) initiated 40 sports and recreation programs in 25 different skill areas, including sports, swimming, judo, guitar, ballet, baton twirling, and scouting. Working out of an office in the housing complex's community centre, two staff members reached out to more than 70 percent of the youth, involving them in a five-step process. The process involved gaining initial participation, fostering continued involvement through a high level of staff contact and recognition, concentrating on developing skills so the youth could participate on an equal footing in mainstream community programs, moving them into a recreation program in the larger community, and incorporating the entire strategy into the larger community's recreational programs. Other noteworthy design elements of PALS include the absence of any financial or administrative barriers to participation (e.g., intake procedures and forms), the evaluation of each child's skill level before and after joining an activity, and program accountability to its funders in the forms of cost analysis, attendance records and gains in skill development.

PALS recognized that economically disadvantaged children and youth are not served or poorly served by mainstream recreational programs and, therefore, do not have the same opportunity for skill development and recognition as their more advantaged peers. The program aimed to upgrade skills and integrate youth into the mainstream recreation programs. The program planners hypothesized that, with improved skills, the youth would also improve their academic performance and self-esteem, and engage in less antisocial behaviour.

A formal evaluation, comparing PALS participants with a control group that matched the age and sex of PALS participants, and from a similarly sized housing complex, revealed no significant changes in self-esteem, school performance or behaviour at home for PALS participants (Jones and Offord 1989). However, observation and archival data revealed that PALS participants averaged significantly fewer police charges during the 36-month course of the intervention, than during the 24 months preceding the program. Unfortunately, after the intervention ended, there were significant rebound effects, possibly because only a small number of youth (mainly the hockey participants) became integrated into the leagues of the larger community.

Finally, PALS was one of the few programs that attempted to document the cost savings resulting from a decrease in charges against youth and a reduction in the number of security reports involving youth. Based on analyses of police, housing authority and city expenditures, savings far exceeded costs.

In an interesting follow-up report, Jones and Offord (1991) discuss why the program did not continue in the community after the demonstration period. Despite their success, many model demonstrations are not replicated or incorporated into education, health and welfare, or parks and recreation agencies. Or, if they are adopted, the program blueprint is modified so dramatically that it bears little resemblance to the original, often because funding has been cut and staff lack appropriate training, motivation or resources. In the case of PALS, Jones and Offord observed that the City of Ottawa cut program funding, failed to engage in the necessary outreach activities, charged a user fee, virtually ignored the skill development thrust, and did not monitor the attendance and progress of individual children. These modifications reveal how a successful demonstration can be subverted, leaving only a shadow of the original program and obviating its potential contribution to youth development.

Characteristics of Effective Youth Development Organizations

After reviewing numerous examples of after-school youth programs, the Carnegie Council on Adolescent Development (1992) issued a report called *A Matter of Time*. The report made the following recommendations for effective after-school programs:
- programs should be based on research concerning adolescent development, including evaluation of the effects of youth development programs;
- programs should emphasize social relationships among peers and between youth and responsible, caring adults;
- programs should encourage parental involvement by creating structures and roles for parents;
- programs should be developed for and by youth;

- programs should be fun, flexible, culturally relevant and linked to activities that interest adolescents;
- programs should offer food to attract youth and as an occasion for relaxing and socializing;
- programs should set clear rules for members to follow, such as no drinking, drug use or gang membership;
- programs should be safe and accessible; and
- programs should provide links to schools as well as to personal and family health and mental health services.

Community Service Initiatives for Older Adolescents

Programs that enlist youth in community service are particularly good for developing skills, leadership and a sense of self-worth among older adolescents. As Schine (1989) observes, community service gives youth the opportunity to assume meaningful roles, to meet society's need for volunteers in health and human services, to apply academic learning to real-life community problems and needs (promoting career experimentation), and the chance to gain support, guidance and recognition from adults. Volunteer youth give the lie to the stereotype of the idle, self-indulgent teenager by demonstrating compassion, respect, and eagerness to take some responsibility for the welfare of others. Paid or unpaid community service can help youth become responsible, productive adults, understand society and themselves, earn the respect of the community, develop self-respect, and learn job skills such as cooperation, decision making and goal setting.

In Canada, in 1986, the Special Senate Committee on Youth issued a report titled *Youth: A Plan of Action*, which proposed a Young Canadians' Community Service Program, modelled on the Katimavik program. It called for teams of unemployed and out-of-school youth aged 17 to 24, to be recruited from all regions of Canada, all socioeconomic levels, both English- and French-speaking backgrounds and rural and urban communities. Participants' living expenses would be paid by the program and they would receive a nominal wage for community service work. After completing the nine-month program, they would receive $1,000 to help them enter the labour market or $3,000 toward postsecondary technical or academic studies. Steps would also be taken to give academic credit to students who attended the program.

In addition to their human services work, the youth would also complete an apprenticeship to equip them with basic skills in areas such as forestry, carpentry, horticulture and construction. The program costs were assessed at $10,000–$9,000 per participant for a nine-month period after the total number of participants reached 10,000. However, this figure does not account for cost savings from unemployment insurance and welfare that the youth might otherwise draw upon.

In April 1994, the federal government introduced a youth service corps and an internship program, although on a much smaller scale than originally proposed. Participants received a stipend paid in weekly instalments to a maximum total of $10,000, as well as a program completion bonus of $2,000 to help pay for books or training or to provide a basis for a business development loan. Opposition to the program was swift, however; critics argued that the program was too small to have a significant impact on youth unemployment, which had swelled to 400,000 (youth aged 16 to 24). Critics to the program, however, observed that the youth unemployment problem needed to be addressed with meaningful jobs, not with more government programs.

The 1996 Speech from the Throne announced a new jobs program for youth that promised to double the number of federal summer student jobs, and challenged the private sector and provincial and municipal governments to do likewise. Although details were not disclosed, the government promised to help youth find their first jobs and gain work experience. At the time of writing, the government had not yet proceeded with the initiatives.

Such community service programs should enhance personal development and give youth career training and some hands-on experience. Strong partnerships between secondary schools and employers are necessary so that the entire cycle of career training, advising, practical experience and apprenticeships is smoothly completed.

Local examples of community service programs include the Early Adolescent Helper Program at the City University of New York's Center for Advanced Study in Education. The Early Adolescent Helper Program involves junior high school students as interns in local senior centres, and in child care programs for preschool and school-age children. By providing a structured after-school program for unsupervised youth, the program motivates youth to stay in school and teaches them about the work world. Studies of program impacts show an improvement in participants' social and self-understanding, and in a sense of making a valuable difference in other people's lives. The work in seniors centres also gives youth a better understanding of the similarities between the generations and emphasizes the importance of good communication skills.

In Atlanta, Georgia, all students are required to perform 75 hours of community service to graduate from high school. At least 200 community agencies host the students. In Kansas City, high-risk 14- to 17-year-olds have been involved in full-time summer service projects. Program advocates suggest that the experience can be maximized by including a reflective component, particularly for middle school students. Program methods include discussions with staff members, written journals and diaries, videotapes and recognition ceremonies.

A third community service program trains and assigns teen volunteers to befriend children with severe handicaps, and provide opportunities for disabled children to participate in community activities (Cooley, Singer, and Irvin 1989). The children had diagnoses ranging from moderate to severe mental retardation and many had additional disabilities, such as cerebral palsy, autism, Down syndrome and sensory impairments. Volunteer training involved three hours of instruction about basic behaviour management concepts and techniques, tips for fostering enjoyable interaction and suggestions for activities. The idea was not to professionalize the volunteers but to teach them enough to make them comfortable with their tasks.

After training, the volunteers met the children and their families in the company of a project staff member. During these sessions, the volunteer would ask standard questions about the child's interests, needs, capacities, adaptive equipment and safety considerations. Each volunteer also had the option of meeting the child's classroom teacher and observing how the teacher handled behaviour problems. Finally, the volunteers and the children began to meet individually, usually three hours a week for a minimum of six months. Each volunteer received support through monthly group meetings and from the staff member who attended their first outing with the child. The meetings focused on problem solving, normalization issues and perspective-taking skills.

Both parents and volunteers evaluated the program. The volunteers reported high levels of satisfaction with their training, involvement with families and level of staff support. Virtually all the volunteers remained involved well beyond the minimum six-month period. Parents reported that the volunteers were reliable, adequately trained, respectful of the family's ideas and suggestions, and creative in finding enjoyable activities in which their child could participate. The parents' sole concern was that termination was difficult for the child, and that the volunteer should be withdrawn gradually. However, even with an incremental termination, it is always difficult for such a friendship to end.

Another program in which youth offer support to others is the Teen Host Program of Newfoundland's Association for New Canadians. In this program, local youth befriend teenagers who have recently immigrated to Canada, involving them in social activities and leadership training. A companion program trains adolescents who have recently come to Canada to serve as peer educators for other ethnic minority youth on use and abuse of intoxicating substances.

Finally, one of the most widely implemented community service activities for youth has been training as peer counsellors and cross-age tutors. Many middle and secondary schools have recruited and trained students to counsel their peers on personal and academic issues, and have assigned senior students as "buddies" or mentors to introduce entrants to a new environment. Peer counselling has also been widely implemented in substance abuse and teen-parent programs. Cross-age tutoring programs in schools throughout both Canada and the United States, enlist youth to upgrade the academic skills of younger children, and often boost the academic performance of the tutor even more than that of the student.

Peer counselling programs are more likely to attract and retain adolescents if they provide opportunities for mutual rather than unidirectional aid and recruit participants on the basis of their abilities rather than their handicaps or deficiencies. Universal strategies are more likely than targeted strategies to be productive. Both the training and the counselling should be introduced as jobs, and retention rates tend to improve if friends are included and wages are paid. However, if the program is designed to help the volunteer as much as the targeted clientele, a variety of helping activities must be available to suit trainees' preferences and talents. Peer counselling is only one of several community service activities that deserves more systematic study, particularly with respect to the develop-mental gains produced by helping others.

Support Interventions

Social support from family or at least one important adult has been found to serve as a source of resilience for youth, buffering them from the impact of painful life events and chronic stress. In a study of 18 male and female adolescents who functioned well despite their parents' major affective disorders, Beardslee and Podorefsky (1988) found that the subjects valued close, confiding relationships. Nine of them identified another person they contacted when their parent was acutely ill to explain the experience or comfort them. Other factors, such as constitutional strengths, self-understanding and self-regard contributed to the resilience of these adolescents, but such factors are more difficult to alter than the quality and availability of social support. Therefore, social support interventions are most promising in work with adolescents.

Social support has sometimes been summarized in the three As: aid, affection and affirmation. Aid is practical assistance—goods, services and money. Affection is emotional support, including opportunities to confide in others and receive compassion, understanding and protection. Affirmation is validation of one's worth and positive feedback about performance.

Programs that marshal, augment or specialize the informal mutual support of adolescents take many forms. These programs vary in structure and content according to the developmental level and psychosocial needs of the clientele. Programs also take place in a variety of settings, most of them at school and at home. Most programs concentrate on either altering the structural features of the school or home environment, or on building more supportive relationships. Almost all of the programs deliver extra support to youth at risk, either to stabilize them when they experience social upheavals or to steer them onto an adaptive path when their behaviour begins to deteriorate.

The literature on support programs for adolescents suggests that most operate with dyads (pairs) and groups, to emphasize strategies to help youth make new ties rather than to specialize the support extended by the ties that already exist in their networks.

One-to-One Support: Mentoring and Being Mentored

The most widely known dyadic (pair-based) program is Big Brothers/Big Sisters, which is the prototype for many intergenerational support programs designed to improve life chances for at-risk youth. Adult participants are called by a variety of names (e.g., foster grandparents, mentors, coaches, home visitors and preceptors), and the frequency, duration and intensity of supportive contacts also vary.

Most dyadic programs (including Big Brothers/Big Sisters) offer diffuse support and rarely prescribe the content, frequency or focus of interaction, or the settings in which contacts should take place. Because they are designed to compensate for a lack of appropriate adult attachments, dyadic programs usually concentrate on developing the kinds of support that are gained from such relationships. A few dyadic programs limit activities, settings and occasions of participants' meetings, or specify formal contacts such as supervision of academic or employment activities or, as with teenage parents, teaching parenting skills. Because adult participants in these latter programs offer specialized support to youth, they are usually trained or selected for the knowledge they have gained through experiences similar to those faced by the youth participants. In most dyadic programs, however, the relationship itself is the end, rather than a means of improving specific coping mechanisms. At best, these primary mentoring relationships take on the qualities of kinship ties, reflecting attachment, closeness, importance, pleasure and trust.

In *The Kindness of Strangers*, Freedman (1991) describe mentoring programs (many pioneered by businesses and corporations), ranging from national initiatives such as Career Beginnings and Big Brothers/Big Sisters to local initiatives such as the Black Male Youth Health Enhancement Program in Washington, D.C., and Proctor and Gamble's partnership with Woodward High School in Cincinnati, Ohio. The latter program matches 100 students from a high school with an 85 percent minority enrolment with the same number of Proctor and Gamble employees. The mentors are asked to commit to a relationship with their protégé for at least five years and to help them develop the attitudes necessary to succeed in an academic program and to provide routes to personal development and success.

The mentoring philosophy is perhaps best expressed by a recommendation offered in *Turning Points*, the Carnegie Council on Adolescent Developments' study of middle schools. It states that "every student should be known well by at least one adult." Similarly, a brochure for the

Philadelphia Futures mentoring program states: "There is at least one teenager in this city who may not make it to college...without you." In short, mentoring offers direct, personal support in a socially sanctioned, individual relationship. In some circumstances, it complements educational and health services and, in others, it supplements or replaces public services.

When mentors and protégés are well matched, especially if their social distance is minimized; when the mentors are committed to their role and prepared to make a long-term commitment to the protégé, and when the mentors have the support of other mentors and of experienced staff, then the relationship can do much for both parties. For the protégé, the mentor can offer guidance on major decisions such as sexuality, education and life goals, while helping to shape values and develop character traits that favour developmentally healthy outcomes. Mentors can help protégés connect present behaviour with later success, and involve protégés in activities that promote competence and widen horizons. The mentoring process teaches both parties about forming and developing relationships and, as the resilience literature shows, the relationship can be a powerful protection in times of crisis and chronic stress. As one mentor of a Washington, D.C.-based program observed:

> These kids, they really do need somebody to talk to. Not so much somebody to hug and hold them necessarily. But somebody to bounce their thoughts off of and to know they're not the only ones feeling desperate and sorry and pitiful today, that this boyfriend who broke their heart is not the absolute end to their lives. They can't get that kind of feedback from other 15-year olds. (Freedman 1991, 46)

Mentoring can be useful in specifically preventive youth programs, such as programs to prevent unwanted pregnancy and early school termination, and in programs to ease the transition from school to work. Hamilton (1994) describes an exemplary British program for unemployed youth that capitalizes on the guidance of mentors recruited from private companies. This program, called Transition to Working Life (TWL), assigns youth aged 16 to 19 who have left school or plan to leave to a working coach. The coach spends two to four hours per week for six months with small groups of eight to ten youth discussing schooling, plans, lifestyle and employment issues, and periodically arranging field trips to explore job opportunities. The coaches' central mission is to motivate the youth, help them persevere in their search for employment or other productive activity, and to inculcate a work ethic. The payoff for employers, who grant the coaches time off work, was that the employees received supervision training from professionals who met the coaches weekly to solve problems and advise them on decisions.

Coaches are nominated by managers and union leaders. The TWL staff ask for nominees who give their coworkers informal guidance and support, master new techniques and equipment quickly, and are good at teaching others to do the same. Interestingly, the TWL staff found that managers and employees with previous experience as youth group leaders were less desirable coaches. The managers were too socially distant from the unemployed youth, and the experienced employees had too many preconceptions about relating to young people.

TWL's results were impressive, especially considering the state of the British economy when it was implemented. Most of the youth participants completed the program and found jobs, returned to school, joined the armed forces or found other constructive activity. The program staff acknowledge that TWL's impact would be stronger if it combined mentoring with training. However, Hamilton (1994) maintains that TWL does not address the systemic barriers facing economically disadvantaged youth, and does not increase the demand for workers.

In general, mentoring guides and champions individuals rather than creating social change for all youth or for youth at special risk of maladjustment, discrimination or marginalization. One confiding, long-term relationship cannot mitigate the combined effects of problems such as poverty, poor housing, family disruption, conflict and inadequate nutrition. In a life of chronic adversity, mentoring is as effective as a toy axe to fell a giant sequoia.

Evaluation research on the effects of mentoring is rare. Little is known about the components of lasting, mutually attractive matches, and youth development outcome criteria have not been developed. Most research consists of reports from youth and mentors about their satisfaction with the experience.

A study of the Adopt-a-Student program in Atlanta, Georgia, found that students with mentors were more likely than students in a comparison group to enrol in postsecondary education. In this program, volunteers from 40 local businesses were paired with underachieving high school students. They meet weekly and attend a monthly job preparation workshop. However, Freedman (1991) cites other mentoring programs that have had mixed results in terms of the academic achievement of the protégés and their rates of early school leaving. The impact of mentoring must be judged in the context of other conditions and supports in the lives of youth.

Experience shows that mentoring is most likely to succeed when it follows certain practices. Freedman (1991) summarized his insights on mentoring programs as follows:
- Prepare youth for their mentor so they understand what to expect.
- Select only mentors who can commit to a long-term relationship and are prepared for the difficulties that can accompany the relationship formation process.
- Base matches on ethnic, racial and class backgrounds.

- Schedule enough time for the relationship to develop, especially when the mentor is replacing or supplementing a parent.
- Find a task or activity as the initial focus for the two parties, to dispel initial nervousness, provide a conversation topic, and mask the helping aspect of the relationship.
- Develop a support mechanism for the mentors by forming mentoring teams or support groups.
- Choose field staff who can relate to both youth and mentors, who can explain the program to parents and school authorities, and who can solve problems when relationships are failing.

Group Support: Creating Transitional Support Systems

The support group is the most popular way to help older adolescent substance abusers, victims of domestic sexual abuse and very young parents. Typically, support groups are organized and led by professionals who combine mutual aid skills with expert knowledge about the stressors members face and productive ways of coping with them. Support groups average eight to ten members, who meet for a fixed number of weekly or bi-weekly sessions (Gottlieb, n.d.). The most detailed information about their process, structure and outcomes comes from reports of groups created for adolescents whose parents have separated or divorced (Kalter et al. 1988; Pedro-Carroll et al. 1986). The findings reveal that the groups speed the adjustment process by normalizing members' feelings and family status, by counteracting self-blame for the separation, and by teaching coping skills for troublesome family interactions and new emotional experiences.

For example, the support group model used in the Children of Divorce Intervention Program at the University of Rochester involves 12 to 16 one-hour group meetings during which children play age-appropriate games designed to help them express feelings and channel anger appropriately, distinguish between problems they can and cannot control, disengage from parental conflict, identify and strengthen their coping skills, and gain a true picture of their role in their parents' divorce (Pedro-Carroll et al. 1986). The group format eases their feelings of stigma and isolation. Educational sessions are also offered to the children's parents and teachers.

Developmental Facilitation Groups, another program, used by the University of Rochester for children of divorced parents, is designed to intervene early in a separation to reduce the incidence and severity of aggressive and depressive symptoms. Separate program modules target youth in the first to third grades, the fourth to sixth grades, and the seventh to ninth grades. The group participants are presented with common stressors encountered during the course of divorce, by means of a displacement technique that involves group stories about imaginary children and role playing of typical divorce conflicts and tensions. Using a manual, the group leaders are trained to issue universal responses to the participants' questions and worries, so that no child is put on the spot.

Both of these support groups have been rigorously evaluated, using delayed-treatment control groups. Both programs show significant impact in many areas. The Developmental Facilitation Groups reduced depression symptoms, aggressive behaviour, anxiety and socializing problems; increased openness to discussing divorce concerns; and improved the participants' mood. Long-term follow-up, as late as four years after the program concluded, revealed that youth who attended the groups had higher self-esteem, better grades, fewer behaviour problems, and fewer referrals for psychological services than the control youths (Kalter et al. 1988).

The Rochester model showed that, relative to youth who did not participate in the program, group participants were described by teachers as better adjusted in the classroom and displaying better frustration tolerance, task orientation and peer relationships. Teachers also observed that program participants were less anxious, withdrawn or disruptive. Parents reported improved communication with their children, more age-appropriate behaviour, and an improved ability to deal with problem situations. Most importantly, participants reported that they were less anxious, and more able to accept and understand changes in their families (Pedro-Carroll et al. 1986).

Mobilizing Support through Policy and Environmental Changes

In addition to individual and group support programs, it is important to alter policies, procedures and environmental factors that impede social support. For example, hospitals now promote family contact by expanding visiting hours, allowing newborns to stay with their mothers and parents to sleep in the room with a hospitalized child, and permitting immediate family members to attend and assist with labour and delivery.

One example of a successful systems-centred support intervention (Gottlieb 1988) for middle school students is presented by Felner and colleagues (1982). To smooth students' transition to junior high school, they gave homeroom teachers guidance and administrative responsibilities such as maintaining contact with students' families. Student relations were stabilized by allowing sets of students to attend all four core academic subjects together. Students not assigned to the demonstration followed the usual system of rotating through classes as individuals.

Empirical data on the program's capacity to encourage peer and adult support revealed that, relative to a matched control group of students in another urban school, students in the demonstration group had significantly better academic and attendance records, and developed more positive self-concepts. They viewed the school's social climate more favourably, perceived its expectations and structure more clearly, and rated the level of teacher support more highly (Felner et al. 1982).

POLICY IMPLICATIONS

This paper records lessons learned from implementing three types of programs to promote youth mental health and social competence. This section summarizes principles to guide the development of primary preventive initiatives and the policies for government actions.

Community Implementation

- Develop a clear service model from sound developmental principles.
- Involve youth in program design and implementation. Give them a general model that can be adapted to youth interests, cultural backgrounds and needs.
- Train staff in advance and supplement training with ongoing support and consultation during implementation.
- Conduct periodic process (formative) evaluations to ensure that the program follows its original design. Although practice may vary from one community or population to another, the principles of an intervention should not change. To maintain consistency, hold regular assessments in which staff can discuss concerns about aspects of the program that they do not understand or for which they have received inadequate training.
- To avoid stigmatizing participants, design the program along universal lines rather than selective (targeting an at-risk group) or indicated (identifying potential participants through advance screening) lines. Such an approach helps produce a program that is as likely to prevent high-risk behaviours as to reduce them.
- When introducing programs to community organizations and institutions, secure the support of senior administrators. In school systems, it is vital to recruit principals and special education authorities to support and communicate enthusiasm to teachers. These authorities should suggest program modifications, as long as they do not violate program principles.
- Use excited, motivated, committed staff to launch a program, their enthusiasm will promote its process and effects.
- In school-based programs, balance planning and flexibility in scheduling and teacher training. Allow teachers to bring creativity to the curriculum materials.
- Make academic links explicit.
- Ensure that any organized parent groups understand and approve school programs. Let them see it in action and volunteer for training.

- Ensure that program costs (materials, staffing, administration) are reasonable so that the program can become institutionalized and eventually adopted by the private sector.
- Describe program goals and activities in positive language to minimize controversy and fear.
  Program planners should also:
- recruit a committed, diverse group of program stakeholders;
- actively involve top administrators;
- fund training and staff development;
- develop a support system to sustain staff persistence, flexibility and morale;
- combine the program with the agendas of community institutions, such as the school system;
- address knowledge, skills and attitudes as a set; and
- run the program long enough to create durable change.

Marketing Programs to Youth

To make programs attractive to youth, consider the following guidelines:
- treat participants as partners and involve them in major decisions;
- emphasize life skills and other positive concepts rather than deviance and ill health;
- serve the needs and concerns of youth;
- respond to the changing needs of participants, especially ethnic, cultural and racial styles and norms;
- wherever feasible, employ youth as program staff and evaluators;
- make the program materials age-appropriate and responsive to transitional periods;
- ensure program continuity, predictability and membership stability over time;
- introduce the program in familiar, neutral settings; and
- provide opportunities for youth to demonstrate skills and earn recognition for accomplishments.

Actions for Government and Youth-Serving Institutions

Policy implications and recommendations directed to schools, youth-serving agencies and government decision makers include:
- Reduce the number of school programs specifically concerning health and social development. Too many independent targeted programs can have negative effects. Schools lack the organizational structure and resources to implement, monitor, evaluate, and revise a plethora of independent programs. Schools do better with single, multiyear, coordinated, comprehensive health education and social competence

programs focused on physical, mental, social and emotional health (Weissberg and Elias 1993). Provide process and outcome evaluation of such initiatives, and adapt program language and content to the community.

- Work with education officials to review and approve all mental health and social development curricula brought into schools. Create scientific standards to ensure that programs are acceptable, effective, and culturally and developmentally appropriate. Valid standards will prevent schools from wasting time and money on materials that use endorsements, packaging and psychological jargon to promise more than they can deliver.

- Offer incentives to communities to create after-school youth development organizations that meet specific demand from youth and have governing structures that include parents, educators and youth-serving agencies. Identify businesses that are interested in the quality of community life and, through time-off or flextime arrangements, help their employees volunteer in community organizations. Provide guidelines for building coalitions of youth-serving agencies, parents and youth who can share resources, and own and promote the program (Children and their Prospects 1995).

- Announce a competitive funding program at least five years long for the establishment of networks of excellence for creating and testing primary prevention programs for adolescents. These "Networks for the Promotion of Adolescent Social Competence and Well-Being" would comprise youth, parents, educators, researchers and health and community service practitioners to develop model programs and evaluate their effects in various community contexts. When advertising the funding program, provide a generic model that can be adapted to local contexts rather than a rigid set of program specifications.

- Ask education authorities and national community service and health organizations about implementing options for community service internships, including options that would earn academic credit. Offer a variety of service opportunities ranging from in-school tutoring to practicums with the elderly, wildlife and conservation programs, and recreation and child care. Create a registry of community volunteer opportunities for youth, and allow groups of volunteer youth to reflect on, gain feedback about, and share their experiences with peers and an adult facilitator. Consult Bachelor of Social Work (B.S.W.) programs for the mechanics and quality control of such internship opportunities. Ensure that cooperative work placements in service settings are available for middle and high school students.

Government Policy Initiatives

- Ask the office of the Secretary of State for Training and Youth and Human Resources Development Canada about grants to foster mentoring programs, particularly for at-risk youth. Such mentoring programs could be sponsored by ethnic and cultural organizations, such as the Black Business Professionals Association or Kiwanis or Rotary Clubs, but always in partnership with youth-serving agencies (e.g., the YMCA) or education institutions. The mentoring context could relate to work development (e.g., banking), academics (e.g., reading or mathematics), or leisure skills (e.g., sports), providing a range of ways for adults and youth to interact. Mentors would contract to mentor youth for a fixed period of time and would receive honoraria, recognition certificates and reimbursement for expenses. Guidelines for planning and implementation (e.g., screening and matching mentors and protégés) would be generated by a panel composed of people experienced in mentoring initiatives, public servants (e.g., administrators of Youth Internship Grants at Human Resources Development Canada), education authorities, national youth-serving organizations, parents and youth.
- The Conference Board of Canada (perhaps through its Work and Family Council) and appropriate branches of the federal government (e.g., Human Resources Development Canada, Health Canada, Secretary of State for Training and Youth) should meet with business, labour, education authorities and youth-serving agencies to discuss the introduction of employer-based mentoring programs. These programs would either enrich existing cooperative learning high school programs by involving mentors, or send mentors from the workplace to meet with protégés in the community. The meeting should be chaired by an influential business leader who has encouraged employees to become involved in youth service activities. For example, Courtney Pratt, the CEO of Noranda, has made community service part of all employees' professional development and an essential component of employee performance appraisals. Pratt is currently chairing a mentoring initiative launched by the Learning Partnership in Toronto, Ontario.
- Secondary school co-op programs are ideal recruiting and deploying adult mentors because students are often placed in large workplaces with many potential mentors. Mentors should not be supervisors because evaluation and support are often antagonistic processes. Instead, a protégé needs both a supervisor and a mentor. Co-op teachers should offer orientation sessions in the workplace for interested mentors, negotiating arrangements with employers so mentors can work with protégés on company time. For example, in an Ontario program called

Reading Partners, volunteer employee-mentors spend two paid and two unpaid hours a week reading to protégés.

- Public and private sector employers and labour unions should encourage retirees to become youth mentors. Retiree organizations can target schools, youth organizations or at-risk youth, and provide retiree-mentors with resource materials, recognition, space and ongoing support. Such a program should allow mentors to choose how they want to get involved and contract with them for a minimum period of involvement to ensure that protégés can form stable, satisfying, confiding relationships with their mentors. Intergenerational mentoring initiatives can be important to elderly retirees because they offer them a public and meaningful social role while capitalizing on their personal strengths and job skills. For protégés, mentoring ties can enhance intergenerational communication and understanding.

- Local Chambers of Commerce and school boards should receive incentives to create company "adoption" or sponsorship programs in which middle and high schools serve as contexts for focused mentoring and job experience. With strong partnerships between secondary schools and employers, the cycle of career training, advising, practical experience, apprenticeship, permanent employment and occupational adjustment can be completed more smoothly.

- Establish a youth mentoring registry through the school board. Offer various mentoring opportunities for qualified adults. Recruit, screen and match mentors to youth, offer mentors ongoing group support, and reimburse mentors for their expenses (up to a maximum). A school official would advertise and promote the program's benefits, risks and challenges through civic organizations, employers and school-community councils.

- Because all mentoring programs must control risks to protégés, program funding should cover police and reference checks for all adult partici-pants. Police community relations or youth divisions may be willing to perform this necessary task. If even one protégé is harmed by a mentor, or if the public believes that a mentor could harm a protégé, the entire enterprise is in jeopardy.

Benjamin H. Gottlieb *is a professor in the Department of Psychology at the University of Guelph. He obtained a joint Ph.D. in psychology and social work from the University of Michigan, and is a fellow of both of the American and Canadian Psychological Associations. Dr. Gottlieb has authored and edited several volumes on the subject of coping and social support, of which the most recent is* Coping with Chronic Stress *(1997).*

Acknowledgements

The author gratefully acknowledges the generosity of the following persons who provided rapid information about the programs and issues addressed in this paper: Robert Brown, Toronto Board of Education; Gordon Cressy, The Learning Partnership, Toronto, Ontario; Steven Danish, Virginia Commonwealth University; Bob Gifford, The Vanier Institute of the Family; Kathleen Guy, The Healthy Child Development Project; Colin Maloney, Catholic Children's Aid Society of Toronto; Sandra J. McElhaney, National Mental Health Association; Dan Offord, Centre for Studies of Children at Risk, McMaster University; Ruby Takanishi, Carnegie Council on Adolescent Development; Jen Tipper, Canadian Institute of Child Health; Roger Weissberg, University of Illinois, Chicago Circle; Betty Yung, Wright State University.

BIBLIOGRAPHY

ASSEMBLY OF FIRST NATIONS. 1988. *Assembly of First Nations Initial Response to Task Force Report on Child and Family Services in Canada.*

BAUMRIND, D. 1971. Current patterns of parental authority. *Developmental Psychology Monographs* 4 (1, pt. 2).

BEARDSLEE, W.R., and PODOREFSKY, D. 1988. Resilient adolescents whose parents have serious affective and other psychiatric disorders: Importance of self-understanding and relationships. *American Journal of Psychiatry* 145: 63–69.

CANADA. SENATE. SPECIAL SENATE COMMITTEE ON YOUTH. 1986. *Youth: A Plan of Action.* Ottawa: Minister of Supply and Services Canada.

CANADIAN FITNESS AND LIFESTYLE RESEARCH INSTITUTE. 1990. STEPHENS, T., and CRAIG, C. L. *The Well-Being of Canadians: Highlights of the 1988 Campbell's Survey.*

CANADIAN INSTITUTE FOR ADVANCED RESEARCH AND CENTRE FOR STUDIES OF CHILDREN AT RISK. 1995. *Healthy Children, Healthy Communities: A Compendium of Approaches from across Canada.*

CANADIAN INSTITUTE OF CHILD HEALTH. 1994. *The Health of Canada's Children: A CICH Profile.* Ottawa: Canadian Institute of Child Health.

CAPLAN, M., WEISSBERG, R., GROBER, J., SIVO, P., GRADY, K., and JACOBY, C. 1992. Social competence promotion with inner-city and suburban young adolescents: Effects on social adjustment and alcohol use. *Journal of Consulting and Clinical Psychology* 60: 56–63.

CARNEGIE COUNCIL ON ADOLESCENT DEVELOPMENT. 1992. *A Matter of Time: Risk and Opportunity in the Nonschool Hours.* New York: Carnegie Corporation of New York.

_____. n.d. Task force on education of young adolescents. *Turning Points: Preparing American Youth for the 21st Century.* Washington: Carnegie Council on Adolescent Development.

COMPAS, B. E. 1993. Promoting positive mental health during adolescence. In *Promoting the Health of Adolescents*, eds. S. MILSTEIN, A. PETERSEN, and E. NIGHTINGALE. New York: Oxford University Press.

CONSORTIUM ON THE SCHOOL-BASED PROMOTION OF SOCIAL COMPETENCE. 1994. The school-based promotion of social competence: Theory, research, practice, and policy. In *Stress, Risk, and Resilience in Children and Adolescents*, eds. R. J. HAGGERTY, L. R. SHERROD, N. GARMEZY, and M. RUTTER. New York: Cambridge University Press.

COOLEY, E. A. SINGER, G. H., and IRVIN, L. K. 1989. Volunteers as part of family support services for families of developmentally disabled members. *Education and Training in Mental Retardation* 52: 207–218.

ELIAS, M., and CLABBY, J. 1992. *Building Social Problem-Solving Skills: Guidelines from a School-Based Program.* San Francisco: Jossey-Bass.

FELNER, R. D., GINTER, M., and PRIMAVERA, J. 1982. Primary prevention during school transitions: Social support and environmental structure. *American Journal of Community Psychology* 10: 277–290.

FREEDMAN, M. 1991. *The Kindness of Strangers: Reflections on the Mentoring Movement.* Philadelphia: Public/Private Ventures.

GARMEZY, N. 1983. Stressors of childhood. In *Stress, Coping, and Development in Children*, eds. N. GARMEZY, and M. RUTTER. New York: McGraw Hill.

GOTTLIEB, B. H. 1988. Support interventions: A typology and agenda for research. In *Handbook of Personal Relationships*, ed. S. DUCK. Chichester, U.K.: Sage Publications. pp. 519–541.

_____. In press. Support groups. In *Encyclopedia of Mental Health*, ed. H. S. FRIEDMAN. San Francisco: Academic Press.

HAMILTON, S. 1994. Social roles for youth: Interventions in unemployment. In *Youth Unemployment and Society*, eds. A.C. PETERSEN, and J.T. MORTIMER. New York: Cambridge University Press.

HAMMOND, R., and YUNG, B. 1991. Preventing violence in at-risk African American youth. *Journal of Health Care for the Poor and Underserved* 2: 359–373.

———. 1993. *Evaluation and Activity Report: Positive Adolescent Choices Training*. Unpublished grant report. Washington: U.S. Maternal and Child Health Bureau.

HEALTH AND WELFARE CANADA. 1992. KING, A., AND COLE, B. *The Health of Canada's Youth: Views and Behaviours of 11, 13, and 15 year olds from 11 Countries.* Ottawa: Minister of Supply and Services Canada.

JONES, M. B., and OFFORD, D. R. 1989. Reduction of antisocial behaviour in poor children by non-school skill-development. *Journal of Child Psychology and Psychiatry* 30: 737–750.

———. 1991. After the demonstration project. Paper presented at the annual meeting of the American Association for the Advancement of Science, Washington (DC).

KALTER, N., SCHAEFER, M., LESOWITZ, M., ALPERN, D., and PICKAR, J. 1988. School-based support groups for children of divorce. In *Marshalling Social Support: Formats, Processes, and Effects,* ed. B.H. GOTTLIEB. Newbury Park: Sage. pp. 165–186.

PEDRO-CARROLL, J., COWEN, E., HIGHTOWER, D., and GUARE, J. 1986. Preventive interventions with latency-aged children of divorce: A replication study. *American Journal of Community Psychology* 14: 277–290.

RICHARDSON, J., DWYER, K., HANSEN, W., DENT, C., JOHNSON, C., SUSSMAN, S., BRANNON, B., and FLAG, B. 1989. Substance use among eighth-grade students who take care of themselves after school. *Pediatrics* 84: 556–566.

RUTTER, M. 1983. Stress, coping, and development: Some issues and some questions. In *Stress, Coping, and Development in Children,* eds. N. GARMEZY, and M. RUTTER. New York: McGraw Hill.

STATISTICS CANADA. 1994. *Suicide in Canada.* Ottawa: Minister of Supply and Services Canada.

SCHINE, J. 1989. *Young Adolescents and Community Service.* Washington: Carnegie Council on Adolescent Development.

THE LAIDLAW FOUNDATION NEWSLETTER. 1995. *Children and Their Prospects.* Toronto: The Laidlaw Foundation.

THE MCCREARY CENTRE SOCIETY. 1993. *Adolescent Health Survey.* Province of British Columbia.

U.S. DEPARTMENT OF EDUCATION, OFFICE OF EDUCATIONAL RESEARCH AND IMPROVEMENT, NATIONAL CENTER FOR EDUCATION STATISTICS. 1990. *National Education Longitudinal Study of 1988: A Profile of the American Eighth Grader.* Washington: U.S. Government Printing Office.

WARRY, W. 1991. Ontario's First People. In *Children, Families and Public Policy in the '90s,* eds. L. JOHNSON, and D. BARNHORST. Toronto: Thompson Educational Publishing, Inc.

YUNG, B., and HAMMOND, W. R. 1995. *PACT: Positive Adolescent Choices Training.* Champaign: Research Press.

Making the Transition from School to Employment

PAUL ANISEF, PH.D.

Professor of Sociology
York University

SUMMARY

Empirical research has produced the data required to identify the predictors of early school leaving, but its models do not address the overall complexity of the issue. In fact, the current models, such as frustration–self-esteem, frequently lead to finger pointing and victim blaming, and have little to contribute to an understanding of the situation of today's youth. One fact is clear: youth unemployment is high and rising, but Canadian schools do not prepare students for today's job market.

Current research clearly indicates that youth at risk of dropping out of school understand and accept the importance of formal education; true dropout rates are lower than past research has suggested, and they continue to decline. Moreover, many dropouts realize that the severe labour market disadvantages they face arise from their lack of credentials, and return to school. However, it is clear that Aboriginal youth and young people from socioeconomically disadvantaged backgrounds, visible minorities and remote rural areas are especially vulnerable to marginalization during their transition to adulthood. Although field studies show no significant gender-related variations in dropout rates, some important gender-related variations are not revealed by statistics on early school leaving. For example, girls are more likely than boys to leave school because of impending parenthood, and boys are more likely than girls to drop out because they dislike school or have behaviourial problems. Also, girls are less likely than boys to enrol in general or basic courses, in which dropout rates are highest.

The underlying factor in early school leaving is frequently socioeconomic status. For example, poor academic performance, remote rural location and Aboriginal ethnicity—powerful predictors of early school leaving that are even more significant in combination—are very likely to indicate low socioeconomic status. The 'dropout problem' can, therefore, be viewed as the problem of perpetuating social and cultural inequality in Canada.

Policymakers need an inclusive analytical framework that includes interrelated individual, family, school, community and government policy factors that affect the school-to-work transition for early school leavers and dropouts who return to school. Success stories about transition programs available in Canada do not meet this need.

A review of the literature on the school-to-work transition for contemporary Canadian youth reveals important changes. Transition patterns are more complex and less linear today than at any time in the past. Despite the uncertainty of their future, most youth are hopeful; a very large proportion of Canadian youth and their parents aspire to postsecondary education, especially university, during the high school years. Unfortunately, the proportion of youth who can realize their aspirations for higher education will decline significantly.

Very few school-to-work transition programs have been formally evaluated, and there is not enough evidence to gauge the effectiveness of alternative approaches. When using the program evaluations that are available, we must account for variations in program type and evaluation methodology. For example, who was asked to judge program effectiveness—staff or client? When comparing results, are all time frames more or less equivalent? Students who report short-term benefits from a transition program may have grave difficulty finding or keeping jobs—a negative outcome that would be revealed only by a long-term assessment.

Experts on current school-to-work transition programs related to student retention were contacted, and two Ontario programs—Change Your Future and the Ontario Youth Apprenticeship Program—chosen for effectiveness and variety of strategies, were profiled. A recent two-year Ontario Ministry of Education and Training project, Education-Work Connections was also chosen for review.

The 'stay-in-school' approach of the late 1980s and early 1990s is giving way to a school-to-work transition approach in Canada. This new approach has significant policy implications for both educators and employers; handled with leadership, cooperation and commitment to covering the true costs, however, school-to-work transition programs could meet the needs of youth for employment and employers' needs for skilled workers.

TABLE OF CONTENTS

PART 1 – FORMULATING THE ISSUE

STATEMENT OF POSITION

For many young Canadians, the transition to adulthood is prolonged and difficult. Difficulties arise from significant economic, social and cultural changes. Economic restructuring has adversely affected the job market for youth and, over the past several decades, unemployment rates have increased substantially. From the perspective of health determinants, ignoring the needs of youth could lead to serious consequences, such as increased youth crime, loss of human capital and erosion of citizenship (Looker and Lowe 1995, 3).

Average real wages for young people have dropped. Although most people believe that postsecondary education is required to enhance job opportunities, a significant minority of high school students in Canada leave school early without graduating. They are either 'pushed out' by factors related to their school environment, factors related to social structure (e.g., social class, culture, racism) or choose to leave for personal reasons. Dropping out of school is no longer considered a single act but as part of a long, gradual disengagement from school.

It is important to treat early school leaving as an interactive transition or process involving relationships among students, families, schools and communities. By defining early school leaving as a transition or process of disengagement, I suggest that it is reversible; many young people who leave high school without a diploma return later to complete their studies. Whatever the case, if we are to identify interventions that offer positive alternatives to early school leaving, we must learn why students disengage. Early school leavers share many of the values of high school graduates but, because of their handicaps in today's competitive, polarized job market, they are marginalized in Canadian society.

Furthermore, I contend that early school leavers are not a homogeneous group. Many could benefit from the school-to-work intervention strategies described in this paper. However, a significant minority of youth are functionally illiterate and alienated, and at high risk of substance abuse and involvement in crime. At a time when governments are cutting back spending in an effort to balance budgets, vulnerable groups stand to suffer most. The needs and problems of Aboriginal youth, disadvantaged visible-minority youth, working class youth and youth from remote rural areas are particularly pressing.

No quick fix or recipe for success will work for all youth. Interventions must respond to unique needs and problems, and build on the good will and motivation of the community, school officials and other partners. These caveats will help policymakers prepare to forge strategies to enable youth to deal with an uncertain social and economic environment and reduce fragmented or fractured transitions.

INTRODUCTION

A research and policy symposium on youth in transition to adulthood, held in Kananaskis, Alberta, April 25–29, 1995, discussed preparation for the world of work, particularly for youth. The gathering agreed that recent policy reports from government and nongovernment organizations signalled a rethinking of the best ways to develop individual potential at school and at work. Two assumptions underlie this mode of thought. The first is that many graduates do not find suitable employment; the second is that research reveals a poor fit between education system outputs and employer needs (Looker and Lowe 1995). The core research issues raised at the symposium concerned how the education system fails those who drop out.

In addition to presenting methods to ease the transition between school and work, this paper will discuss social and cultural change and its effect on the development of youth in Canadian society. In addition to emphasizing strategies to maximize school attendance, we must also address the task of providing effective strategies for smoothing the transition to work for Canadian youth. The school-to-work transition has become increasingly complex and often involves multiple entries and exits. Canadian society has changed. New strategies are needed.

Almost 20 percent of Canadian youth cannot find jobs, and those who do are frequently stuck in entry-level positions because the competition from older workers for better jobs is so fierce (Canada. Human Resources Development Canada 1995). The workforce participation rate of youth throughout Canada dropped from 70 percent in 1990 to 62.6 percent in April 1995, mainly because of discouragement factors and the "jobless recovery." In real numbers, there are about 400,000 unemployed youth in Canada, and it costs about $4.5 billion to maintain them on social assistance (Canada. Human Resources Development Canada 1995). Moreover, people aged 15–24 now form a smaller proportion of the population and of the labour force than ever before. In 1980, this group made up 27 percent of the labour force, but only 19 percent in 1990 (Kerr 1992).

A recent study by the Canadian Federation of Youth used focus group interviews to document the employment experiences of Canadians between the ages of 15 and 29. The study sample included a social cross section, including middle-class, Aboriginal, immigrant and street youth. Despite variations, common themes were expressed across the range of groups. Most of the study subjects saw themselves as "occupationally challenged" despite their best efforts to find good, long-term employment (Canadian Federation of Youth 1995b, 1). All participants coped with unemployment as well as they could, but they expressed frustration, particularly around the feeling that institutions, such as schools, could do more. For example, participants claimed, schools do not offer enough apprenticeships and practicums, or provide youth with enough information and counselling at ages early enough to move them to the labour market effectively.

A cautionary note is in order, however. As Levin indicates, high youth underemployment does not indicate that Canada suffers from serious job shortages. The evidence seems to suggest that total skill level requirements have increased slightly (Levin 1995, 10). Indeed, Canadian studies show that a secondary school diploma does not guarantee the holder a meaningful full-time job. Recent high school graduates without postsecondary education have approximately the same labour market outcomes (i.e., wages) as high school dropouts (Levin 1995, 16). But, because graduation is the key to further education and better career paths, the gap between high school graduates and dropouts widens in the long term.

FRAMING THE PROBLEM

Allyson Holbrook (1993), an Australian scholar, provides useful insights on school-to-work transitions:

> In the contemporary discourse, 'Youth Transition' refers to a range of issues raised by the current prolonged experience of youth unemployment. At another level, transition is conceptualized as a positive transformation or conversion from one state of being to another. Progression, and hence linearity, is implicit. Transition from school to work involves an institutional shift and a concomitant change in experience and expectations. Given the 'desirability' of a close relationship between schooling and work, it has generally been assumed that the best and most effective transition is a 'smooth' one, i.e., the young person finds the job that they are suited for quickly and stays there long enough to satisfy the demands of their employer and to ensure their own and society's stability (p. 3).

Although youth in the 1990s face life course transitions that are no more disorderly and stressful than youth in earlier decades, it is safe to assume that the nature of life course transitions, and particularly school-to-work transitions, has changed dramatically in recent years. In the 1950s, starting a full-time job, leaving home, getting married and having children were fairly well-connected transitions for young people. Today, economic restructuring, globalization and other social changes mean that these transitions are frequently longer and more difficult. According to Statistics Canada labour force data, the number of youth holding part-time jobs has doubled in the last decade. At present, 43 percent of all employed 15–24-year-olds work part time (Canadian Federation of Youth 1995a, 15). Of this group, 55 percent are female. This increase in part-time employment signals a lack of full-time jobs, not a lifestyle change. Young people today encounter a more transient employment pattern and a more difficult school-to-work transition.

It is important to examine the school-to-work transition as a process that has become increasingly complex, nonlinear and uncertain (Anisef and Axelrod 1993). School systems designed to socialize young Canadians for an industrial society now must adapt to an age of technological communication (Anisef 1994a).

Buchmann's study of two American cohorts—one from the 1960s and the other from the 1980s—established that job market factors, such as a decline in full-time employment opportunities, caused the school-to-work transition experienced by the 1980s cohort to be longer than the transition of the 1960s cohort. Buchmann concludes that, for the 1980s cohort, the school-to-work transition was "a process of gradual integration rather than clear demarcation" (Buchmann 1989).

In Canada, too, researchers have found longer transitions. One reason for the blurred transition from student to worker is that, unlike Britain and especially Germany, Canada permits individuals to leave and reenter the education system without institutional or social penalty (Krahn and Lowe 1991, 130–170).

Macmillan's research indicates the social cost of a prolonged transition to adulthood that is directly related to job opportunities for youth (Macmillan 1995, 51–79). Social changes, including increased youth unemployment, and older age at first marriage and parenthood, prolong the transition to adulthood. These factors and the decrease in average real wages for young workers also tend to prevent the formation of social bonds between individuals and in society at large. Crime is a significant consequence of a lack of social bonds.

The effects of changes in family composition and structure, youth culture, and the job market suggest that Canada needs new education and learning policies that respond to a dynamic model of health. Although the National Forum on Health recognizes that a wide range of factors beyond health care affect the health of Canadians (e.g., physical environment, genetics, and social and economic circumstances), it is equally important the Forum adopt a dynamic model of health that reflects the effects of significant social, cultural and economic changes in Canadian society. Furthermore, the Forum must understand the need for forging strategies to help youth move into adulthood in an uncertain social and economic climate. The frontier between school and employment has become increasingly blurred for students, and this trend will probably become more pronounced. One example of this blurring is the trend for high school students to hold part-time jobs (Anisef 1994a, 131–154).

In advanced postindustrial societies, the family gives way to large corporations and bureaucratic schools. Often the interests and goals of schools and families are contradictory, and young people's lives tend to be segmented by opposing influences (Anisef 1994, 13). As a result, youth are particularly vulnerable to rapid social and economic change.

The conclusion of this position paper includes recommendations for action on public policy principles to give policymakers a basis for practical advice on school-to-work transitions and student retention.

KEY FACTORS IN EXAMINING SCHOOL-TO-WORK TRANSITIONS AND STUDENT RETENTION

In examining the transition from school to work and its relationship to student retention, we must keep in mind several key factors, including gender, socioeconomic status, race, ethnicity and location. Canadian youth come from families with a wide variety of cultural and economic backgrounds, and many speak languages other than English and French. Regional diversity strongly influences the experiences and learning needs of Canadian students, and gender differences further increase the range of student needs. The education system has not kept pace with the increasing diversity of its student population.[1]

Gender

At a general level, the transition to adulthood varies by gender, although studies as recently as the mid-1980s have focused exclusively on male experience (Hogan 1981). Studies have found that males are more likely than females to drop out of school (Tanner, Krahn, and Hartnagel 1995). Also, successful transition is more critical to the perceived adult status of men, while marriage is more critical to the perceived adult status of women (Green and Wheatley 1992, 667–686).

As a concept, gender both operationalizes biological sex and represents socialized and institutionalized patterns of behaviour specific to males and females. Thus, the educational achievement of females, which is linked to their career trajectories, is based not only on individual choices, but also on socially sanctioned and influenced opportunities. In Canada, the differences in labour market outcomes for male and female graduates are attributable to sex-segregated labour market structures, union and profession membership, and specific job conditions (Hughes and Lowe 1993). According to Mandell and Crysdale (1993), an informal curriculum in schools has served to exclude and misrepresent women's experiences for decades.

Young males presume that parenthood will propel them into the labour market, while young females presume that parenthood will push them out of the labour force. The traditional images of the male breadwinner and the

---

1. Region of residence (i.e., whether youth live in urban, rural or remote rural areas) is important, and will be discussed in the next section.

female homemaker remain intact, despite the substantial educational attainments of women in recent years (Looker 1995).

In Schneider's 1994 examination of young people's ideas about future occupations, schools were found to encourage the formation of distinct gender identities. She notes that teachers and friends of both genders tend to discourage female students from enrolling in advanced courses. Unfortunately, teachers and guidance counsellors influence the course of action of young adults in gender-specific and sometimes detrimental ways.

Males tend to derive greater economic benefits from their education than females, and this difference becomes more pronounced as education increases (Willits 1988). Parallel results were reported in a recent study of British and German youth, which showed that males and females are not equally rewarded for extended education (Evans and Heinz 1994).

Socioeconomic Status

The relationship between individual socioeconomic status and career outcomes is also gender specific. Research documents an indirect relationship between socioeconomic status and occupational attainment and earnings, as mediated by the strong relationship between socioeconomic status and educational achievement (Krahn and Lowe 1991). Moreover, the development of career aspirations is related to the socioeconomic status of an individual's family of origin, and the role of career aspirations is frequently contingent on labour market conditions (Empson-Warner and Krahn 1992). Researchers have also noted a decreasing effect of socioeconomic origins on individuals' outcomes as they move through life.

People born with class advantages tend to maintain them, however. Krahn and Lowe discovered:

> … a disintegration of the traditional boundary between student and worker roles. But changes in the school-to-work transition have not altered the structure of inequality in Canadian society…young people from higher socioeconomic backgrounds are still more likely to stay in school. Class differences in postsecondary educational attainment persist despite rising educational levels. Yet youth continue to value higher education (cited in Levin 1995, 15).

In their study of British and German youth, Evans and Heinz report that individuals from middle-class origins have longer domestic transitions than people from working-class origins, and that this stretching of transitions is accompanied by a dissociation of transition stages. For example, it is no longer necessary to exit from one status before beginning another (e.g., student worker). Evans and Heinz also find that working-class youth seek sources of identity stabilization other than employment when they cannot find jobs (Evans and Heinz 1994, 62).

Race and Ethnicity

Canadian research on the school-to-work transition includes only a limited examination of the effects of race and ethnicity on occupational attainment or earnings after leaving school. Some work has been done on Aboriginal and immigrant youth experiences in the school system. Jones (1994) notes that Aboriginal youth are more likely to drop out of school than other students. Aboriginal youths' experiences in the white, middle-class school system, and the resulting damage to their self-image, help to explain why Aboriginal students have lower completion rates.

James' longitudinal study examines the relationship between social conditions and the experiences of black youth. In this study, black youth in Canada see themselves as disadvantaged, and use strategies such as self-confidence, determination and hard work to improve their social situation (James 1994). In a recently released report, George S. Dei and colleagues indicate that black African Canadian students and parents are deeply concerned about the structural schooling processes that tend to disengage black students. This study suggests that the structures of learning, teaching and administration in our schools are at fault, not parents (Dei et al. 1995).

Examining the experiences of immigrants in the Canadian education system, Lam states that Jewish and Chinese youth are two to three times more likely to complete a university degree than other Canadians. Most Canadians of West European and East European descent have about an average probability of completing university, while Canadians of South European descent have the least chance. Lam is also quick to point out that high educational attainment does not necessarily result in success in the labour market. "Census data have indicated that people from black, Chinese and Greek communities face the most discrimination in employment because of their ethnic origin" (Lam 1994, 123). Lam also notes that, although Asian immigrant youth are usually associated with high educational attainment, Indochinese youth often quit school and take jobs to help support their families.

Hogan (1981) finds a variety of patterns among racial and ethnic groups. For example, black Hispanic males with four years of high school experience a higher rate of school interruptions than average, but at higher levels of education they have lower rates of school interruption and are more likely to take longer to complete school. In contrast, men of East European and Russian origin have fewer school interruptions than average when they have less than a high school education, but more interruptions if they have four or more years of college; they also tend to take longer to complete school. Hogan finds that, although blacks, Hispanics, East European and Russian males complete school at comparatively late ages, they adhere to normative patterns when family resources are taken into account.

MAJOR CONCLUSIONS FROM THE DROPOUT LITERATURE RELATING TO SCHOOL-TO-WORK TRANSITIONS

A vast array of literature deals with school dropouts, but this literature is more confusing than enlightening. Recent work in the field indicates that dropping out arises from a complex assortment of factors that, when taken together, make the overall problem very difficult to define (Canada. Human Resources Development Canada 1994). Dropping out is frequently conceptualized in terms of unfavourable educational outcomes that result from individual choice and hold negative consequences for the economic well-being of individuals, communities and the nation. Policymakers often adopt a deficit approach that defines schools and students as "broken" and research attempts to isolate the faulty parts. By treating dropping out as a single or final act and omitting distinctions between dropping out, stopping out and fading out, this approach defines leaving school as an exit rather than as part of a transition (Bellamy, Ross, and Anisef 1994). The interrelationship of students, families, schools and communities is not well understood, and the various theories that have been offered (e.g., frustration–self-esteem, participation-identification, deviance) do not provide a model extensive enough for examining all educational outcomes, including early school leaving (Andres and Anisef 1995).

Another school of thought, described by Kelly (1994, 1), defines non-completers as pushouts. Researchers employing this framework see the factors emphasized by the dropout model as symptoms rather than causes. This model focuses on unequal economic, political and social structures, and school practices, such as tracking and expulsion, that combine to discourage, stigmatize and exclude children. The 'dropout' concept blames the individual, and the 'pushout' concept blames institutions that purge unwilling victims.

It is increasingly clear that dropping out of school, like the school-to-work transition, is a process that occurs over time and varies from person to person. Recent work on early school leaving places more emphasis on a mutual process of rejection or what can be called disengagement (Kelly 1994, 2). This term suggests a long-term, interactive process that may be reversible, encouraging researchers to "connect events in students' lives over time and look for cumulative effects" (Kelly 1994, 3). Renihan notes, "Whatever the case, it is important that we recognize why students disengage, in order to accommodate the interventions most likely to furnish positive alternatives to early school leaving" (Renihan and Associates 1994, 11).

METHODOLOGICAL ISSUES

Before summarizing the major conclusions from a review of dropout literature, we must point out several methodological problems in this field of enquiry. First, there seems to be no single definition of "dropout." In some Canadian school districts, students who marry, transfer to another school, are expelled, fail a grade or take a job are counted as dropouts but, in other districts, none of these students would be counted as dropouts (Renihan and Associates 1994, 12). This inconsistency of definition is compounded by such methodological inconsistencies as: different time frames for calculating and reporting data; different ways of counting students who drop out during the summer; different baseline populations (e.g., K-10 and K-12); different ways of counting special education students; different ways of adjusting the count when students return to school; and counting only full-time students. These methodological problems must be resolved.

MAJOR CONCLUSIONS[2]

Major conclusions gleaned from reviewing the extensive literature on dropouts in North America are summarized under eight headings.

Dropout Rates

Contrary to popular belief, repeated by journalists, politicians and educators, that 33 percent of young Canadians drop out of high school before graduation, recent Statistics Canada studies show that the rate is closer to 18 percent. Examination reveals that the dropout rate has been declining slowly for several decades, and the current, hostile labour market has encouraged even more to stay in school. Many young people who leave school early choose to return months, or even years, later. The 1991 School Leavers' Survey estimated that about 25 percent drop out of high school at some stage, but about 50 percent of early leavers return to school, sometimes at a different type of institution, and many stay until they graduate.

Importance of Demographic, Family and Social-Cultural Background

Virtually all studies establish a strong link between family background (i.e., income level, occupational status, level of education) and early disengagement

---

2. The primary sources for these conclusions are Tanner, Krahn & Hartnagel (1995); Anisef (1994a); Anisef (1994b); Dei (1995a) and Canada. Human Resources Development Canada (1994).

from high school. Family background has a wide range of both direct and indirect effects, including: intellectual stimulation in the preschool years, communication of high educational expectations, interest in school-related activities, parenting style, and children's aspiration levels. Since lack of secondary and postsecondary schooling makes it very difficult to land a job, the tendency for members of disadvantaged groups to drop out of school contributes to persistent familial patterns of social inequality.

Family structure and support seem to be important influences on academic achievement and the eventual decision to drop out. Students from single-parent households and large families are much more likely to drop out. Teachers are more likely to assess students from mother-headed households as having conduct, personality or immaturity problems.

Dropout rates are higher in rural areas and small communities, especially Aboriginal communities. Research indicates that urban students are more likely to recognize the importance of a high school diploma. American studies show a strong link between race and ethnicity and dropping out of school, but there is less evidence of this relationship in Canada.

More males (60 percent) tend to drop out of school than females (40 percent), and studies indicate that males are more likely than females to disengage because of behaviour problems (e.g., suspension or expulsion for failing to cooperate with the teacher) and economic reasons (e.g., being offered a job or helping to support the family). Females are more likely to leave due to impending motherhood. Studies indicate that pregnancy frequently indicates other problems, such as low self-esteem, poor academic achievement and lack of options.

Impact of School-Related Factors and Reasons for Dropping Out

School-related factors are significant to a young person's decision to drop out. Therefore, the size and organization of a school, its resources, and its unique social and educational climate influence its dropout rates. Early disengagement frequently arises not only from problem students, but also from problem schools. Some structural factors have a social class component, since children of prosperous families usually attend schools with more resources.

As dropouts see it, they leave school because they are treated badly there, or because school programs do not meet their learning needs. They see themselves as forced, streamed or pushed out. Schools contribute significantly to the decision to drop out by signalling poor students and students with discipline problems that leaving is an option. Academic failure, boredom and dropping out are frequently linked to streaming or tracking. General and basic-level programs are apparently not challenging or rewarding enough to keep students engaged.

The quality of a school is a major influence on the dropout rate. Teachers' attitudes and practices in the classroom are key determinants of students' perception of success or failure. Teachers can inadvertently "label" students from observing their dress or grooming habits, and the attitudes arising from these labels can affect academic results.

Most research indicates that dropouts most frequently cite school-related reasons for quitting. Difficulty with school work, problems getting along with teachers, boredom, and general alienation from school culture and the education system are common reasons.

Employment-related reasons are mentioned less often, and few dropouts leave school to work full time out of financial necessity. Dropouts seem to be attracted to full-time employment because of adult status and the freedom and money that come with it, particularly if they feel rejected or frustrated at school.

Personal reasons, including problems in getting along with family members, emotional difficulties, poor health and pregnancy, are cited less frequently than school- or employment-related reasons. Problems at home, the most frequently cited, can upset or distract students, causing their school work to suffer, their self-esteem to drop, and their interest in school to decline.

Dropping Out as a Process

Dropping out cannot be seen as a single act. It is an event in a long process of gradual disengagement from the education system involving many interrelated factors at the individual, family, school, community, job market and government policy levels. The process perspective reveals some of its complexities (e.g., the many dropouts who 'drop back') and suggests interventions that might help raise graduation rates.

Dropouts and the Job Market

Studies in the past decade demonstrate that high school dropouts earn less than graduates and are more likely to be unemployed. The negative consequences of leaving school early are even more acute in today's rapidly changing job market than they were 10 or 20 years ago. As unemployment rates remain high, especially among youth, and part-time employment becomes more common, the job market is becoming more polarized. Better-educated people compete for a limited number of high-skilled, well-paid jobs, dislodging the less-educated from a declining number of middle-level jobs. High school dropouts, at the tail of the job seekers' lineup, must accept work at the lowest levels of the secondary job market.

Dropouts' Coping Techniques[3]

Most dropouts cope with poor jobs and frequent unemployment. They prefer work over unemployment, but at times must accept support from family and friends to ride out the worst effects of unemployment and underemployment. More than 50 percent live with parents or siblings, and only a few are truly isolated—i.e., living on the street or in shelters—and they suffer no more than others in the same situation.

Dropouts have several psychological coping strategies—e.g., gratitude even for poor jobs ("It's better than no job at all") or for pleasant relationships with co-workers when other rewards are conspicuously absent. The most important coping strategy is a conviction that they will someday return to school to obtain the diploma they need to get a better job.

Dropouts and the Dominant Value System

In comparisons of dropouts and graduates, the most important difference is the higher level of crime and drug use noted among dropouts. On the other hand, many dropouts look back on leaving school early as a bad decision, remain committed to the value of education, and firmly believe that they will return to school some day. Faced with marginal jobs and/or unemployment, dropouts cope by clinging to a conviction that further education will liberate them from the secondary job market. Research indicates that almost 50 percent of those who leave school without a diploma attempt to return.

The label 'dropout' conjures up an image of highly alienated, disaffected, rebellious youth, but studies show that most dropouts are well integrated into the dominant North American value system. Like high school graduates, dropouts believe in education, want interesting and well-paid jobs, and would like to marry and start families. They may have dropped out for school-related or other personal reasons, but they're not alienated either from school or society as a whole.

Dropouts as a Social Problem

The recent focus on the economic problems of dropouts tends to deflect attention from their social and human problems. Dropping out is a serious social problem, not because dropouts are a threat to society, but because of the damage they do to themselves. Evidence indicates that dropouts constitute a disadvantaged underclass, but there is little evidence that they are ready to explode. Most dropouts share the values and goals of high

---

3. This section on coping is drawn from Tanner, Krahn and Hartnagel's 1995 study of Edmonton dropouts.

school graduates, and their higher levels of deviant behaviour (drugs, alcohol, minor crime), while problematic for society as a whole, simply indicate their social marginalization. This marginalization, which arises from their relegation to the secondary job market, is the real social and human problem of contemporary dropouts.

In today's competitive, polarized job market, opportunities for young people without credentials are very limited, and dropouts are, consequently, severely handicapped. Since children from less-advantaged families are more likely to drop out, a high dropout rate represents a continuing familial pattern of social inequality. The dropout problem is a social problem of individual disadvantage and class inequality.

PART 2 – SUCCESS STORIES

In keeping with the mandate of the Determinants of Health Working Group, we investigated strategies for uncovering and documenting successful methods for facilitating the school-to-work transition for Canadian youth, particularly youth at risk of dropping out of school. After consulting a wide range of experts[4], we profiled two intervention programs. The two programs, both located in Ontario, are *Change Your Future* (CYF) and the *Ontario Youth Apprenticeship Program* (OYAP). OYAP incorporates the Ontario Co-op program in its approach to the transition to work.

As well as profiling these intervention programs, we will summarize a recent Ontario Ministry of Education and Training (MET) project called *Education and Work Connections* (EWC). EWC is MET's effort to coordinate Ontario's community-based transition-to-work programs. We will also review one transition-to-work intervention program. A TVOntario film on EWC gives some valuable insights on strategies for facilitating the school-to-work transition for early school leavers.

We chose CYF and OYAP because:
- experts recommended them;
- they represent a range of strategies and models used in 'best practices' programs; and

---

4. Officials from the Ontario Ministry of Education and Training, including Aryeh Gitterman, Grant Clark and Margaret Murray, were contacted. Robert S. Brown of Research Services, Toronto Board of Education, provided key insights, as did Tom Tidy, a field program evaluator with the National Stay-in-School Initiative. Other contacts for insights and information on transition interventions were: Lorie Cranson, of the school-business organization Learning Partnerships; Susan Wayne, Manager of the Toronto Centre for Career Action, Toronto Board of Education; and Caroline Aubichon and Joanne Lamoth of Youth Services, Human Resources Development Canada.

- we wanted to reflect the complexity of the transitions Canadian youth face—especially youth at risk of dropping out.[5]

But first, we discuss the strategies or models on which interventions are frequently based.

Mentoring and Helping

Mentoring and helping are frequently used with at-risk youth to give individual role model intervention addressing topics such as social and emotional aspects of school, academic requirements and career counselling. Mentors can be community volunteers (especially seniors) who advise and maintain a nonacademic focus; fellow students who help with doing academic work, resisting peer pressure and coping with everyday difficulties; and local business people working in formal partnerships with the school to offer at-risk students positive role models, opportunities to try out career options, and opportunities to apply knowledge and skills acquired in the classroom.[6]

School-to-Work Programs

School-to-work programs generally involve business-education partnerships and can be subdivided into programs that involve only out-of-school activities and programs that combine in-school and out-of-school programming. The former usually involve a work placement under an employer's supervision; such placements vary in length and may include a wage. Almost all school-to-work programs permit students to earn credits for their work placement. In-school programming typically includes a pre-placement workshop on skill assessment, employer expectations, time and money management, job search techniques and goal setting, and seminars to reinforce concepts by relating them to on-the-job situations. A school-to-work program coordinator usually supports students and ensures things go

---

5. Aryeh Gitterman gave me an unpublished report by The ARA Consulting Group, Inc. entitled *School-to-Work and School Retention: Best Practices Research Project, Final Report* prepared for the Ontario Ministry of Education and Training, March, 1993. This report helped me choose programs to profile and offers a good discussion of underlying models or strategies.

6. Robert S. Brown, Research Services, Toronto Board of Education wrote a draft report entitled "Mentoring At-Risk Students: Challenges and Potential," dated October 1995. This report is an excellent overview of mentoring programs, pointing out that the apparent simplicity of the concept of mentoring at-risk students can disguise the enormous complexity of applying it; a great deal more needs to be done before we can see the true picture.

well on the job. The greater the risk of dropping out, the more attention a student usually gets.

Curriculum and Program Modification

This type of program rests on the assumption that teaching must accommodate students' individual learning styles. It is most often seen in alternative school programs such as those established for Aboriginal youth. Alternative school programs focus on selecting course content, teaching methods, educational materials and performance evaluation procedures that apply to the specific needs of the students.

School Organization

The primary focus of this strategy is alternative school programming, emphasizing policies that improve school climate, improve student services such as peer counselling, and recognize attendance and academic achievement. It also focuses on facilitating communication between students, parents, teachers and schools. Alternative schools are generally used to meet the needs of special students (e.g., students with above-average intelligence who have difficulty in regular schools because they are not sequential learners). Highly specialized curricula, special care, individual attention and strong group dynamics are characteristics of effective school organization programs.[7]

SUCCESS CRITERIA

The research literature associates these and other program strategies with success. These findings are not based on formal program evaluations because evaluations are rare.[8]

- Individual attention tends to motivate students. Many early school leavers do so because they think nobody cares. The mere perception that special attention is directed to their needs can improve attitude and behaviour.

---

7. This list of strategies for youth at risk of dropping out of school is not exhaustive. Career conferences, educator training programs, life skills, personal development, and home-and-life support are other useful strategies. However, the strategies outlined here are primary elements of school-to-work and student retention programs.

8. These findings pertaining to program success are reported in The ARA Consulting report (1993, 18) and the Renihan and Associates report (1994, 98).

- Students become frustrated and discouraged when they fall behind their classmates; catch-up programs are often helpful.
- The earlier the intervention, the more likely the student's success.
- Effective programs build on students' academic and life skills.
- Effective programs involve students in every aspect of school life, making them useful contributors to school society.
- Effective programs include activities to show students what will be expected of them in the workplace.
- Activities and objectives that increase students' self-confidence and employability are helpful.
- Involvement of parents and the community contribute significantly to program effectiveness.
- Whatever its specific objectives, a program will get good results if students believe that it supports their efforts toward relevant goals (e.g., graduation, acquiring job skills).

CHANGE YOUR FUTURE

We have several reasons for profiling CYF. First, experts frequently mention CYF as an effective program. Second, CYF includes a variety of intervention strategies (e.g., in-school transition-to-work program, unofficial mentoring, alternative schooling). CYF operates in seven Ontario school boards, but most of our information came from the Toronto Board of Education. This board has an excellent research services department that produced detailed information on CYF.

Target group – CYF's target population has always been visible minority students, although various terminology has been used since 1991. The Toronto Board of Education found that visible minority (mostly black) students selected for CYF were definitely at risk according to their marks and accumulated credits.

Jurisdiction – CYF is funded by the Ontario Ministry of Citizenship Anti-Racism Secretariat and administered by the Ontario Ministry of Education and Training (MET).

Background – The Toronto Board of Education launched its CYF in the spring of 1991. This was one of seven CYF pilot projects.

CYF targets visible-minority students considered to be at risk of dropping out of school. The idea for CYF arose from the Radwanski Report, which indicated a relationship between low levels of academic achievement and visible-minority status. At the time, there was no valid information on Canadian dropout rates.

The original blueprint for CYF included a work component for at-risk minority students, and individual and group counselling sessions to help these students complete their studies. Only students capable of completing secondary school were selected.

The CYF pilot was scheduled for one school year, but funding was extended for a second year. The program had an almost complete turnover of both schools and students from Year 1 to Year 2, so each year is seen as a separate intervention program.

Program purpose – CYF targets visible-minority students identified by teachers and guidance counsellors as at risk of dropping out of school. Individual counselling and group sessions are used to improve students' marks and interest in school, and reduce dropout and transfer rates.

People involved – The program depends on its counsellors. Each counsellor is assigned to a specific school for all or part of each school day. Coordinators, who, for the past two years, have come from MET, are also involved. CYF expanded to 12 boards by 1995. Each board runs its CYF program more or less autonomously.

Program features – Mentoring and alternative schooling are the program's essentials. Individual counselling and group meetings allow students to discuss personal, school-related and employment problems in a supportive environment. Although transition to work is the program focus, many students in the program actually derive the most benefit from individual and group counselling sessions. This mentoring element makes school more socially welcoming for visible-minority students.

Attendance at most of the weekly sessions is the main student requirement.

Student selection – Teachers and guidance counsellors select CYF candidates, although word of mouth has brought requests from many at-risk students. Final selection is made by guidance counsellors and the CYF counsellor.

Numbers served – Approximately 50 students are selected each year for CYF.

Funding – CYF was initially funded by the Ontario Ministry of Citizenship Anti-Racism Secretariat and supported by the MET. Individual boards have contributed some funds in the intervening years, and the MET has provided administrative support. Recently it has been suggested that school boards should support the program entirely.

Difficulties encountered – The most significant difficulty CYF faces is uncertain funding. From one year to the next, no one knows whether the program can continue.

Another important barrier was the economic recession. The program's preliminary objective was securing employment for at-risk students but, in the early '90s, not enough employers could be found to participate in the program. However, employers have recently begun to show more interest in the program.

The third significant barrier is a conflict of priorities within schools. CYF requires students to attend sessions, and CYF sessions are structured so that students miss, at most, two classes a month per subject. Some teachers seem to think that CYF students, who are often not doing well in school, should not miss classes to attend CYF sessions.

Evaluation – Most boards do not conduct formal evaluations, but the Toronto Board of Education does them yearly. In 1994, the Toronto Board of Education released a two-year evaluation of CYF, entitled "A Two-Year Evaluation of the Change Your Future Program at the Toronto Board of Education" (Brown 1994). Although the results of the evaluation were positive, the evaluation made no difference to CYF funding. MET completed an in-house evaluation of CYF but did not publish it.

Program success – CYF participants' comments and academic results indicate that the program has been moderately successful, considering the difficulties of interventions with at-risk students in secondary schools. The Toronto board indicated specific effects on the dropout rate over two years (1991–92 and 1992–93):

> When data from both years are combined, 9% of *Change Your Future* students dropped out during the school year, compared to 19% dropout for the two comparison groups. This is important because, with an average age of 17 years, many students were at a stage when dropping out would become a serious option. The 9% annual dropout rate, while somewhat higher than the Board annual rate of 8%, was probably lower than the annual dropout rate for 'at risk' students (Brown 1994, 15).

Although CYF was not designed as a mentoring program, many program participants' comments indicate that mentoring, in the form of individual counselling and peer group discussions, was considered a benchmark of success. Participants identified several specific benefits, including: the advantage of a supportive group environment for discussions; the opportunity for students to identify with the CYF counsellor; the opportunity to discuss personal problems and how they relate to school; and advice about what to do about school and jobs.

Programs like *Change Your Future* signal the importance of understanding the transition to work as a process, rather than simply placing youth in jobs. For youth, and in this instance visible-minority students at risk of dropping out, this means close attention to the school as a social setting and the quality of the interactions in schools that encourage students to stay or disengage. Programs like CYF, that use a variety of interventions (e.g., mentoring and alternative schooling) could probably be replicated elsewhere. In fact, most visible minority CYF participants believe that the program should include all students, pointing out that the program has much to offer that does not apply only to a special target population. Students who have participated in *Change Your Future* believe that it would work for all students.

ONTARIO YOUTH APPRENTICESHIP PROGRAM

OYAP was selected for two reasons. First, this program builds on a transition-to-work strategy known as the Co-operative Education Program, which coordinates school to work strategies with out-of-school cooperative job placements. Most Ontario school boards offer cooperative education, and more than 60,000 students use the Co-operative Education Program. Also, OYAP represents an effort to implement the best features of European apprenticeship models, particularly the German "dual system." The success of the dual system is well known, and it is instructive to explore how Ontario has adapted it.

Target group – In school boards and sections where the program is approved, students may apply to OYAP in Grade 10, and they begin in Grade 11 or when they reach the age of 16. OYAP participation does not guarantee an apprenticeship placement.

Jurisdiction – OYAP is administered by MET and the Ontario Training and Adjustment Board (OTAB).

Background – OYAP began in 1988 as the School Workplace Apprenticeship Program (SWAP) and became the Ontario Youth Apprenticeship Program in 1994. The Ontario Ministry of Skills Development and MET launched the program because, although Ontario's high schools provide good opportunities for the 40 percent of students who are university bound, they do not fare as well for the 60 percent who are headed directly for the labour market. An education model suitable for these students was clearly needed. After some exploration, the German dual system was chosen for Ontario. Before proceeding with a profile of OYAP, I will briefly describe this European model of apprenticeship.

An old German adage says *Handwerk hat goldenen Boden*—a trade in hand finds gold in every land.

Theory and practice are the cornerstones of the dual system and, in 1993, fully 90 percent of all German youth attending secondary general schools or intermediate schools applied for vocational training.[9] After completing high school, German youth can select from among 380 job-training programs recognized by the government, in the areas of skilled trades, business and industry. While taking job training, students must also attend business school once or twice a week for general education and a theoretical background to promote and expand their practical training. Two-thirds of instruction is job training and one-third is business school. This system gives students formal education while they learn a trade on the job. Apprenticeships usually last two to two and a half years, and are subject to the state education code.

---

9. Information on the dual system was supplied by the Consulate General of the Federal Republic of Germany in Toronto.

Companies employing apprentices bear the greatest share of program costs, and their share amounts to approximately 2.5 percent of German wages and salaries. Business schools receive substantial state support (i.e., about DM 8 billion), and trainees receive wages. Master artisans and business people view program costs as an investment in the future, and believe that apprenticeship is the best way to meet their need for trained workers. No company is required to offer apprenticeships; in fact, only companies with trained, qualified employees and appropriate facilities may take on apprentices. When they qualify, apprentices are not obliged to work for the company that trained them, nor is the company required to hire them.

Some advantages of the dual system are:
- trainees use up-to-date equipment, and learn technological innovations and developments;
- companies are subsidized to train and educate their employees;
- companies can count on a good supply of trained workers; and
- the workforce of the nation benefits from more general education, higher social standing and better prospects for career advancement.

Program purpose – In 1988–1989 the Ontario government recognized that it needed a program for young people who were not planning postsecondary studies. Such a program would also address shortages in Ontario's workforce by attracting students into careers in the skilled trades. While the major objective of OYAP is to give students an opportunity to finish high school while learning a trade, many school boards also see OYAP as particularly valuable to youth who are at risk of dropping out. As an apprenticeship program, OYAP offers financial rewards to young people who become registered apprentices. Students are employed at apprenticeship rates while they complete the requirements for the Ontario Secondary School Diploma (OSSD). This formal combination of paid work and supervised study makes both apprenticeship and high school more accessible and appealing to young people.

MET is inclined to shift the focus of OYAP to make the program cover a wider range of occupations. In its original form, the program concentrated on industrial trades in which apprenticeship is traditional. However, new information technologies and career areas require the expansion of apprenticeship. MET, following the advice of the Royal Commission on Learning, wants to adjust school curricula to make technology training more prestigious. High schools are adapting to meet the needs of the 60 percent of students who are not going to university by providing a more effective school-to-work transition. MET also wants to encourage girls and other student target groups to explore careers in the skilled trades. It should be noted that in 1992–1993, the OYAP gender breakdown was 538 males and 96 females.

MET would probably like to expand the co-op program because it teaches work skills. In 1995, 60,000 to 65,000 Grade 11 and Grade 12 students—20 to 25 percent of all Grade 11 and Grade 12 students in Ontario—were in co-op programs. People think the co-op program should be expanded even further to give more young people a chance for jobs in the future.

People involved – OYAP's success depends on the commitment, motivation and effort of principals, vice-principals, and technology and co-op teachers, who are most likely to locate apprenticeships for students. Apprenticeships are also located by OTAB staff. There is a fair amount of variability by region.

Parents are also important to the apprenticeship program, sometimes taking on students as apprentices.

Program features – Not all OYAP participants are successful in securing a formal apprenticeship. Each participant begins with an unpaid work placement as a cooperative education student. After 90 days, the employer decides whether to retain the student as a paid apprentice. Apprenticeship is governed by the *Trades Qualification and Apprenticeship Act*, which defines the relationship between an employer and an apprentice. The 90 unpaid days count as a probationary period for the apprenticeship and for credit in a high school co-op program. Once an apprenticeship is offered, both the employer and the apprentice sign a formal agreement. The apprentice is committed to three or four years with the employer, and the employer is responsible for training and paying the apprentice.

OYAP is very closely tied into Ontario's cooperative education program. Students receive cooperative education credits for work experience in OYAP, in accordance with the requirements of *Co-operative Education, Policies and Procedures for Ontario Secondary Schools 1989*, and schools must monitor the cooperative education activities offered in the workplace. The 90-day trial period qualifies the student to receive co-op work experience credits. Student apprentices can accumulate enough credits for the OSSD in two to two and a half years beyond Grade 10. After completing the OSSD, apprentices may be within two years of achieving a Certificate of Qualification in a trade.

Student apprentices must be employed with a qualified journey person and must be registered as apprentices with the OTAB. Students may also accumulate additional apprenticeship hours by working during vacation and holiday periods.

Student apprentices must fulfil all the requirements of the apprenticeship program and the in-school and out-of-school portions of the co-op program. Sometimes the academic curriculum is modified to contain some of the in-school components of the apprenticeship program; however, this can be done only if the teacher is also a qualified journey person. Apprenticeship training in the workplace is usually monitored by OTAB training consultants.

The most common model is a full-time co-op placement in semester II of Grade 11 followed by a full-time co-op–apprenticeship placement for the entire semester II of Grade 12.

The procedures for developing an OYAP program include:
- assessing the need for apprenticeships in a community;
- obtaining commitment from employers for apprenticeship placements;
- determining whether school boards can provide programs to meet employers' needs;
- consulting with local companies, unions and community colleges;
- ensuring that students may easily move back to the regular school program; and
- developing a wide variety of schedules.

Student selection – OYAP participants are often selected by technology co-op teachers.

Numbers served – Since 1992, approximately 600 students per year have participated in OYAP, and this number has been relatively steady. It should also be noted that OYAP participants constitute only a small fraction of the 60,000 students in Ontario co-op programs. The program has expanded from five school boards in 1989 to more than 50 school boards in 1995–1996. The severe economic recession of the early 1990s, which made it difficult for employers to hire apprentices, is largely responsible for the low rate of student participation in OYAP.

Funding – OTAB funds OYAP through MET. Each approved school board is eligible for a start-up grant of $25,000.

Expenses arise mostly from time spent by technology teachers, school board officials and OTAB staff finding apprenticeships. School boards sometimes have trouble getting OTAB representatives to help them obtain placements.

Difficulties encountered – Employers willing to take on an apprentice are very selective, and are reluctant to hire at-risk students. They tend to prefer motivated, committed students. The recession has reduced the number of apprenticeships available and made employers even choosier. Employers must hire back laid-off apprentices before taking on new apprentices, and this has limited apprenticeships still further. Some collective agreements limit apprenticeship to workers with seniority, and employers are generally reluctant to accept high school students because of their youth—especially in trades in which apprenticeship is traditional.

Implementing OYAP in high schools also has drawbacks. Some teachers of academic subjects resent promotion of vocational training, and scheduling problems arising from the placements are very common.

Evaluation – The Sunset Review showed important variations from region to region and school to school in OYAP effectiveness. Unfortunately, the Sunset Review has not been published, and MET has not released its results, because of procedural errors. Statistics are compiled annually, but do not constitute a formal review.

Program success – OYAP is successful because it really helps students learn work skills in real jobs, and it allows them to earn wages, high school credits and apprenticeship hours all at the same time. The program is designed to keep doors open, and students who find that they are not suited to a trade after one semester can return to a regular school program without penalty. These students may return to OYAP later in their schooling and, even if they do not, what they learn may eventually prove valuable. Participating schools also benefit. Teachers are exposed to training methods used in industry, and schools can forge partnerships with local colleges and promote apprenticeship as an exciting career path for students not inclined toward postsecondary education. OYAP tends to promote high school technology departments and to strengthen co-op programs. The proportion of female participation is still low, but OYAP does steer girls into non-traditional occupations.

For employers, OYAP is a good source of apprentices, particularly because the program allows them to look over students before accepting them as apprentices. The program links employers to local schools, so they can contribute ideas and training suggestions. Finally, the program reduces employers' recruiting and training costs substantially.

OYAP-like programs are available in other provinces (e.g., Youth Strategy Linkages in Newfoundland-Labrador; Registered Apprenticeship Program in Alberta; and Passport to Apprenticeship in British Columbia). These programs improve both student retention and employment prospects. However, the lack of published, formal evaluations prevents us from offering proof of program success.

EDUCATION-WORK CONNECTIONS

Jurisdiction – MET administers EWC.

Background – The report of the Royal Commission on Learning emphasized lifelong learning and the need to ensure that the paths between high schools, colleges, universities and the world of work remain open and effective. This vision can be realized through effective community-based partnerships.

The two-year EWC project was designed to prepare students for adulthood and working life, help them make informed career transitions, and launch them on a lifelong course of personal development, education and training. Community involvement, individual initiative and community partnerships help bring learning and working together, offer students better opportunities to make successful transitions from school to work, and improve student retention rates.

Project purpose – Although many students are enrolled in cooperative education programs, the total number of participants, compared with the general student population, is still relatively small. All students need to make successful decisions and transitions from high school. The process requires commitment not only from students, but also from parents, teachers and the community, all of whom must believe in the programs. EWC's mandate was to find schools and communities that already work together to provide school-to-work transition programs and activities for students. EWC assumes that, if schools are to become effective centres for community services for children and youth, they must take the initiative in building a community of concern.

EWC has four elements:

- eight two-year demonstration projects, representing a variety of activities, in different parts of Ontario;
- *Ontario Prospects*, a tabloid on careers distributed to students;
- service sessions, workshops and four-day training sessions for teachers and community partners throughout the province; and
- an Internet newsgroup to keep people connected after the end of the project to continue the discussion electronically.

Project features – MET did not create the projects. School principals and teachers, parents and employers created EWC projects, usually drawing other people in. MET sponsored or funded the demonstration projects. EWC sponsored mentoring programs, peer-helping programs, community work experience programs, teacher internship programs, career activities programs and curriculum development programs.

The Eastwood Comprehensive Alternative Education Program Model is an EWC demonstration project in the Waterloo County Board of Education. The Eastwood project was developed to mobilize school services—guidance, special education, library, cooperative education and administration—and find ways to bring community partners into the school to support learning. The objective of the project is to engage students in acquiring the knowledge, skills and attitudes they need to succeed in the twenty-first century.

The project requires participants to combine academic study with a graduated cooperative education program and to work with mentors, most of whom are seniors. The mentoring component connects students with experienced, understanding people who are not teachers, and who will listen attentively. The project also includes transition year co-op placements, corporate mentoring, community tutoring and job shadowing.

The project aims to improve students' attitude, self-knowledge and understanding of the surrounding world. It has been very successful—90 percent of participants since 1990 have continued their education or have taken full-time employment.

Future of EWC – Although EWC has formally ended, the demonstration projects and other activities continue. The report of the Royal Commission on Learning validated the school-community partnership in the school-to-work transition. MET plans to build on the success of EWC and the Royal

Commission's comments on schools cooperating with communities by introducing initiatives to carry on the work of EWC.

PART 3 – CONCLUSIONS AND POLICY IMPLICATIONS

Dropping out is a process, not a single event. This notion is seldom recognized by researchers and policymakers, but it must be, if we are to avoid the trap of seeing dropping out as an outcome of schooling. In many young people, disengagement is seen as early as primary school. Early school leavers frequently disengage for valid reasons, and not because they are academic failures. Indeed, most studies indicate that dropouts offer school-related reasons (e.g., boredom, alienation, rejection by the school system) for wishing to leave early. Given that disengagement from school is an interactive process that is frequently seen in primary school, it makes good sense from a health perspective to promote research and interventions to facilitate reengagement of students with school when they are still very young.

This research could be done in conjunction with the National Longitudinal Survey of Children (NLSC), which is being conducted by Human Resources Development Canada. The primary objective of NLSC is to develop a national database on the characteristics and life experiences of Canadian children as they grow from infancy to adulthood (National Longitudinal Survey of Children 1995, 1). The information generated will be made available to policymakers and researchers interested in developing policies and strategies to make children's lives healthier, more active and more rewarding. The data will help policymakers most by providing a firm basis for initiatives that enhance children's engagement with school.

Canadians' belief that the school-to-work transition is more disorderly and wasteful than it used to be may exaggerate the orderliness of the old days, but youth unemployment and part-time work are, indeed, on the increase. Indirect entry to paid employment is certainly more typical today than a direct transition from school to work. Moreover, employers claim that early school leavers lack competencies and general skills—a problem some policy analysts attribute, at least in part, to Canada's university-driven high school curriculum. The powerful university influence is reinforced by parents' ambition for their children (King and Peart 1995). Also, high school academic courses simply cannot and do not teach the knowledge and skills required for effective multiple transitions to work. Alan King's view of the situation in Ontario is particularly pessimistic:

> In our present system, the imprecise sorting procedures in secondary schools encourage some students to retain the hope of attending a postsecondary institution long after the likelihood of gaining admission has dimmed. What this means for secondary school programming is that the vast majority of students in grades 10 and 11 continue to take university-bound courses

(over 70 percent) leaving little opportunity to develop viable secondary school-to-work programs because of the small numbers who would select such programs (1994, 21).

Even cooperative education, which is endorsed and supported by teachers and students alike, has been less than successful in providing a broad range of school-to-work programs. There is a conspicuous absence of apprenticeships and co-op placements in union shops, and the transition programs are successful in direct proportion to the goodwill they earn from teachers, principals, and participating companies and organizations. The support and commitment of both employers and unions must be secured before broad-based school-to-work programs can become reality.

This situation is particularly hard on youth at risk of dropping out of school. These youth need the most help in making smooth, effective transitions. It is increasingly clear that the boundaries between school and employment have blurred for most high school students. Surveys show that, by the time most of today's students leave secondary school, approximately 75 percent of them will have held part-time jobs (Anisef 1993, 31). As I have said elsewhere, it is possible to take advantage of these blurred boundaries:

> At present, except for a restricted implementation of the co-operative education model, the learning place and the workplace are set apart. School activities appear to have little direct bearing on what occurs in the workplace. Skills required on the job do not appear to be reflected in the curriculum of the school. The relevancy of one to the other must be made clear to the secondary school student. One approach would be an initiative directed at drawing the part-time workplace and the classroom together in a mutually valued and supportive network (Anisef 1993, 35).

It makes good sense for schools to harness community resources to help students. It also make sense that students want to understand how to apply what they learn, and are highly motivated by clear connections between their formal education and their future career.

A recent Toronto Board of Education report recommends several noteworthy ways to strengthen partnerships between educators and employers.

> [To] improve the impact of part-time jobs on school performance, the employer community can work in partnership with the schools to co-develop curricular programs and activities that impart transferable and up-to-date technical and business skills and knowledge that are applicable to a wide range of occupations (Cheng 1995, 23).

In addition, teachers could be trained to "integrate" students' work experiences into classroom activities and lesson content to make learning more relevant, and guidance counsellors could place students in jobs that will help them develop useful, transferable skills. By emphasizing collaborative relationships between educators, employers and parents, the disadvantages of part-time work can be limited and the advantages maximized (Cheng 1995, 22–23).

The ambitions of early school leavers may be lower and less clearly defined than those of graduates of high school or postsecondary institutions, but they still outstrip the low-level jobs they obtain. This gap indicates they learned high aspirations in school. It is clear that most young Canadians will need more education or training to realize the aspirations of their school years. Studies indicate, however, that most early school leavers do not reject education, but remain committed to conventional social values. They usually decide to leave school because of courses, teachers or social aspects of school life. Their negative experiences outweigh their awareness, which frequently becomes more urgent as they get older, that completing their education would prepare them better for a smoother, effective transition to adult, working life.

Early school leavers are more likely than high school graduates to experience an uneven job history, unemployment and low pay. Understandably, they are also more prone to depression and feelings of failure. Still, most remain optimistic about the future and tend to blame themselves for not trying hard enough, for not getting the credentials they need, and so on. Their reactions tend to be more conventional than political—they blame themselves, not society, for their lack of opportunity and personal difficulties in the job. This is particularly true of men.

Early school leavers form a underclass lacking the skills required for meaningful employment in today's highly competitive job market. Canadian high schools evidently do not offer the education required to gain entry to many occupations (Anisef 1993, 31). Policymakers should, however, be aware that emphasis on transition-to-work programs has a downside; it may disadvantage high-risk subgroups—the functionally illiterate, the disengaged disconnected from school, the alienated, and those prone to substance abuse and crime (Anisef 1994, 103). Employers do not see these youth as desirable candidates, and cooperative education-apprenticeship programs may not help them much. Students who apply to programs like OYAP do so because they see apprenticeship as the high road to a good job. Potential apprentices are not high-risk youth, however.

A recent study entitled *Our Children At Risk* by the Organization for Economic Co-operation and Development argues that children and youth already at risk may be the biggest losers as governments cut spending to balance budgets (Crane 1995, B2). The term "at risk" is optimistic, suggesting that preventive action and early childhood, school and school-to-work transition interventions can improve chances for a healthy, productive life, but governments are cutting programs and interventions that target children and youth at risk. These economic policies will eventually marginalize youth, particularly those already at risk.

Effective transition programs are very important in today's polarized, competitive job market, but we must note the human and social aspects of early disengagement from school. Dropping out is a process that must be understood as part of a prolonged, nonlinear process of moving from school to employment and back again. School-to-work transition programs, desirable as they are, cannot replace efforts to meet students' special needs— for example, about 75 percent of immigrants who settle in Canadian cities belong to visible minorities.

All the dropout studies reviewed in this paper clearly indicate that disengagement must be understood as a phenomenon linked to class and other social and cultural factors. At the same time, however, many of the studies reviewed seem to generalize findings to a "dropout" category. This tendency invites a certain degree of desensitization to the variation among students who either leave school early voluntarily or are pushed out for a variety of reasons. Even high school graduates frequently find their education inadequate. Whether students drop out, are pushed out or disengage from school, we must not forget power and status factors, such as social class, ethnicity, race, gender and community type (urban or rural) when examining the early leaving process. To think of such youth simply as dropouts, pushouts or disengagers may cause us to overlook these very important factors. Aboriginal youth, disadvantaged visible-minority youth, working class youth and remote rural youth all have their special needs and problems. For example, George S. Dei (1995), in describing black students' encounters with authority in Toronto schools, writes:

> Students further describe struggles to construct self and group cultural identities in a school environment that does not adequately highlight their cultural presence, heritage and history in the official and hidden school curriculum. The students thus powerfully link issues of identity and representation with schooling. They attest to the intersections of race, gender, class and sexuality in their school and off-school lives (p. A31).

In designing interventions, we must remain attuned to the very specific needs and problems experienced by student groups, in school and out of school (e.g., at work). Our review of school-to-work transition interventions indicates that there is no quick fix or recipe for success that will work for everyone. Success principles and criteria can be applied, but the effectiveness of any intervention depends on the goodwill and motivation of the community, school officials, employers and other partners.

As Benjamin Levin writes, the framing of the policy issue of dropouts is crucially important:

> Much less prominent in the discussion are human considerations—the frustration and despair of students who see no future for themselves in our schools or our labour market. Equity issues play a much smaller role in the public policy discussions of dropouts. There is no mention in the Canadian government documents of the link between social class and educational attainment, even though this connection is firmly established in Canadian research (Radwanski 1987). [Levin 1992, 260]

Policies and programs that encourage returning to school make sense because early school leavers recognize that they need to finish school to get better jobs. The National School Leavers' Survey shows that almost 50 percent of early school leavers attempt to return and complete their studies (Tanner and Krahn 1995, 157). Moreover, dropout and school-to-work transition literature reveals early school leavers are much more likely to complete their studies if appropriate community-based alternative schooling programs are in place.

The recent literature on school-to-work transitions clearly shows that Canadians make multiple entries and exits during the first third of their young adult lives. Although many early school leavers have relatively poor academic records, many more have quite satisfactory marks. Enough at-risk students do not drop out that the total at-risk population of Canadian secondary schools is dangerously high (Levin 1992, 262). It is, therefore, more beneficial to discuss the total activity of Canadian schools than to focus on at-risk students. We need to know more about school activities and their importance for and effect on students. At the same time, we cannot wait for schools to solve their problems, especially since many of these problems are part of the interaction of students, schools, parents, communities, culture and society at large. We can, however, make entry and re-entry into school easier and more acceptable for young people, and facilitate partnerships between students, schools and other potential contributors to a helpful system, such as employers, unions and training institutions. Schools can help students understand the world of work, but they should not be the only source of knowledge.

A careful review of educational reform in Canada over the last 50 years reveals that some initiatives worked extraordinarily well while others were quickly forgotten, victims of political disfavour or inappropriate evaluation standards. It is relatively easy to formulate reforms, but it is much harder (but essential) to develop a framework for reform so that useful initiatives do not get overlooked or misclassified (Anisef 1993, 36). Frequently, inappropriate evaluations are used or no evaluations are done at all when considering the effectiveness of intervention programs. The literature on student retention and the school-to-work transition indicates that formal evaluation based on experimental and scientific methodology was conspicuously absent. Canada needs careful, formal program evaluations in this area, over longer periods of time.

The literature and programs reviewed for this paper strongly suggest that the effectiveness of school-to-work transition programs for youth disengaging from school hinges not on cogent public policy, but on the goodwill and commitment of educators, employers, parents and community-based organizations. A strategy is therefore needed to sustain and, in many instances, to increase the general health of Canadian youth. Government organizations should advocate and facilitate student retention programs designed to smooth what has become an increasingly difficult transition process (Human Resources Development Canada 1994, 104). Mechanisms such as an Internet home page are also needed to enhance access to the bewildering variety of intervention programs and research on student retention and the school-to-work transition. Good evaluation research is particularly important. My literature review and discussions with experts in the field demonstrated that formal evaluations are infrequent. the use of formal evaluation is of fundamental importance to build up a more objective assessment of "best practices" programs. Ways to facilitate access to formally evaluated programs for school boards, educators, youth and student organizations are needed in every province.

Paul Anisef *is a professor of sociology in the Department of Sociology at York University. He received his Ph.D. degree in Sociology from Cornell University. His major research interests include the transition from adolescence to adulthood, and various issues relating to educational equality. Recent publications include* The Learning and Sociological Profiles of Canadian High School Students *(1994);* Transitions: Schooling and Employment in Canada, *(1993) and* "Post-secondary education and underemployment in a longitudinal study of Ontario baby boomers", *Higher Education Policy (1996).*

BIBLIOGRAPHY

ANDRES, L., and ANISEF, P. 1995. The Stay-in-School Initiative: Social construction of a national crisis? Unpublished paper.

ANISEF, P. (Ed.) 1994a. *Learning and Sociological Profiles of Canadian High School Students: An Overview of 15 to 18 Year Olds and Educational Implications for Dropouts, Exceptional Students, Employed Students, Immigrant Students and Native Youth.* Lewiston (NY): The Edwin Mellen Press.

_____. 1994b. *A Learning Cultures and Learning Styles Framework for Addressing the Issue of Drop-Outs in Canada.* Ottawa: Prosperity Secretariat.

ANISEF, P., and AXELROD, P. Eds. 1993. *Transitions: Schooling and Employment in Canada.* Toronto: Thompson Educational Publishing.

BELLAMY, L., ROSS, J., and ANISEF, P. 1994. Breaking the fingers of blame and recasting the problem of dropout. Paper presented at the Southwest Social Science Meetings, San Antonio (TX). March 30–April 3.

BROWN, R. S. 1994. *A Two-Year Evaluation of the* Change Your Future *Program at the Toronto Board of Education, 1991–1993.* No. 208. Toronto: Toronto Board of Education Research Services.

_____. 1995. Mentoring at-risk students: Challenges and potential. Unpublished paper. Toronto: Toronto Board of Education Research Services.

BUCHMANN, M. 1989. *The Script of Life in Modern Society: Entry into Adulthood in a Changing World.* Chicago: University of Chicago Press.

CANADA. HUMAN RESOURCES DEVELOPMENT CANADA. 1995a. *Youth Face Tough Times.* Internet http//hrdc.gc.ca.

_____. n.d. Proposed research themes for a human resource development agenda, *The World of Learning.* Ottawa.

CANADA. HUMAN RESOURCES DEVELOPMENT CANADA. YOUTH AFFAIRS BRANCH. 1994. *Taking Stock: An Assessment of the National Stay-in-School Initiative.* Prepared by Fred Renihan & Associates. Ottawa: Human Resources Development Canada.

CANADIAN FEDERATION OF YOUTH. 1995a. *Youth Unemployment: Canada's Hidden Deficit.* Ottawa: Canadian Youth Foundation.

_____. 1995b. *Youth Unemployment: Canada's Rite of Passage.* Ottawa: Canadian Youth Foundation.

CHENG, Maisy. 1995. *Issues Related to Student Part-Time Work: What Did Research Find in the Toronto Situation and Other Contexts?* No. 215. Toronto: Board of Education Research Services.

CRANE, D. 1995. Children face the biggest losses when budgets are cut back. *Toronto Star,* Saturday, December 30, 1995.

DEI, G. S. 1995. Report's critics can't ignore student alienation. *Toronto Star,* Friday, December 8.

DEI, G. S., HOLMES, L., MAZZUCA, J., MCISAAC, E., and CAMPBELL, R. 1995. *Drop Out or Push Out? The Dynamics of Black Students' Disengagement from School.* Toronto: Ontario Institute for Studies in Education.

EMPSON-WARNER, S., and KRAHN, H. 1992. Unemployment and occupational aspirations: A panel study of high school graduates. *Canadian Review of Sociology and Anthropology* 29 (1): 38–54.

EVANS, K., and HEINZ, W. R. 1994. Transitions in progress. In *Becoming Adults in England and Germany,* eds. K. EVANS and W. R. HEINZ. London: Anglo-German Foundation. pp. 1–16.

GREEN, A. L., and WHEATLEY, S. M. 1992. I've got a lot to do and I don't think I'll have the time: Gender differences in late adolescents' narratives of the future. *Journal of Youth and Adolescence* 21 (6).

HOGAN, D. P. 1981. *Transitions and Social Change: The Early Lives of American Men.* New York: Academic Press.

HOLBROOK, A. 1993. Key issues in the historical analysis of youth transition. ANZHES (Australian and New Zealand History of Education Society) Conference, Melbourne, Australia, December 1993.

HUMAN RESOURCES DEVELOPMENT CANADA. National Longitudinal Survey of Children. 1995. Developments, *Newsletter* 1 (1).

HUGHES, K. D., and LOWE, G. S. 1993. Unequal return: Gender differences in initial employment among university graduates. *Canadian Journal of Higher Education* 23 (1).

JAMES, C. E. 1993. Getting there and staying there: Blacks' employment experience. In *Transitions: Schooling and Employment in Canada*, eds. P. ANISEF and P. AXELROD. Toronto: Thompson Educational Publishing, Inc. pp. 3–20.

JONES, A. 1994. Native youth. In *Learning and Sociological Profiles of Canadian High School Students: An Overview of 15 to 18 Year Olds and Educational Policy Implications for Dropouts, Exceptional Students, Employed Students, Immigrants, and Native Youth*, ed. P. ANISEF. Queenston (ON): Mellen Press. pp. 105–120.

KELLY, D. M. 1994. School dropouts. In *The International Encyclopedia of Education*, 2nd ed., eds. T. HUSEN, and T. N. POSTLEWAITE. Oxford, U.K.: Oxford Pergamon Press.

KERR, K. 1992. *Labour Market Development.* Ottawa: Library of Parliament.

KING, A. J. C. 1994. Restructuring Ontario secondary education, part 2: A background paper for the Ontario Royal Commission on Learning. Royal Commission on Learning, Toronto (ON).

KING, A. J. C., and PEART, M. J. 1995. Factors inhibiting the transition of youth to work and adulthood. Paper prepared for the National Research and Policy Symposium on Youth in Transition to Adulthood, Kananaskis (AB), April 25–29, 1995.

KRAHN, H., and LOWE, G. 1991. Transitions to work: Findings from a longitudinal study of high school and university students in three Canadian cities. In *Making Their Way: Education, Training and the Labour Market in Canada and Britain*, eds. D. ASHTON, and G. LOWE. Toronto: University of Toronto Press.

LAM, L. 1994. Immigrant students. In *Learning and Sociological Profiles of Canadian High School Students: An Overview of 15 to 18 Year Olds and Educational Policy Implications for Dropouts, Exceptional Students, Employed Students, Immigrants, and Native Youth*, ed. P. ANISEF. Queenston (ON): Mellen Press. pp. 121–130.

LEVIN, B. 1992. Dealing with dropouts in Canadian education. *Curriculum Inquiry* 22 (3): 257–270.

––––––. 1995. How can schools respond to changes in work? *Canadian Vocational Journal* 30(3): 8–20.

LOOKER, D. E. 1995. Transitions to adult life. Paper presented to the Youth 2000 Conference, Middlesbrough, U.K., July 1995.

LOOKER, D. E., and LOWE, G. 1995. Theme 2—Preparation for the world of work. Research and Policy Symposium on Youth in Transition to Adulthood, Kananaskis (AB), April 25–29, 1995.

MACMILLAN, R. 1995. Changes in the structure of life courses and the decline of social capital in Canadian society: A time series analysis of property crime rates. *Canadian Journal of Sociology* 20 (1): 51–79.

MANDELL, N., and CRYSDALE, S. 1993. Gender tracks: Male-female perceptions of home-school-work transitions. In *Transitions: Schooling and Employment in Canada*, eds. P. ANISEF, and P. AXELROD. Toronto: Thompson Educational Publishing, Inc. pp. 21–41.

RADWANSKI, G. 1987. *Ontario Study of the Relevance of Education, and the Issue of Dropouts.* Toronto: Ministry of Education.

RENIHAN, F., and ASSOCIATES. 1994. *Taking Stock: An Assessment of the National Stay-in-School Initiative.* Hull: Youth Affairs Branch, Human Resources Development Canada.

SCHNEIDER, B. 1994. Thinking about an occupation: A new developmental and contextual perspective. In *Research in Sociology and Education*, ed. A. M. PELLAS. 10: 239–259.

TANNER, J., KRAHN, H., and HARTNAGEL, T.F. 1995. *Fractured Transitions from School to Work: Revisiting the Dropout Problem.* Toronto: Oxford University Press.

Youth, Substance Abuse and the Determinants of Health

PAMELA C. FRALICK, B.A., M.A., M.A.P.,
AND BRIAN HYNDMAN, B.A., M.H.SC.

Canadian Centre on Substance Abuse
*Ottawa, Ontario** *

SUMMARY

Examining any application of the determinants of health framework is challenging. As a relatively new means of conceptualizing health issues, this perspective is not yet particularly well reflected in the extant literature. Focusing on youth, within the broader realm of substance abuse, presents additional difficulties, given that most of the research conducted to date reflects an adult world, investigating such key determinants as income, social status, employment and working conditions. There is no doubt that these factors do affect young people through their caregivers and households, but the long-term effects may be different from those determined in studies assessing adult populations.

This paper is an overview of the relationship between the substance abuse problems experienced by young people and the primary determinants of health. In particular, it attempts to apply these determinants to the youth population, investigating the effects of factors such as peer group forces, self-esteem, household relationships and educational achievement. The literature on links between health and substance abuse, substance abuse and the determinants of health, and resiliency, is examined.

* With contributions from: Alberta Alcohol and Drug Abuse Commission, Kaiser Youth Foundation

To illustrate how these youth-specific concerns can be addressed through substance abuse prevention efforts, the paper reviews six examples of community-based prevention programs for young people in Canada. These initiatives deal with a range of substances, including alcohol, tobacco, inhalants and licit and illicit drugs. To allow for a better understanding of the factors associated with the success of these initiatives, the paper analyzes the rationale underlying the projects, key players, funding sources and evaluation results, where available. The potential replicability of each initiative is also analyzed.

Unfortunately, many of these programs do not have a strong evaluation component, or they have not been operating long enough to draw reliable conclusions about their effects. However, they are still worth considering, given the overall dearth of information in this area.

Although the nature and scope of these initiatives vary, all their activities were guided by the recognition that health-promoting behaviour does not occur in isolation from healthy environments. Through a variety of strategies addressing the broad determinants of health—including skills training, regulatory policies, employment opportunities, social network building and intersectoral planning—these initiatives fostered healthy environments that helped young people to be more able to make health-promoting choices about the use of alcohol and other drugs.

The following areas need further attention:
— *research on youth, rather than adult, populations;*
— *research on how determinants interact;*
— *use of both quantitative and qualitative methodologies;*
— *evaluations of community-based programs;*
— *effective, appropriate research questions for these assessments;*
— *involvement of youth in all stages of research and program design; and*
— *demonstration projects based specifically on a determinants of health model.*
  Three underlying principles should guide policy development:
• *recognizing a role for both health promotion and population health;*
• *increased intersectoral collaboration; and*
• *community-based approaches.*

Finally, several concrete policy recommendations were made, based on these principles and the findings of the literature review and project analyses.

TABLE OF CONTENTS

The goal of the working group on the Determinants of Health of the National Forum on Health is to foster debate among Canadians on the best ways of investing scarce resources to improve the health of our population. One approach it has chosen is the development of exploratory papers on a number of key, relevant issues and target populations. These expert papers will assist the working group in identifying what can be done to act on the physical, psychological, social, cultural and economic determinants of health.

As part of this process, this paper focuses on the prevention of substance abuse in youth, within a determinants of health framework. A summary of relevant literature will, first, establish the link between health and substance abuse (including use of tobacco) and, secondly, explore the links between substance abuse and the determinants of health. The latter will include a discussion of the unique position of alcohol, which has both risks and benefits.

Of equal importance is the need to establish the position of substance abuse within a determinants of health framework. Although a definitive statement on this issue is not yet possible, the results of the literature review can point us in the right direction and set the stage for subsequent theoretical analyses.

The third element to be covered in the literature review will be the body of literature concerning resiliency, an area with great relevance to the study of youth substance abuse. Finally, a summary will identify those determinants believed to be most important for this population and issue, according to research available today.

After setting the stage with key conclusions, a selection of recent and current projects that seem to embody the principles of the determinants of health, although the initiative might have been planned without this theoretical underpinning, are analyzed. The goal of the analysis is to identify scenarios that have led to enhanced physical and mental health, and that could be replicated to benefit the public.

The paper concludes with recommendations based on the combined findings of the literature review and project analysis. The recommendations deal with both research gaps and policy directions.

CLUES FROM THE LITERATURE

The quest for the ideal policy to maximize the health of Canadians is not new. As modern medicine developed, it focused on biomedical approaches— provision of the best health services possible. This view prevailed from mid-century until the 1970s, when a noteworthy shift to preventive activities occurred (Pinder 1994). This shift in thinking was influenced to a great extent by the government's need to contain escalating health care costs. Since the 1970s, health status has been increasingly associated with individual lifestyle (Lalonde 1974). Unhealthy habits, such as smoking, and the misuse of alcohol and other drugs were referred to as self-imposed risks, believed to result from personal choices.

Although this approach evolved to recognize the concomitant role of the environment in health, it is only very recently that research has focused primarily on the importance of social, economic and cultural environments to population health (Evans, Barer, and Marmor 1994). New research has taken the study of health away from the compartmentalized medical-model perspective, and acknowledged the broader determinants of health outside the health care system. Accordingly, this approach has been embraced at the highest political levels (Premier's Council on Health Strategy 1991; Federal, Provincial and Territorial Advisory Committee on Population Health 1994). This is the model that will influence Canada's health policy in the immediate future.

Within the existing body of research on population health and the determinants of health, however, little attention has been paid to the role of substance abuse. This is not surprising, given the recency of the research. Nevertheless, it is critical that this issue not be ignored as policy develops, given its broad impact on the health of Canadians. Whether or not it can be definitively given the status of a "determinant of health" in its own right, there is no doubt that substance abuse plays a pivotal role in health, and has tremendous impact on other health determinants. Substance abuse can result from a deficit in the basic prerequisites for health and well-being, such as lack of nurturing, absence of supportive parents or caregivers, or unemployment. Conversely, preexisting substance abuse can diminish access to the social, economic and environmental prerequisites for health, and inhibit an individual's ability to improve his situation. In summary, the importance of this crosscutting issue cannot be ignored.

Substance Abuse and Health

In establishing the importance of substance abuse in the determinants of health model, it is first crucial to clearly identify the nature of the relationship between the various substances and health. This document includes alcohol, tobacco and illicit drugs within its framework. Although these substances are all abused, they cannot be treated similarly, because of the pharmacological and social differences in their use and effects.

The health costs associated with *tobacco* are well known, generally accepted, and increasingly indisputable. According to 1991 data, an estimated 36,325 deaths in Canada were indirectly attributable to smoking. These deaths were due primarily to chronic bronchitis, asthma and emphysema, as well as neoplasms, stroke, hypertension and heart disease (Canadian Profile 1995).

National data are available from this report for young people aged 15 to 19, indicating that 25 percent of young women and 19 percent of young men smoke either occasionally or daily. Fifty-one percent of smokers aged 20 to 24 reported having started smoking before the age of 16, and 63 percent of all daily smokers started to smoke daily before the age of 18. Although they may experience few immediate health effects because of smoking, the mortality statistics quoted earlier indicate their possible future.

Harms caused by *illicit drugs* affect fewer people, and vary to some extent from one drug to another. In general terms, 510 drug-related deaths were reported in Canada in 1991 and 21,746 drug-related cases (78.2 per 100,000) were handled at general and psychiatric hospitals. Young people aged 15 to 19 had the highest admission rates (162.5 per 100,000) for medical problems caused by drug abuse.

It is impossible to obtain a reliable estimate of the drug use by street youth, given the transient nature of the population, as well as their natural reluctance to respond to data gathering. In terms of harm, with approximately two-thirds of these young people involved in drug use, they are constantly exposed to a variety of dangers, including HIV infection through needle-sharing, unsafe sex practices, lack of resources and poor hygiene. They also run the risk of becoming involved in criminal activities such as burglaries, robbery with violence, drug trafficking and prostitution (Anderson 1992).

Perhaps most complex is the relationship between *alcohol* and health, given that it has both health risks and benefits. Attempting to find a balance between risks and benefits (how much is too much? for whom? under what circumstances?) has become an overriding concern for alcohol researchers. What is the net effect of alcohol on health?

It is now accepted beyond a reasonable doubt that moderate consumption of alcohol can have health benefits, particularly in its association with reduced rates of heart disease. Other areas of research for health benefits include cancer, weight management, gastrointestinal disorders, insomnia, stress reduction and social facilitation, where positive effects have been reported more frequently than negative ones.

Although it is important to recognize that alcohol can have health benefits, research currently limits this claim to one major area (coronary disease), and to specific subpopulations (men over 45 years of age, postmenopausal women). The harms to health from alcohol are much better known and documented. We know that alcohol causes many problems (English et al. 1995), exacerbates others (Rice 1993), can have a negative impact on family income and marital stability, and can increase spouse and child abuse. These factors are closely related to key determinants of health (Edwards et al. 1994).

The most recent data to focus on problems related to alcohol consumption come from Canada's 1993 General Social Survey. One in 10 respondents reported that drinking had adversely affected his social life, physical health, happiness, home life or marriage, work, or finances (Single et al. 1995). In addition, two in five reported having experienced problems because of other people's drinking.

If death can be described as the ultimate health impact of alcohol, then the statistics are significant—in 1993 at least 3,183 deaths could be directly attributed to alcohol, and 15,980 indirectly. In addition, there were 38,261 alcohol-related hospital admissions (Canadian Profile 1995). Although these statistics may pale in comparison to the equivalent figures for tobacco, the numbers cannot be ignored.

In the 1993 General Social Survey, 57 percent of respondents aged 15 to 17 and 79 percent of those aged 18 to 19 reported being current drinkers. The situation is even more extreme for street youth. A national study indicated that 88 percent of street youth reported using alcohol, with 9 percent drinking daily (Radford 1989).

The links between damage to health and alcohol, tobacco and illicit drug use are inescapable. These effects are pervasive; they are felt by too many Canadians, in all social strata. The next step in the literature review will be to examine the links between substance abuse and the identified determinants of health, although the question still remains as to whether substance abuse itself should be accorded "determinant" status and investigated on its own merit.

Substance Abuse and the Determinants of Health

Income and Social Status

Income and social status are perhaps the most important determinants of health. Epidemiological surveys have consistently shown significant inequities in the health status of people in lower socioeconomic positions. Simply stated, well-off people appear to lead longer, healthier lives than their disadvantaged counterparts (National Council of Welfare 1990).

When the relationship between *alcohol* consumption and income level is examined, survey data generally indicate that alcohol use is more predominant among high-income groups. As a predictor of the frequency and volume of alcohol intake, however, income level has yielded mixed results. Canadian surveys show that individuals from high-income households drink more frequently and consume more alcohol than people in other income groups, but lower-income respondents tend to consume greater amounts of alcohol on the occasions when they do drink (Health and Welfare Canada 1990; Adlaf 1993).

The 1993 General Social Survey provided a profile of the individual most likely to have a drinking problem: a young adult male, single or divorced, who is unemployed or has a relatively low income.

There is no clear relationship between the drinking habits of young people and the socioeconomic status of their families. Martin and Pritchard (1991) found that young men from upper-middle-class and wealthy backgrounds tended to drink more frequently, while the results of other studies indicate higher levels of consumption among males from lower socioeconomic classes (Sieber 1979; Parker and Parker 1980).

Although the consumption of alcohol is generally greater among persons of higher socioeconomic status, the incidence of alcohol-related problems appears to be more prevalent among the economically disadvantaged. For example, impaired drivers responsible for collisions tend to be lower in socioeconomic status (Macdonald 1989), even though high-income earners are more likely to drive after drinking (Wilkins 1988).

There is a strong negative relationship between socioeconomic status and *tobacco* use. Canadian survey data consistently show that low-income groups are significantly more likely to report that they smoke than respondents in higher-income groups, although the gap in tobacco use between these extremes has narrowed somewhat in recent years (Wilkins 1988; Pederson 1993).

Young people from lower socioeconomic backgrounds are generally more likely to smoke than their more economically privileged peers (Boyle and Offord 1986). Burton (1994) speculates that the rate of people starting to smoke after high school may actually rise as smoking increasingly becomes a habit of lower socioeconomic classes:

> ...if the student leaves a relatively heterogenous school environment and enters a more homogenous workforce primarily composed of persons from lower socioeconomic environments, smoking may be reinforced and even promoted by group norms (1994, 97).

Low income is a significant contributing factor to the abuse of *illicit drugs* among young people. In a metanalysis of etiological research studies on the causes of adolescent drug abuse, Hawkins, Catalano, and Miller (1992) found that children who come from areas of economic deprivation, and who experience behaviour and other adjustment problems early in life, are more likely to have drug-related problems later on.

Street youth use drugs at a high rate to cope with the effects of a violent home life and the day-to-day hardship of living on the street—they also find it easy to get drugs on the street (Canadian Profile 1995). A full 71 percent had used cannabis in the past year, 31 percent cocaine (including crack), and 44 percent LSD. Twelve percent reported injecting drugs, exposing them to the additional risk of serious infection (HIV, hepatitis).

Recap: Low-income status is generally related to higher use of tobacco, the abuse of illicit drugs, and the development of alcohol-related problems among youth. Street youth, in particular, exhibit extremely high levels of both consumption and related problems.

Social Support Networks

Support from friends, families and communities is associated with positive health outcomes. A California study, for example, found that people with more social contacts tend to live longer (Berkman and Syme 1979).

A related but separate social determinant of health is community cohesion or attachment, the extent to which community members feel a collective sense of responsibility for the health and well-being of their fellow residents. Areas where residents have little attachment to the community, and where there are few strong social institutions, are more likely to experience alcohol- and drug-related problems (Hawkins et al. 1993).

Community-level interventions can help to foster stronger social networks among socially isolated individuals. Assessments of community interventions to strengthen social networks have demonstrated a number of positive health effects, including enhancing the capabilities of untrained or volunteer workers, greater participation in health activities, and the activation of social support (Cohen and Syme 1985; Israel 1985; Gottlieb 1987; Wallerstein 1993).

Social networks are a predisposing factor in the use of *alcohol and illicit drugs* by young people. Favourable parental and peer attitudes toward alcohol and drug use are significant risk factors for drug abuse among adolescents (Hawkins, Catalano, and Miller 1992; Glanz and Pickens 1993). Several longitudinal studies have found a number of consistent social predictors of drug initiation and drug use among young people, including peer alcohol and drug use, parental alcohol and drug use, parental sociopathy, and lack of social conformity (Chassin 1984; Kaplan 1985; Jessor 1986; Sadava 1987).

Overall, the social environment, and especially the influence of social networks, is thought to be the single most important determinant of *smoking* onset among young people (Anderson 1995). This relationship is substantiated by Canadian data; according to the Ontario Health Survey (1990), adolescent smokers (12 to 17 years of age) were more likely to report, at a statistically significant level, that they lived in households with at least one other smoker, and that they had a higher proportion of friends who were smokers (Badovinac 1993).

A study by van Roosmalen and McDaniel (1989) found that friends played a highly significant role in affecting the smoking habits of adolescents, especially females. Eighth-grade female smokers had a larger proportion of friends who smoked than their male counterparts, and there appeared to be more indirect peer pressure on females to smoke.

Just as social networks can be a risk factor for the onset of tobacco use by young people, etiological research has consistently revealed that healthy family and peer influences are primary protective factors against the adoption of smoking (Flay et al. 1983; McNeill et al. 1988; Charlton and Blair 1989; Conrad et al. 1992). For example, a U.S. national survey of youth revealed that teenagers were three times as likely to abstain from smoking if no one in their household smoked. Teenagers seldom smoked themselves if none of their best friends of the same sex smoked (Moss et al. 1992).

Recap: Family and peers are key predictors of adolescent use of alcohol, tobacco and illicit drugs. These influences can be both positive/protective or negative/facilitating in regard to the behaviour.

Education

As with income level, there is a strong negative relationship between *smoking* and degree of educational attainment: individuals with lower levels of educational attainment are significantly more likely to report smoking (Ontario Health Survey 1990; Pederson 1993). A number of studies indicate that adolescent smoking is related to poor academic achievement and dissatisfaction with school (Skinner et al. 1985; Krohn et al. 1986; Newcomb et al. 1989). Research by Hill (1989) suggests that an orientation toward scholastic achievement may be a protective factor against smoking initiation and maintenance.

The relationship between educational attainment and the use of *alcohol* and other *drugs* is less clear, although survey data generally reveal a positive relationship between educational attainment and alcohol consumption (Single 1995). Etiological research generally finds that early school drop-outs have higher rates of drug use (Smart and Blair 1980; Mensch and Kandel 1988; Smart et al. 1992).

Education is an important factor in deterring the abuse of alcohol and other drugs by young people, the majority of whom are in school. Schools have long served as the primary venue for educational interventions aimed at preventing or delaying tobacco, alcohol and drug use by young people. Although the results of these initiatives are mixed, school-based drug education programs are generally successful in increasing knowledge of the negative consequences of substance abuse and, to a lesser extent, sustaining healthy attitudes and behaviour (Bremberg 1991; Tobler 1989). Given the aforementioned relationship between educational attainment, income security and perceived sense of control, one could assume that educational attainment serves as an important protective factor against substance abuse in later life.

Even so, is it really the programming provided by schools that reduces the likelihood of drug use, or just the general setting itself? Based on an extensive review of available literature and evaluations, Edwards et al. (1994,

208) conclude that "there is no present research evidence which can support their deployment (school-based education public education, warning labels, and advertising restrictions) as lead policy choices or justify expenditure of major resources on school-based education (or mass media public education campaigns), unless they are placed in a broader context of community action." Given that so many other environmental forces will be in action concurrently, the potential for focused impact is slight, and long term at best. These findings have significant implications for policy development, which will be discussed later in this paper.

Recap: The educational environment is critical in deterring use of alcohol, tobacco and illicit drugs by young people. This is not, however, relevant to those youth who do not respond well to a traditional educational setting, and end up on the street or in low-paying jobs.

Employment and Working Conditions

Given the psychosocial stress associated with unemployment, it is not surprising that the unemployed tend to be at greater risk for problems associated with the abuse of alcohol and other drugs. Studies conducted by the Addiction Research Foundation, for example, found a higher incidence of drinking, alcohol-related problems and psychotropic drug use among unemployed workers (Smart 1979; Groeneveld, Shain, and Simon 1990).

The impact of employment and working conditions on the substance use of young people has not been studied intensively, as most youth in western, industrialized nations like Canada have not yet been absorbed into the workforce. Young people who drop out of school and seek employment opportunities despite their limited skills and experience are more vulnerable to psychosocial stress, which, in turn, predisposes them to the abuse of alcohol and other drugs. A study of street youth in Toronto supported this view of the relationship between employment, stress and substance abuse among young people (Smart and Adlaf 1991). As family members, the psychosocial health of young people is also affected by the employment status and working conditions of their parents and caregivers.

Recap: Employment, per se, does not appear to be as critical a determinant for youth as for adult populations. However, the importance of the parents' employment situation cannot be underestimated, as it will determine the relevance of other determinants, such as income status.

Physical Environment

Factors in the biophysical environment, such as air, water and soil quality, are key influences on health and well-being. Factors in the human environment, including housing, workplace safety and road design, are also important determinants of health (Evans et al. 1994).

When considering the impact of the physical environment on the use of alcohol and other drugs by young people, it is important to note the relationship between physical living and working conditions and socio-economic status. In Canada, the physical environment (e.g., neighbourhood or community) in which an individual lives is often a function of his socioeconomic status (i.e., economically disadvantaged people are more likely to live in poor-quality housing in congested, polluted neighbourhoods). For economically disadvantaged young people, poor living conditions are a symptom of the economic and social deprivation that puts them at greater risk for drug- and alcohol-related problems (Hawkins, Catalano, and Miller 1992).

Street youth are also at a particular disadvantage when it comes to physical environment, since they often must rely on shelters designed for adult needs. They are also influenced by exploitive older youths and adults, intent on attracting them to lives of prostitution and drug dealing. Their environments will be unsanitary and unsafe, putting them at risk of disease and personal injury, as well as providing opportunities for significant substance abuse.

Recap: It is the relationship between income and physical environment that has the greatest impact on young people, as poor living conditions create greater opportunities for contact with a drug-using population.

Personal Health Practices and Coping Skills

A large body of research has revealed that factors related to a deficit of coping skills (e.g., low self-esteem) are major determinants of **tobacco** use among young people. Burton and colleagues (1989) found that young people who had strong intentions to smoke were more likely to have relatively positive images of smokers and low images of themselves, a finding that supports the notion that smoking may appeal to young people with low self-esteem. A review of gender differences in the smoking behaviour of young people revealed that low self-esteem was related to teenage smoking among boys, but not girls (Clayton 1991). Similarly, Allen and colleagues (1994) found male adolescent smokers to be more lonely, shy and unsociable than nonsmokers, while female smokers scored lower on shyness but higher on sociability than nonsmokers. These studies suggest that coping skills training and self-esteem enhancement may not be appropriate for young female smokers.

Personal health practices and coping skills are also related to the use of *alcohol* and other *drugs* by young people. Factors such as self-image, degree of alienation, beliefs about and attitudes toward drugs, and response to peer pressure have been cited repeatedly as key influences on substance abuse by young people (Flay et al. 1983; Glanz and Pickens 1992; Anderson 1995).

Society attaches great importance to these individual-level attributes in the prevention of substance abuse among young people considering the overwhelming majority of preventive interventions that target coping skills and personal health practices, rather than broader social and environmental determinants. While many of these efforts have, to varying degrees, been successful in preventing the onset of experimentation with alcohol and other drugs, the determinants of health framework articulated in this paper underscores the need to simultaneously address the broader social and environmental factors contributing to substance abuse among young people.

A large body of research is developing concerning the character trait of "resiliency," which is closely related to coping skills. Resiliency will be examined more fully in a subsequent section, but it must be taken into consideration when discussing substance abuse—why are some youth at risk while others appear not to be? Part of the answer lies in resiliency, and how one develops this protective quality.

Recap: Self-esteem is a recurring theme in assessments of youth substance abuse—it is a key influence on and predictor of the use of tobacco, alcohol and other drugs. However, while most intervention programs have focused on targeting coping skills, they have not given equal attention to the reasons for the lack of self-esteem, which appear to be grounded in the more broad-based determinants of health, such as income status and education.

Healthy Child Development

One of the most serious preventable consequences of substance abuse is Fetal Alcohol Syndrome (FAS). The result of in utero exposure to ethanol, FAS is characterized by pre- and/or postnatal growth retardation, central nervous system damage and facial abnormalities (Sokol and Clarren 1989). Estimated incidence rates suggest that FAS is a main contributor to the known causes of mental handicap (Robinson, Conry, and Conry 1987; Abel and Sokol 1991). Individuals affected by FAS experience permanent disabilities and require a lifetime of supportive services to deal with the problems arising from their condition (Streissguth et al. 1991).

As a consequence of alcohol abuse, the incidence of FAS in newborns is related to an array of behavioural, social, economic and environmental determinants. Accordingly, a wide range of comprehensive, preventive actions addressing the fundamental determinants of health is necessary to prevent this condition (Loney, Green, and Nanson 1994).

Summary of the Literature

Five key findings that should ultimately direct additional research and policy can be summarized thus:
- low-income status is negatively correlated to the use of tobacco, alcohol and illicit drugs, and their concomitant problems;

- family, caregivers, friends or peers wield perhaps the greatest influence (positive and negative), and are the best predictors, of adolescent substance abuse;
- the educational setting is protective—it deters and delays the onset of substance abuse;
- the physical environment for low-income people can encourage substance abuse; and
- coping skills, such as self-esteem, connection to or alienation from a group or community, and beliefs and attitudes toward drugs, are strongly related to substance abuse, but not in isolation from other factors such as income status and educational environment.

Resiliency

The concept of resiliency has been receiving increased attention of late. It is not a new concept, but it is being newly applied to health promotion, and it has relevance to the determinants of health. Resiliency can be defined as "the capability of individuals, families, groups, and communities to cope successfully in the face of significant adversity or risk. This capability changes over time, is enhanced by protective factors in the individual system and the environment, and contributes to the maintenance and enhancement of health" (Mangham et al. 1995).

Resiliency theory makes three key assumptions: resiliency can be influenced and enhanced; resiliency is dynamic, changing over time; and, through its relationship to positive functioning and ability to use supportive resources, resiliency is conducive to health. Most recently, resiliency theory has moved from the realms of the individual and family, and been applied to communities, although this application is somewhat more abstract. Mangham and colleagues (1995) found several factors that contribute to resiliency in communities: mutual support, collective expectations of success in meeting challenges, a high level of community participation, and a sense of control over its policies and choices.

Resiliency theory also outlines the cyclical nature of the effect, in that communities that respond well to adversity seem to gain the strength to repeat this process, becoming ever more empowered. On the other hand, a community can also move in the opposite direction. If unable to respond positively to adversity, it can become increasingly weakened and powerless, and less able to meet future challenges.

There are several observations from the Mangham and colleagues discussion paper that relate to, and support, a determinants of health approach. Their theory suggests that groups should be targeted rather than populations—that enhancing protective factors among high-risk individuals will pay the greatest dividends. However, while skills are emphasized as protective factors, a supportive environment is recognized as essential—social support. Finally, specific situations may respond better to interventions: for example, divorce, chronic disease or unemployment. Certainly, substance abuse fits here as a "situation." Underlying these observations is the recognition that more research is needed to augment the theoretical base.

Unfortunately, when it comes to substance abuse in particular, the addition of resiliency to the equation raises as many questions as it might answer. Why are some individuals and communities resistant to the effects of their environment while others are not? How can resiliency be fostered in those who do not naturally show this characteristic? Can it be taught, or is the experiential process the only effective one? Although the research base on this concept is limited, it has identified three broad categories of protective factors: individual, familial and support. These are worth repeating from the Mangham and colleagues (1995) paper, as they apply to the work being done in determinants of health, despite the generally broader focus on populations in determinants of health research. Individual factors include a sense of personal competency, the ability to plan, cognitive skills, a sense of meaning, problem solving ability, optimism, internal locus of control, skills in coping with stress, and resourcefulness in seeking support.

At the family level, protective factors include effective parenting, warmth and affection, strong family support, and family cohesion. Support factors · include the presence of caring, supportive individuals, such as teachers, extended family members, or people outside the immediate family. Also of importance are supportive environments that encourage autonomy, responsibility and control. All of these indicators should be considered as health policy is developed.

Implications for Theory

The literature is fairly clear in showing links between youth substance abuse and the determinants of health. Low socioeconomic status, deprived social support systems, poor education, parental unemployment, street life and low self-esteem are all significant predictors of the use of alcohol, tobacco and illicit drugs. But what are the implications of these findings for addressing the problem?

At present, a comprehensive theory outlining the relationship between the determinants of health and the misuse of alcohol, tobacco and other drugs by young people has not been developed. There are still too many gaps in the research to allow such a theory to be presented. However, we are able to advance some ideas in this direction. Some understanding of the relationship between these variables can be gained through two different, and sometimes contradictory, approaches to understanding the impact of life experiences on the health and well-being of young people.

The *latency* model emphasizes that particular events that tend to occur early in life, will have a strong independent effect in later life, regardless of other events in later life. For example, early exposure to cancer-causing agents may result in cancer decades later, even without intervening exposure.

In regard to the relationship between substance abuse among young people and the determinants of health, the latency model contends that deprivation of the prerequisites for health at an early age may place young people at increased risk of addiction in later life. For example, an infant deprived of adequate nutrition and positive opportunities for social interaction may be more susceptible to a range of health and social problems in later life, including the misuse of alcohol and other drugs. The effectiveness of particular prenatal and early childhood intervention programs in changing the life paths of disadvantaged children lends support to the latency model (Weikart 1989; Martin, Ramey, and Ramey 1990).

The *pathways* model, by contrast, emphasizes the cumulative or additive effect of life events on the development of young people, and the ongoing importance of conditions conducive to healthy living throughout the life cycle. The pathways model is traditionally associated with the complex range of findings from longitudinal studies, which demonstrate the enduring effect of particular life events on health and well-being over the entire life span (Hertzman 1993).

The pathways model thus implies that the extent to which young people have positive exposure to the determinants of health (e.g., education, income, a strong social support network) in their present situations will affect the degree to which they are able to realize an optimal level of health and well-being. Any deficits in these determinants place young people at increased risk of substance abuse, which, in turn, may contribute to deficits in the determinants of health (e.g., limited employment opportunities).

Thompson (1995) notes that the latency and pathway models may be viewed as complementary to one another in one respect. Any early life event that could exert a *latent* effect in adulthood could also be the first step along a lifelong *pathway* with implications for health, well-being and competency in the future.

As theories for guiding the development of responses to address the predisposing causes of substance abuse, the latency and pathways models have different implications for policy and program decisions. If the pathways model applies, then a "cradle-to-grave social contract"—programs and policies aimed at ensuring equitable access to the fundamental determinants of health throughout one's life—is most relevant, given the cumulative effect of life events. If, however, the latency model applies, then policies and programs promoting optimal conditions for early childhood health are the most relevant interventions. Perhaps, policy focusing on youth should address the key related factors identified in the literature review above, while more general health and related policy could be based on the pathways model.

In this light, Thompson's review of the literature (1995) provides a summary of key, concrete interventions that should be considered in attempt-

ing to affect the childhood risk factors that may expose the developing individual to a higher probability of substance abuse as an adolescent:
- reducing early childhood aggressiveness, particularly in males;
- developing competent parenting and family management styles;
- reducing parent-child conflict and marital conflict;
- increasing positive parent-child involvement; and
- reducing parental substance abuse, criminality and antisocial behaviour.

These recommendations still leave the issue of operationalization to be addressed, but do point the programmer and policymaker in the right direction. Interventions such as parenting programs and daycare programs focused on social skills are indicated, as are programs based in educational settings that provide opportunities for positive socialization and for meeting positive role models and mentors.

ILLUSTRATIVE PROJECTS

Introduction

Regardless of the explanatory framework one chooses to adopt, there is clearly a need for preventive interventions to go beyond the mere dissemination of educational information or the enhancement of coping skills. We have already highlighted the need for a multifaceted approach, which takes into account the individual, the family and the environment, and fosters resiliency at both the individual and community level.

In recent years, a growing awareness and acceptance that a broad-based approach to substance abuse is essential has led to a number of innovative, community-based interventions focusing on the social, economic and environmental causes of substance abuse among young people. Although the innovators may not have been aware of the determinants of health framework, they unconsciously incorporated many of the concepts now accepted in this context. The interventions described in this section illustrate the ways that a determinants of health perspective can guide the development of community-level responses to the "root" causes of substance abuse by young people.

The following six projects were selected from 15 initiatives reviewed for the preparation of this report. Four main criteria guided the selection of projects:
1. They were community-based (as opposed to institutional programs and services);
2. They focused on the prevention of tobacco, alcohol and other drug use;
3. They explicitly identified young people (up to age 21) as the priority group for project interventions; and
4. They incorporated activities that, directly or indirectly, addressed the social, economic and environmental determinants of health.

Although this report attempts to include a range of projects from across Canada, several initiatives based in Ontario seem to provide the best examples of "retrofitting" the determinants of health model to existing projects. Since the "fit" was deemed more important than geographical positioning, these projects were selected over others.

When considering the usefulness of the following interventions in addressing the social and environmental factors placing young people at risk of substance abuse, two limitations should be noted. First, most of these initiatives have not been subject to a rigorous evaluation. The absence of assessment data on the planning and implementation of these initiatives is, in part, a reflection of the low priority of, and limited capacity for, evaluation among community-level sponsors.

The second limitation that should be kept in mind when reviewing these projects is the absence of an explicit adoption of the determinants of health framework. While the activities initiated under these projects addressed the broader determinants of health, none of the initiatives embraced the determinants of health approach as a rationale for their efforts. Accordingly, the positioning of these projects within the determinants of health framework represents a "retrofit", as mentioned above, that enables the reader to better understand how community-level interventions can address the underlying causes of substance abuse by young people.

In spite of these limitations, the following interventions represent unique and innovative approaches to addressing the myriad of causal and protective factors related to the use of alcohol and other drugs by youth. As such, they merit further consideration as examples of practical, community-level responses to substance abuse that are equivalent to the determinants of health approach. None of the projects dealt with only one drug—nicotine, alcohol and illicit drugs were targeted together. Although each substance has a different consumption pattern and harm associated with its use, the underlying issues concerning the use of all of these substances are similar enough to be reached through multifaceted approaches.

Finally, it should be mentioned that community-based initiatives were deliberately selected over other approaches (such as legislative). The rationale for this decision will be elaborated on in the section on policy principles.

The Projects

The Media Arts Program

The Media Arts Program is an ongoing skill-building initiative for young people living in Regent Park, a low-income community in the east end of Toronto. Sponsored by the Regent Park Focus Community Coalition, one of nine community-based substance abuse prevention projects funded by the Ontario Ministry of Health's Health Promotion Branch, the program provides a range of learning experiences for young people in the media arts field (e.g., photography). Participants apply their new skills to develop videos and print materials focusing on substance abuse and related problems in the Regent Park area. The innovative approach adopted by the Media Arts Program was recognized in 1995, when it won the Toronto Mayor's Anti-Drug Task Force Award.

The goal of the Media Arts Program is "to use media technology to stimulate discussion, share information and inspire action around substance abuse." The objectives of the program are "to provide youth and young adults with a forum to interactively learn about substance abuse; to teach youth to teach others about substance abuse; and to use print, media and video presentations to present strategies that individuals, families and communities can use to prevent substance use and promote health," (Ontario Government 1995, 2).

A needs assessment conducted by the local community health centre guided the development of the program. Informal discussions and interviews with young people in Regent Park revealed a dearth of accurate information about drug use and its consequences. Most young people did not read the local newspapers. All of the youth interviewed in the needs assessment, however, reported watching television and videos, a finding that led to the identification of the Media Arts Program as a means of engaging their interest in substance abuse prevention.

The program also emerged from the work of the local youth centre coordinator, who saw that many of the young people he was trying to attract to after-school activities were "hanging out" in bars, video arcades and pool halls. In these settings, they were coming into contact with drugs as well as individuals engaged in illegal activities, many of whom were befriending the young people and providing negative role models. The Media Arts Program was conceived as an appealing alternative that would dissuade young people from spending time in high-risk settings that increased their vulnerability to drug- and alcohol-related problems.

The Media Arts Program comprises a number of individual projects, including six collaborative efforts with local schools and community agencies, where young people work in small production teams to research and present information through video. Another ongoing program intervention is the media arts camp project, a 13-week activity offered each summer for young people aged 14 to 21.

Components of the program include media awareness training (i.e., watching TV and reading the papers), media skills training (learning how to produce a video and a newspaper), and the development of videos and newspapers by the program participants. In addition, the Media Arts Program offers an ongoing peer education program for youth, weekend and after-school employment opportunities for youth, and ongoing promotion and outreach to the community.

Future activities planned for the program include working with Rogers Cablesystems to televise completed videos, and producing a minimum of two videos promoting healthy lifestyle alternatives and the Regent Park community. Both of these videos were broadcast in 1996. Program leaders are also investigating the possibility of developing a youth video business cooperative to provide video services to agencies and institutions.

Since its inception in 1991, more than 200 youths and young adults have participated in the Media Arts Program. Topics addressed in the videos include parental substance abuse, peer pressure, tobacco use and racism. Program participants have created a total of 23 videos. *Catcha Da Flava*, a youth-oriented magazine produced by participants, was initiated in 1995.

At present, two videos are being used as drug education resources and are being disseminated through a variety of venues, including local festivals and events, Drug Awareness Week, the Toronto School Board, the North York School Board, the Toronto Department of Public Health and Rogers Cablesystems' community channel. An estimated 2,000 children in Toronto's public and separate schools have seen the videos.

Evaluation forms distributed at viewings indicate that the videos have been successful in informing youth about drug and alcohol abuse: after watching the videos, most young people reported learning something about substance abuse they did not know before. Many of the teachers at participating schools reported using the videos to stimulate discussion of peer pressure and other issues related to the use of alcohol and other drugs. In general, teachers, students, public health officials, parents and community workers who have seen the videos feel they are a highly effective, culturally appropriate means of communicating information and motivating action on substance abuse.

Participants in the Media Arts Program report increased levels of skills and knowledge related to accessing drug education resources and information. As a direct result of the program, many participants are more aware of the consequences of drugs and alcohol and are, therefore, in a better position to make healthy choices. Moreover, the activities offered through the program provide the young participants with healthy recreational alternatives to drug use, as well as marketable skills that can be applied to pursue future educational or career opportunities.

The annual cost of running the Media Arts Program in 1994 is estimated at $37,000, including $16,400 for the media arts camp and $14,492 for the after-school program. In spite of the expenses involved, components of the Media Arts Program are highly generalizable and could be replicated by other community agencies, schools and organizations. Much of the media technology used by the program, such as the video-editing equipment, was donated by community sponsors. The dissemination of substance abuse prevention videos could easily be implemented in other communities with a local access cable TV station.

In summary, the Media Arts Program is an innovative multicomponent initiative that has direct and indirect impacts on a range of nonmedical determinants of health. Through collective participation in a range of activities requiring cooperation and group work, the *social support networks* of the young people are enhanced. The information on substance abuse and related issues conveyed through the media arts program enhances the *personal health practices and coping skills* of participants, by better enabling them to make healthy decisions about the use of alcohol and other drugs. Lastly, participants can apply the practical skills learned through the program to pursue future educational and career opportunities, which may, over the long run, positively affect their *income, educational and social status.*

Alexandra Park Residents' Association

A Residents' Association formed in the Alexandra Park area of Toronto illustrates the positive impact of community development efforts addressing the fundamental determinants of health. Through the efforts of the Residents' Association, Alexandra Park has undergone a transformation, from a centre for drug trafficking, where residents were plagued by crime and violence, to a vibrant, cohesive community where residents of all ages are involved in community life.

The Alexandra Park Residents' Association underwent an extensive reorganization in 1990, when local residents became fed up with the poor quality of life in their neighbourhood and began a series of initiatives toward renewal. A new association executive strengthened the association's ties with other community organizations, seeking assistance from local politicians, schools, the police, the Metropolitan Toronto Housing Authority (MTHA), city departments, and other local agencies.

With the assistance of the MTHA and City of Toronto officials, the Residents' Association removed walls and shrubs that hid drug dealers, and improved lighting in the community. The association worked with the police and the MTHA to evict tenants operating crack houses and increase the frequency of patrols to discourage gangs of drug traffickers.

In addition to these enforcement measures, the Residents' Association worked with the MTHA and the City of Toronto Mayor's Task Force on Drugs to develop a prevention program for young people. Through this project, a youth coordinator worked with a group of young people at high risk for drug abuse and drug trafficking. Fifteen young people, who had previously been denied access to recreational facilities participated in recreational programs, organized a youth conference, developed resumés, attended job readiness training workshops, and applied for and found jobs. As a result of the project, the young participants received positive directions and opportunities for personal growth and economic advancement.

The original youth project ended in 1992, when funding ended. Since that time, however, the Residents' Association has continued to devote resources to activities aimed at preventing substance abuse among young people. Current initiatives include: an economic development project to help young people create small businesses and access job readiness training; children's recreational programming (e.g., basketball); and youth dances and other social events at the community centre.

In keeping with its philosophy of empowering youth, the Alexandra Park Residents' Association actively involves young people in association activities. Two young people are members of the association's board of directors, which is made up exclusively of community members. In addition, the local community centre, which serves as the venue for association activities, maintains a policy of hiring local youth for jobs at the centre. Over the past year, eight young people have been employed in part-time or seasonal positions at the centre.

The work of the Residents' Association has resulted in tangible changes in the community. Local residents are reportedly less suspicious of strangers in the community. The gangs of drug traffickers have been dispersed, and most of the crack houses have been eliminated (Alexandra Park Residents' Association 1996). Local residents are currently negotiating with the MTHA to have their units turned into cooperative housing. In recognition of the positive changes its activities have fostered in the community, the Alexandra Park Residents' Association received the Canadian Centre on Substance Abuse (CCSA) Award of Distinction in 1995.

Funding for the youth program and other activities is generated by the Residents' Association, which raises over $30,000 a year through activities such as bingo hall rentals and bake sales. A network of community partners also provides ongoing support for programming efforts. For example, the recreational programs for youth are offered in collaboration with a local school, which provides gym space, and the local housing authority, which provides staff and supplies.

The activities of the Alexandra Park Residents' Association are generalizable to other economically disadvantaged communities: the low cost of its program activities, its high degree of community involvement and extensive reliance on local support, and its focus on practical, achievable solutions that address the felt needs of community members, are attractive features of the Residents' Association that could be incorporated by similar initiatives.

In summary, the activities of the Residents' Association have had a positive impact on some of the fundamental determinants of health. The *physical environment* of the community has improved through an increased police presence, and through changes aimed at increasing safety and deterring drug sales (e.g., better lighting). Young people taking part in the program benefit from practical *education* (job readiness training), enhanced *social support networks*, and improved *personal health practices and coping skills*. Lastly, the job opportunities and career-related training offered by the program increase the current and, possibly, the future *income and social status* of the young participants.

Town Youth Participation Strategies

Town Youth Participation Strategies (TYPS) is an innovative community-based substance abuse prevention program for young people living in small communities (under 25,000). Sponsored by the Tri-County Addictions Program in Smith Falls, Ontario, the purpose of TYPS is to provide five small towns with ways to involve young people in designing, operating and participating in healthy social and recreational activities. Each of these sites will focus on three specific goals: establishing local youth councils, developing youth centres, and producing a participatory video on issues relevant to local youth (Voakes 1995).

The rationale for the TYPS project emerged from a pilot initiative funded by Health and Welfare Canada under the Community Action Program of the National Drug Strategy in 1991–1992 (now known as Canada's Drug Strategy). A street worker in a small Eastern Ontario town was hired to investigate the issues, problems and needs of local youth, with particular emphasis on substance abuse. The street worker's report revealed that small town youth may be a high-risk population primarily because of the lack of recreational and social opportunities and a lack of awareness of available support services. As a result, some young people in small towns become alienated from their community. This sense of alienation manifests itself in an array of high-risk activities, including alcohol and drug abuse, leaving home prematurely, and dropping out of school (Voakes 1992).

In response to the issues raised in the street worker's report, a number of preventive activities were launched in the pilot community. To actively engage young people in identifying and acting on shared issues and concerns related to drug abuse, a Youth Advisory Council was formed. Young people from the community, representing a diverse range of backgrounds, met regularly to discuss various issues identified by the street worker, who encouraged the young people to ask questions and suggest remedial action. A few adult members, representing various youth service providers in the community, also took part in Youth Advisory Council meetings. The adult members of the council acted in an *ex officio* capacity, answering questions specific to their service and listening to the views of the young people (Voakes 1995).

Because of the short duration of the pilot project, the Youth Council was not developed fully and entrenched into the community. The current, multisite TYPS project plans to create youth advisory councils in each of the participating communities.

The lack of recreational and social opportunities for youth in the pilot community was addressed through the establishment of Midnight Junction, a drug- and alcohol-free teen centre that quickly became a popular hangout for local young people. Following the lead of the pilot initiative, the TYPS project leaders have identified the organization of youth centres in participating communities as a key program priority (Voakes 1995).

A participatory video project, enabling young people to identify and document topics of interest to them, was the third major activity of the TYPS project. Although a video was not completed during the pilot initiative, the idea generated considerable interest among young people, who were attracted by the prospect of expressing themselves through a popular medium.

Although full evaluative data on the impact of this initiative are not yet available, TYPS represents a promising participatory approach to addressing the risk factors for substance abuse among youth in midsized and smaller communities. A questionnaire has been developed to evaluate the impact of the youth centres established in the participating communities. Anecdotal reports from the pilot community indicate a drop in vandalism and alcohol-related incidents among young people since the opening of the teen centre. The young people involved in the pilot project have worked with the street worker to develop evaluation and documentation materials (Voakes 1995).

The total budget for the TYPS project (January 1, 1994 to March 31, 1997) is $305,500. In spite of the costs involved, portions of the project (e.g., the Youth Advisory Council) are easily replicable in other communities where sufficient interest and support exist. Resources in-kind could be sought from community partners to keep direct financial costs to a minimum.

As with similar community-based initiatives, the TYPS project facilitates equitable access to a range of nonmedical determinants of health. Through their involvement in the youth advisory councils and the youth centres, young people can strengthen their *social support networks* and enhance their *personal health practices and coping skills.* By offering young people social and recreational alternatives that reduce the incidence of drug- and alcohol-related problems, the wider community also benefits from a safer *physical environment.*

Out of the Mainstream Youth Project

In the fall of 1993, the Health Promotion Directorate of Health Canada, undertook a series of consultations to develop an operations strategy to address the needs of young people during the second phase of Canada's Drug Strategy. These consultations, which took place at the regional, provincial and territorial levels, involved service providers and youth.

One of the key issues emerging from the consultations was the lack of collaboration between community groups and agencies serving young people, which resulted in service gaps in some areas and duplication in others (Mattar 1996). The problem was particularly evident in midsized cities and smaller communities away from the large urban centres (Toronto, Vancouver) with large street youth populations.

In response to this concern, the Alcohol and Other Drugs Programs Unit (within the Health Promotion Directorate) launched the Out of the Mainstream Youth Community Development Project (OOMY). The goals of the project are "to work with test communities to assist them with the process of community development around youth at risk; to learn from this experience in terms of what works and what doesn't; and to develop sets of learning or models for community development for this target group transferable to other communities." (Anderson 1996).

The OOMY Project is currently under way at five sites across Canada: Halifax, Montreal, Manitoba/Saskatchewan region, Hay River and High Level, Alberta, and Whitehorse and surrounding communities in the Yukon Territory. Project coordinators are responsible for networking with local youth and community service providers to initiate community development activities at each of the sites.

Since its inception in 1994, OOMY project leaders have implemented a number of activities in response to identified community priorities. Some examples include: investigating the ways in which Halifax street youth are portrayed in the local media; coordinating service provision and increasing youth access to existing services in Montreal; organizing a workshop on sustainability for youth service providers in Manitoba and Saskatchewan; and initiating efforts to open a youth centre in Whitehorse (Mattar 1996).

The OOMY project is still in the early stages of development. Because of this, many of the community activities are still in the planning stages, and the impact of the project has not yet been evaluated. However, the OOMY project represents a promising framework for engaging key stakeholders, including young people, to identify and respond to substance abuse prevention priorities. Through its emphasis on intersectoral collaboration, the project is meeting one of the key prerequisites for effective action on the determinants of health (Premier's Council on Health Strategy 1991).

YWCA Crabtree Corner FAS Prevention Project

A community-based project designed to address the issue of Fetal Alcohol Syndrome (FAS), the YWCA Crabtree Corner has gained national recognition as an example of how high-risk communities can deal with addiction issues. YWCA Crabtree Corner is a community service program and resource centre, offering emergency short-term daycare and a variety of support services for women and their families in the downtown Eastside area of Vancouver.

The FAS Prevention Project operating out of Crabtree Corner was developed in 1988 in response to community concerns about the lack of support services available to mothers-to-be in the area. Eighteen community agencies offered strong support for the project, which received a three-year grant from the Health Promotion Directorate, Health and Welfare Canada, in 1990. Community partners include the Vancouver Wife Assault Task Force, the HIV/AIDS Clinic for Women and Children, the Downtown Eastside-Strathcona Coalition, the East Vancouver Nobody's Perfect Steering Committee, and the Child Poverty Action Group.

A community advisory committee, comprising agency representatives and community members with an interest in FAS issues, is responsible for coordinating the project. The committee provides a venue for the multi-sectoral partnerships necessary for the development of comprehensive strategies to prevent problems related to substance abuse.

Activities implemented by the FAS Prevention Project to date include:
- developing a resource library including video, audio and print information on FAS;
- organizing a series of community-based workshops and conferences on FAS;
- facilitating a variety of educational and information sessions on FAS prevention for single mothers, teens, health workers and other community members;
- developing a series of FAS prevention guides in easy-to-understand language;
- developing plain language brochures and pamphlets on FAS prevention; and
- lobbying decision makers for healthy public policies such as bottle labelling legislation, culturally appropriate warning signs, and protocols for pregnant women in alcoholism treatment centres.

In addition to the FAS-specific activities listed above, project participants have access to the ongoing services available at the centre, including child care, food supplements, parenting programs, clothing and information about other support services.

The Crabtree Corner FAS Prevention Project has been well received by the community. As of 1994, more than 600 community members took part in FAS educational sessions. One of the greatest successes of the project is its ability to foster intersectoral collaboration, enabling professionals from a variety of backgrounds to work together on a shared concern while avoiding duplication and issues of territoriality. Project partners include representatives from education, health, the criminal justice system, social services, and local businesses. In recognition of its innovative approach to addressing the underlying causes of FAS, YWCA Crabtree Corner received the provincial CCSA Medallion of Distinction in 1994.

As a broad-based "project within a project", YWCA Crabtree Corner is an innovative means of fostering *healthy child development*. To achieve this objective, it offers a range of activities addressing some of the other fundamental determinants of health, including *income and social status* (food supplements, daycare services and clothing), *social support networks* (through participation in workshops, conferences and the community advisory committee), *education* (easy-to-understand print materials), and *personal health practices and coping skills*.

Compliance for Kids

Compliance for Kids is a community-based project aimed at preventing smoking among young people. Unlike other preventive efforts, which focus on the knowledge, attitudes and behaviour of youth, Compliance for Kids targets a key environmental factor encouraging the uptake of smoking: the sale of cigarettes to minors. The program was originally developed by the Edmonton group Action on Smoking and Health, and has been implemented in several Alberta communities.

The Compliance for Kids program consists of two main approaches: a lobbying effort to enact a city bylaw against tobacco sales to minors, and an educational program aimed at tobacco retailers. The latter initiative is premised on the assumption that merchants' behaviour will be influenced by their familiarity with, and acceptance of, the program. All tobacco vendors in participating communities receive signs, decals, copies of the relevant legislation, a letter from the mayor, staff training materials and other resources designed to curb tobacco sales to minors.

The implementation of the Compliance for Kids program in three Alberta communities (Grande Prairie, Red Deer and Taber) was assessed by Abernathy (1994). The three measures used to evaluate the efficacy of the program were vendor compliance with the legislation, vendor knowledge of the relevant legislation, and the stated willingness of the vendor to sell cigarettes to a youth bearing a note from a parent or another adult.

Results of a pre/post test carried out in the participating communities revealed that only one community, Taber, experienced a significant reduction in the sale of cigarettes to minors. This result may be attributable to the fact that, while in the other communities, vendors received the background material in the mail, Taber vendors received the relevant documentation from a health department official accompanied by an RCMP officer. A lesser degree of success was found in Grande Prairie, and almost no effect was observed in Red Deer, where sales to minors were already lowest at the beginning of the study (Abernathy 1994).

Vendor knowledge of the legislation increased significantly in Taber, where it was initially low (from 42.8 percent to 85.7 percent). Modest increases in knowledge were obtained in the other communities. The pro-gram also yielded significant reductions in the percentage of vendors willing to sell cigarettes to minors presenting a note from their parents or another adult. Merchant satisfaction with the program was high, with over 85 percent of those interviewed rating it as "very good" or "excellent."

The Compliance for Kids initiative is an example of how community-based initiatives can foster *social and physical environments* conducive to the maintenance of health-promoting behaviours. By reducing the availability of cigarettes to minors, the project addressed a key social and environmental determinant of smoking.

Summary

The preceding projects are but a few examples of the ways in which community-based initiatives can prevent drug and alcohol use by young people within the context of the broader determinants of health. Unfortunately, they all suffer the same limitation—lack of evaluation. Although we have referred to moderate successes, this analysis is based on anecdotal information or short-term outcome data. The newness of these multifaceted community-based programs precludes long-term results. Edwards et al. (1994) comment on the same limitation in their extensive literature review in the area of alcohol policy. However, they also find that "the community's acceptance of, or better still its active backing, is a prerequisite for the successful application of any public health policy, and must be integral to alcohol policies. Community action strategies recognize this fact, and aim to mobilize existing community resources and support to this end" (p. 210).

Although the nature and scope of these initiatives vary, all their activities were guided by the recognition that health-promoting behaviour does not occur in isolation from healthy environments. Through a variety of strategies that unconsciously addressed what we now term the determinants of health—including skills training (the Media Arts Program), regulatory policies (Compliance for Kids), employment opportunities (Alexandra Park Residents' Association) and intersectoral planning (Out of the Mainstream Youth)—these initiatives fostered healthy environments that better enabled young people to make health-promoting choices about the use of alcohol and other drugs.

RESEARCH GAPS

By addressing the social, economic and environmental factors affecting the health of young people, community-based projects using a determinants of health framework have begun to gain a degree of acceptance in the field of substance abuse prevention. Support for these initiatives is far from universal, however, as proponents of a determinants of health approach must justify initiatives that address issues such as poverty, social isolation and job skills training, which have traditionally been viewed as beyond the scope of substance abuse prevention efforts.

There is a clear need to demonstrate that a determinants of health approach is an effective and legitimate means of guiding the development of prevention programs for young people. Nevertheless, several research and methodological considerations need to be addressed before conclusions about the efficacy of this approach can be supported with confidence. In a climate of increasing fiscal restraint, the resolution of these research issues is crucial for the continued support of substance abuse prevention programs addressing the broad determinants of health. Fortunately, fiscal restraint can also facilitate increased intersectoral collaboration among key stakeholders that deal with the various determinants of health.

The following issues are of particular importance for the development of effective preventive programming for young people based on a determinants of health framework:
- focusing research on youth, rather than adult populations;
- furthering research on how determinants interact;
- using both quantitative and qualitative methodologies;
- conducting evaluations on community-based programs;
- designing effective, appropriate research questions for these assessments;
- involving youth in all stages of the research and program design; and
- supporting a demonstration project based specifically on a determinants of health model.

Reorientation of Research to Assess the Impact of the Determinants of Health on the Health and Well-Being of Young People

The bulk of the survey research cited in the literature supporting a determinants of health focus (e.g., Mustard and Frank 1991) has been conducted on adult populations. As a result, the extent to which this research can be used to make inferences about the relationship between determinants of health and the health of young people is limited.

While social, economic and environmental factors undoubtedly affect the health and well-being of young people, through interaction with their schools, neighbourhoods, social networks and families, the effects of these determinants (both short- and long-term) may be different from those observed in adult populations. For example, the impact of job loss on a family can be expected to affect young people in a different way than the unemployed parent or caregiver, given the extent to which social norms emphasize employment in defining an adult's sense of self-worth.

To better understand the impact of the determinants of health on the health and well-being of young people, further research focusing exclusively on youth is required. Such research will better inform the development of programs and services aimed at deterring substance abuse among young people by addressing the underlying risk and protective factors (e.g., resiliency).

Research Examining the Interrelatedness of the Key Determinants of Health

Justification for a determinants of health approach to addressing community health priorities, such as substance abuse, rests mainly on social epidemiological studies linking health outcomes (e.g., smoking) to proximate measures of a particular health determinant (e.g., Statistics Canada's low-income cut-off level as a measure of poverty). The extent to which this research can be used to support inferences about the health of populations, however, is limited, as it fails to account for the interrelationships between the key determinants of health.

Simply stated, the determinants of health cannot be isolated from one another. The impact of a drug education program in a school setting, for example, cannot be fully understood without considering a range of social and environmental influences, such as the socioeconomic status of the students, family and parental attitudes toward drug abuse, and the extent to which the school environment fosters or inhibits the development of social networks.

Further research on the interrelatedness of the determinants of health is required to better understand their cumulative impact on substance abuse among young people. This research should afford program planners greater precision in the development of interventions addressing identified health risks. A greater understanding of the relationship between health determinants will, among other things, make it easier to identify protective factors that buffer the impact of social and environmental risks.

Integration of Appropriate Qualitative and Quantitative Research and Evaluation Methodologies

Historically, people in the public health field have relied on quantitative epidemiological studies to identify the risk factors contributing to disease, and to document the impact of preventive efforts (i.e., reductions in the prevalence of communicable and noninfectious diseases). Quantitative approaches to assessment continued to predominate as the locus of preventive efforts shifted to community-based programming.

The extent to which social epidemiology and other quantitative methods should be used to inform and assess interventions addressing the broad determinants of health is an increasing source of contention among practitioners (Frank 1995; Labonte 1995). While quantitative methods are a valuable and necessary means of inquiry, they are not sufficient for under-standing complex, multifaceted relationships, such as the links between the determinants of health and substance abuse. Research methods that combine quantitative and qualitative data collection are preferable for a number of reasons.

First, the decision-making requirements of community-based substance abuse prevention efforts, such as those described in the previous section, place high priority on access to timely, accessible information. Quantitative research and evaluation methods—which usually entail a substantial investment of time for data collection and analysis—risk either prolonging the decision period or yielding results only after the best opportunity for their use has passed (Van Sant 1989). Qualitative research methods are a better way to gather the process-related information needed for the ongoing modification of community-based projects.

The second limitation of quantitative approaches for understanding the relationship between substance abuse and the broad determinants of health concerns the application of the collected information. Qualitative methods are more amenable to the research and evaluation issues of interest to community programmers and the community participants they work with (Stewart-Brown and Prothero 1988). These questions are most often concerned with participant attitudes and perceptions, such as the extent to which participants feel more empowered and capable of addressing their shared health concerns as a result of the program. Because questions of this nature involve how people interpret the importance of specific events or actions, they are better assessed through qualitative methods. Unlike quantitative approaches, which invariably reduce beliefs, opinions and attitudes to a set of numbers for statistical analysis, qualitative approaches generate rich, detailed data that preserves the perspective of program participants (Steckler et al. 1992).

Lastly, quantitative methods can undermine the process of facilitating empowerment, that is, the ability to control one's environment, which is often a key objective of community-based substance abuse prevention projects. A quantitative survey or evaluation can often be an alienating experience for marginalized communities, who are usually the priority groups for preventive activities addressing the determinants of health. People with lower English language or literacy skills, for example, may internalize their inability to comprehend questions as a personal shortcoming prohibiting them from future involvement with a program. Economically disadvantaged individuals may resent quantitative forms of evaluation, as they feel that their lives are already subject to intense scrutiny by government officials and agencies (Labonte 1993).

Qualitative methods, by contrast, overcome some of the "disempowering" aspects of evaluation. Community participants usually view qualitative measures as less intrusive than quantitative approaches. Qualitative methods also tend to be more 'user friendly', incorporating the language and culture of the people involved with a project. Moreover, qualitative methods encompass the immediate concerns and issues of project participants, not just the interests of the sponsoring institutions (Labonte 1993).

For these reasons, research assessing the relationship between substance abuse among young people and the determinants of health should use complementary quantitative and qualitative methodologies. Complementary qualitative information, which uncovers the contextual issues underlying the misuse of alcohol and other drugs, will better enable researchers to understand the true 'significance' of quantitative data.

Comprehensive Program Evaluations of Community-Based Prevention Efforts Addressing the Broad Determinants of Health

The examples of community-based prevention initiatives described in the previous section reflect the paucity of comprehensive evaluations assessing the impact of these efforts. As Goodstadt (1995) notes, evidence for the value and utility of "newer" prevention programs, including those addressing the broad determinants of health, is scarce and largely anecdotal.

Most references on the subject identify two primary types of evaluation (Windsor et al. 1984; Green and Lewis 1986; Posavac and Carey 1989). *Process evaluation* examines what actually happens in an intervention, including all of the planning and implementation steps, while *outcome evaluation* determines the extent to which an intervention was successful in achieving its goals (e.g., reduced incidence of alcohol-related incidents among young people in a community). Both levels of evaluation are relevant for assessing the impact of community-based substance abuse prevention programs using a determinants of health framework.

In addition to providing reliable and valid information on program effectiveness, a thorough evaluation of a community-based prevention program serves a number of purposes. It provides constructive feedback to community participants. It can help to focus attention on aspects of a project that need to be revised, or it could point to the need for new priorities and goals. It could help to clarify existing problems, or identify problems that had gone undetected. Over the long term, an evaluation could serve as a resource for lobbying decision makers, or a promotional resource for raising awareness of the issues a project seeks to address. At a general level, program evaluations should make participants more aware of what is happening, more perceptive of probable project outcomes, and more perceptive of the underlying factors demonstrating a project's success or failure (van der Eyken 1991).

Greater efforts, therefore, need to be devoted to evaluating the process and outcome of community-based substance abuse prevention projects for young people using a determinants of health approach. In addition to the benefits listed above, a thorough evaluation of community-based prevention efforts will enable practitioners to identify the most effective components of these activities in promoting and maintaining the health and well-being of young people. This, in turn, will permit a more cost-effective investment of scarce public resources in future program and service delivery.

Specificity of Research Questions Assessing the Impact of Substance Abuse Prevention Efforts

In assessing the usefulness of preventive interventions, practitioners and program sponsors often adopt a bottom line approach, posing broad questions such as: Do community-based interventions work? How effective is a determinants of health approach to preventing substance abuse? Which, among the many available strategies addressing the determinants of health, is most effective? What works? As Goodstadt (1995) notes, responding to these questions is difficult, as the available evidence is complex, inconsistent and often unconvincing to the sceptic.

In response to the pressure to demonstrate the sweeping effectiveness of interventions across priority groups and communities, practitioners need to recognize that, however reasonable bottom line questions may seem, they are still the wrong questions. They are unidimensional; they fail to account for the complexity of factors influencing the health status of individuals and communities.

Goodstadt (1995, 1) suggests that a more appropriate research question for understanding the effectiveness of preventive interventions is: "Under what circumstances are specific health promotion strategies effective—regarding which health issue, for which objectives, for which populations, in what time frame, using which approaches, measured against which criteria?" The adoption of this approach to understanding the impact of interventions addressing the determinants of substance abuse among young people will, over the long run, yield more effective information for program development than searches for magic bullet solutions that do not exist.

Participatory Action Research Involving Young People at Risk of Substance Abuse

Several of the community-based programs described in the previous section incorporate principles of participatory action research, an approach originally proposed by the social psychologist Kurt Lewin (1946, 1952). Simply stated, participatory action research is "the way groups of people can organize the conditions under which they can learn from their own experience, and make this experience accessible to others" (McTaggart 1993, 66). This approach has both an individual aspect, in which participatory action researchers change themselves, and a collective aspect, in which participatory action researchers work with community groups to achieve social change.

A distinctive feature of participatory action research is that those affected by the outcome of the research (e.g., youth at risk of substance abuse) are responsible for deciding on the course of action suggested by the research (Kemmis and McTaggart 1988).

Since participatory action research often focuses on the social and environmental determinants of health and illness through resolving community health concerns, participants are less likely to feel exploited by the research process. The use of participatory action research also ensures that researchers use appropriate methods that enable disadvantaged communities to address their shared priorities and validate their knowledge and experience.

Lastly, there is some evidence that the health and well-being of community members may benefit from participation in the research process. Research has begun to identify empowerment as a health-enhancing variable. A growing body of community health and social science literature indicates that collective efforts aimed at facilitating the process of empowerment by working with community groups to address their shared concerns can yield tangible health benefits in the form of higher self-esteem, increased self and collective efficacy, enhanced social support, stronger social networks, and greater community cohesion (Wallerstein 1993). This concept was discussed earlier with reference to the literature on resiliency.

Accordingly, participatory action research methods should be given equal priority to traditional research methods when examining the impact of the determinants of health on substance abuse among young people. Where possible, researchers, community change agents and young people should work together to plan, implement and analyze substance abuse prevention projects addressing the fundamental determinants of health.

Substance Abuse Prevention Research Project Based on a Determinants of Health Framework

Although the projects discussed in this paper addressed the fundamental determinants of health, they were not premised on such a framework, per se. Because of the absence of such initiatives, conclusions about the efficacy of a determinants of health approach to addressing health issues, such as substance abuse, tend to be inferred from "compatible approximations" rather than substantiated by direct application. To better understand the implications of a determinants of health approach for the planning and implementation of substance abuse prevention efforts for young people, resources should be allocated to support a community-based initiative specifically developed on a determinants of health framework.

Other Research Questions

- How can we keep young people in an educational setting, to take advantage of the protective effect afforded by this environment?
- How can we foster resiliency, to help young people cope better with their disadvantages in regard to the broader determinants of health?
- To what extent is substance abuse a determinant of health?
- To what extent does substance abuse have an impact on other determinants of health?

IMPLICATIONS FOR POLICY

Underlying Principles

In recent years, policies and program efforts in the field of substance abuse prevention have become increasingly multidimensional, dealing with the immediate problems of alcohol and other drug use, as well as risk and protective factors such as family violence, self-esteem, enforcement and community support systems. With the emergence of a determinants of health approach to addressing health priorities, this trend can be expected to grow. To translate the theoretical underpinnings of the determinants of health approach into practical policies and program efforts aimed at addressing the social, economic and environmental causes of substance abuse among young people, the following underlying principles need to be considered first:

- a role for both health promotion and population health;
- increased intersectoral collaboration; and
- community-based approaches.

Health Promotion and Population Health Must Be Recognized as Complementary Approaches for Action on the Determinants of Health

Health promotion, "the process of enabling people to increase control over, and to improve, their health," (Ottawa Charter for Health Promotion 1986, i), has long recognized the importance of equitable access to the fundamental determinants of health for the health and well-being of individuals and communities. The Ottawa Charter for Health Promotion (1986) lists the following "prerequisites for health": peace, shelter, education, food, income, a stable ecosystem, sustainable resources, social justice and equity. The Charter notes that "improvement in health requires a secure foundation in these basic prerequisites" (1986, i).

To ensure that these prerequisites are available to individuals and communities, the Charter identifies five priority areas for action: build healthy public policy, create supportive environments, strengthen community action, develop personal skills and reorient health services (1986, i-ii).

Since the release of the Charter, a number of health promotion efforts at the national, provincial and community level have been initiated in accordance with these priorities. Health promotion continues to be one of the key approaches guiding the planning and implementation of policies and programs addressing the fundamental determinants of health.

In recent years, however, the concept of population health has become more influential among health planners and policymakers at the federal and provincial level. Examples include: the establishment of a Federal, Provincial and Territorial Advisory Committee on Population Health and the subsequent development of a population health framework; the establishment of a Population Health Issues Unit within Health Canada to replace some of the functions of the Health Promotion Directorate; and the establishment of a Population Health Unit at the Public Health Branch of the Ontario Ministry of Health (Rootman 1995). In addition, the publication of key documents advocating a population health approach to dealing with health priorities (e.g., Evans et al. 1994) have garnered widespread attention and support.

Like health promotion, population health strategies address the entire range of factors that determine health, including social support networks, education, personal health practices and healthy workplace environments. Unlike health promotion, which relies on targeted as well as population-wide approaches, population health focuses exclusively on strategies designed to affect the entire population (Federal, Provincial and Territorial Advisory Committee on Population Health 1994).

The rise of population health as an alternative (albeit a complementary alternative) to health promotion has sparked debate regarding the merits of both approaches. In a critique of the population health approach, Labonte (1995), expresses concern that population health, with its focus on social epidemiology, forces health back into a continuum of disease rather than reinforcing a holistic view of health outside of the medical model. Moreover, population health's focus on the need to contain financial expenditures on health care could "unintentionally undermine the fragile legitimacy for empowerment, community development, qualitative research and political advocacy that health promoters have struggled for two decades to obtain" (Labonte 1995, 167).

It is interesting to note that key documents supporting the adoption of a population health approach (Federal, Provincial and Territorial Advisory Committee on Population Health 1994; Frank 1995) fail to mention health promotion, or describe how health promotion strategies could contribute to the objectives of population health. For example, community mobilization, a key health promotion strategy, is overlooked in population health documents, despite being one of the key approaches used to enable disadvantaged groups to secure equitable access to the determinants of health. Virtually all of the examples of preventive interventions for young people described in the previous section of this paper employed principles of community development and mobilization.

To avoid the possibility of confusion, duplication and tension arising from two competing approaches to addressing the determinants of health, proponents of both health promotion and population health need to be aware of the positive contributions that each of these complementary approaches can make to addressing shared objectives. Ensuring that the entire population has access to the fundamental determinants of health, for example, should not preclude community development, advocacy and targeted health promotion efforts for disadvantaged segments of the community.

Intersectoral Collaboration Addressing the Determinants of Health Linked to Substance Abuse among Young People Must Be Promoted and Increased.

The adoption of a determinants of health approach to preventing substance abuse among young people necessitates the formation of partnerships from a range of sectors, including justice and enforcement, recreation, education, health, community and social services, transportation, and workplaces. The importance of intersectoral collaboration as a means of fostering concerted action on the determinants of health has been identified by a number of key planning and policy documents (Ottawa Charter for Health Promotion 1986; Premier's Council on Health Strategy 1991; Federal, Provincial and Territorial Advisory Committee on Population Health 1994).

All the community-based program efforts described in the previous section relied on intersectoral partnerships. These partnerships strengthened the impact of these projects at the community level, affording them a level of outreach to the priority group they would not otherwise have been able to achieve.

Fralick (1995) notes that the establishment of these partnerships will require some initial groundwork; partners representing sectors outside the purview of health and substance abuse prevention will need to be educated about the determinants of health, the importance of a multidimensional approach to dealing with substance abuse, and the impact of their policies and practices on the health of young people. In addition, the formation of successful intersectoral partnerships requires a fundamental shift in how partners view their work in the context of the determinants of health. Key sectors must be involved at the earliest stage of planning. This is critical to fostering collective ownership of the ideas and the process.

Community-Based Approaches Addressing the Social, Economic and Environmental Determinants of Substance Abuse among Young People Must Be Supported.

The realization of a determinants of health approach to the prevention of youth substance abuse culminates in the development and implementation of comprehensive programs and policies dealing with the broad range of health determinants. Ideally, these programs and policies will result from concerted action by a range of sectors and partners, thereby ensuring that each of the identified priorities (e.g., housing, social support) is addressed comprehensively.

The examples described in the previous section represented a cross section of community-based responses to dealing with the determinants of health related to the misuse of alcohol and other drugs by young people. As a means of ensuring more equitable access to the determinants of health, community-based approaches have several advantages over more traditional population-level responses, such as legislation or social marketing campaigns.

First, the causes of health-related problems faced by young people, such as addiction, are rooted in the social, economic and environmental conditions in their communities. Community mobilization strategies help to reduce health problems by dealing with the underlying causes present in the community (Perry 1986; Bracht 1990).

Second, community-based responses to health concerns help foster social skills and competencies, which are important determinants of health. Unlike population-level communication campaigns, which have been accused of treating young people as passive recipients of information, participatory community-based programs are more effective in equipping young people with the skills they need to maintain an optimal level of health. Community-based programs are an effective means of facilitating empowerment—the ability of individuals and communities to assume control over their own environment—which has been linked to a range of positive health outcomes (Wallerstein 1992).

The third reason favouring community-based programming as a means of preventing substance abuse among young people concerns the ability of community-level interventions to equip participants with an increased capacity for collective problem solving. As the financial resources required for 'top-down' state-sponsored support decrease, the onus for dealing with societal problems, such as substance abuse, will rest increasingly with communities. By enhancing the leadership, negotiation and communication skills of participants, community-based strategies help to increase the collective capacity of young people to address their shared concerns.

Lastly, community-based programming is flexible enough to accommodate the diversity of young people and the communities in which they live. Community-based programs can be tailored to the special characteristics and circumstances of their priority target groups, thereby avoiding the one size fits all mentality that limits the effectiveness of many population-level social marketing campaigns against substance abuse.

For these reasons, community-based programming efforts are effective at preventing substance abuse among young people by providing equitable access to the determinants of health. Federal and provincial governments should allocate a greater proportion of resources to these initiatives, and give priority to community-level initiatives.

Policy Recommendations

The literature and case studies have provided us with many clues as to where to focus our efforts and resources when dealing with youth substance abuse from a determinants of health perspective. We know that low income and poor self-esteem will increase the likelihood that young people will abuse substances. An educational setting can provide protection against their use. Family and peers can influence use and abuse either positively or negatively, depending on the nature of the interactions.

We also know what some of the protective interventions should be: effective parenting; fostering of personal responsibility; dealing with early childhood aggressiveness in males, parent-child conflict, marital conflict and parental substance abuse; improving the quality of parent-child involvement; providing positive role models and mentors; and ensuring that high-quality daycare programs focusing on social skills are available.

The case studies presented in this paper are excellent examples of how the underlying policy principles discussed above have been integrated with these interventions, to deal with the inadequacies in the determinants of health. The following recommendations are offered to further guide the development of health policy for the prevention of youth substance abuse:

- investigate means of fostering positive, healthy home environments, for example, through effective parent training;
- work to decrease socioeconomic inequities among young people by providing income-generating opportunities for disadvantaged youth (e.g., summer job training programs);
- investigate how to keep young people in school and provide appropriate, alternative educational opportunities to disadvantaged or special needs youth;
- increase young people's sense of personal competency by providing learning experiences and opportunities for social interaction that enhance the life skills needed for healthy growth and development;
- provide programs involving positive role models and mentors;
- foster intersectoral collaboration among key community institutions (e.g., schools, recreation centres) to better enable these institutions to provide a healthy, nurturing social environment for young people;
- promote the community-level adoption of policies (e.g., enforcing bans on tobacco sales to minors) aimed at preventing the use of tobacco, alcohol and other drugs by young people;

- ensure that young mothers and young mothers-to-be from disadvantaged communities have equitable access to food, clothing, shelter, primary care facilities and other fundamental determinants of health;
- ensure that small children who are not living in safe, nurturing and stimulating environments have equitable access to the fundamental determinants of health;
- actively involve young people in the development of program and policy development, for example, creative educational interventions (videos, street theatre) promoting healthy drug-free lifestyles;
- ensure that young people have access to healthy sports and recreational activities as alternatives to alcohol and drug use; and
- ensure all programs and services address literacy issues.

CONCLUSIONS

In formulating these recommendations, the author is aware of the current climate of fiscal restraint and the lack of new funding for programs. One strategy for ensuring that communities have the resources they need to prevent substance abuse among young people entails a reinvestment of some of the money currently allocated to population-level social marketing campaigns. An analysis of Health Canada's 1992–1993 expenditures associated with substance abuse revealed that, of all the components of the strategy, with the exception of cost-shared treatment of the performance-enhancing drug initiative, more funds ($4.7 million) were expended to promote public awareness and provide basic information than to conduct any other activity within the Strategy , from national coordination to research.

Investing even a portion of these resources in community-level programs would greatly enhance the ability of local groups and agencies to deal with the determinants of health linked to the use of alcohol and other drugs by young people.

This paper is not intended to be a comprehensive blueprint for the development of substance abuse prevention strategies addressing the determinants of health; rather, it should be viewed as one of the prerequisites for the realization of comprehensive programs and policies that deal with the underlying causes of substance abuse among young people. Greater attention to the implications of a determinants of health framework for substance abuse prevention will, over time, foster the development of more effective strategies that will help us deal with the multiplicity of social and environmental factors affecting the use of tobacco, alcohol and other drugs by young people. The merit of these initiatives will ultimately be measured by the extent to which they foster healthy, supportive environments, families and schools, which, in turn, will support and maintain healthy drug-related choices and behaviour by young people.

Pamela C. Fralick *has worked in the substance abuse field for twenty years, covering research, treatment, education, programming and policy development. During eight years with the Canadian Forces in Europe, she directed an alcoholism treatment facility, was responsible for policy development, and coordinated all health promotion programs. Returning to Canada, she spent two years with Health Canada before accepting the position of deputy chief executive officer with the Canadian Centre on Substance Abuse. In April 1997, she established a consulting service, specializing in health policy and research.*

BIBLIOGRAPHY

ABEL, E. L., SOKOL, R. J. 1991. A revised conservative estimate of the incidence of FAS and its economic impact. *Alcohol Clinical Experimental Research* 15(3): 514–524.

ABERNATHY, T. 1994. Compliance for Kids: A community-based tobacco prevention project. *Canadian Journal of Public Health* 85(2): 82–4.

ADLAF, E. M. 1993. Alcohol and other drug use. In *Canada's Health Promotion Survey 1990 Technical Report*, eds. T. STEPHENS and D. FOWLER-GRAHAM, Ottawa: Health and Welfare Canada. pp. 103–124

ALEXANDRA PARK RESIDENTS' ASSOCIATION. 1996. Personal communication.

ALLEN, G., PAGE, R. M., MOORE, L., and HEWITT, C. 1994. Gender differences in selected psychosocial characteristics of adolescent smokers and nonsmokers. *Health Values* 18(2): 34–39.

ANDERSON, J. 1992. A *Study of "Out-of-the-Mainstream" Youth in Halifax, Nova Scotia*. Ottawa: Health Promotion Directorate, Health Canada.

———. 1996. Personal communication.

ANDERSON, K. 1995. *Young People and Alcohol, Drugs and Tobacco*. WHO Regional Publications. European Series, no. 66. Copenhagen: World Health Organization.

BADOVINAC, K. 1993. A closer look at the adolescent smoker in Ontario: Results of the Ontario Health Survey for teens 12 to 17 years of age. *Public Health and Epidemiology Report Ontario* 4(9): 260–263.

BERKMAN, L. F. and SYME, S. L. 1979. Social networks, host resistance and mortality: A nine-year follow-up study of Alameda County residents. *American Journal of Epidemiology* 109: 186–204.

BOYLE, M. H., and OFFORD, D. R. 1986. Smoking, drinking and use of illicit drugs in Ontario: Prevalence, patterns of use and sociodemographic correlates. *Canadian Medical Association Journal* 135(10): 1113–1121.

BRACHT, N. Ed. 1990. *Health Promotion at the Community Level*. Newbury Park (CA): Sage Publications.

BREMBERG, S. 1991. Does school health education affect the health of students? In *Youth Health Promotion: From Theory to Practice in School and Community*, eds. D. NUTBEAM, B. HAGLUND, P. FARLEY, and P. TILGREN. London: Forbes Publications. pp. 89–107.

BURTON, D. 1994. Tobacco cessation programs for adolescents. In *Interventions for Smokers: An International Perspective*, ed. R. RICHMOND, Baltimore (MD): Wilkins and Wilkins. pp. 95–105.

BURTON, D., SUSSMAN, S., HANSON, W. B., ANDERSON-JOHNSON, C., and FLAG, B. R. 1989. Image attributions and smoking intentions among seventh-grade students. *Journal of Applied Social Psychology* 19(8): 656–664.

CANADIAN INSTITUTE OF CHILD HEALTH. 1993. *Prevention of Low Birthweight in Canada: Literature Review and Strategies*. Toronto: Health Promotion Branch, Ontario Ministry of Health.

CANADIAN PROFILE. 1995. *Alcohol, Tobacco and Other Drugs, 1995*. Ottawa: Canadian Centre on Substance Abuse.

CHARLTON, A., and BLAIR, V. 1989. Predicting the onset of smoking in boys and girls. *Social Science and Medicine* 29: 813–818.

CHASSIN, L. 1984. Adolescent substance use and abuse. *Advances in Child Behavior Analysis and Therapy* 3: 99–152.

CLAYTON, S. 1991. Gender differences in psychosocial determinants of adolescent smoking. *Journal of School Health* 61(3): 115–120.

COHEN, S., and SYME, S. 1985. *Social Support and Health*. Orlando (FL): Academic Press.

CONRAD, K., FLAG, B. R., and HILL, D. 1992. Why children start smoking: Predictors of onset. *British Journal of Addiction* 87: 1711–1724.

DEPARTMENT OF HEALTH AND WELFARE. 1990. *National Alcohol and Other Drugs Survey: Highlights Report.* Ottawa: Minister of Supply and Services Canada.

EDWARDS, G., ANDERSON, P., BABOR, T., CASSWELL, S., FERRENCE, R., GIESBRECHT, N., GODFREY, C., HOLDER, H., LEMMENS, P., MAKELA, K., MIDANIK, L., NORSTROM, T., OSTERBERG, E., ROMELSJO, A., ROOM, R., SIMPURA, J., and SKOG, O-J. 1994. *Alcohol Policy and the Public Good.* Oxford: Oxford Medical Publications.

ENGLISH, D. R., HOLMAN, C. D., MILNE, E., HULSE, G., and WINTER, M. 1995. The quantification of morbidity and mortality caused by substance abuse. Paper presented at the 2nd International Symposium on the Social and Economic Costs of Substance Abuse. October 2–5, 1995, Montebello, Quebec.

EVANS, R. G., BARER, M. L., and MARMOR, T. R. Eds. 1994. *Why are Some People Healthy and Others Not? The Determinants of Health of Populations.* New York: Aldine De Gruyter.

FEDERAL, PROVINCIAL AND TERRITORIAL ADVISORY COMMITTEE ON POPULATION HEALTH. 1994. *Strategies for Population Health: Investing in the Health of Canadians.* Ottawa: Minister of Supply and Services Canada.

FLAY, B., D'AVERNAS, J., BEST, J. R. KERSELL, M. W., and RYAN, K. 1983. Cigarette smoking: Why young people do it and ways of preventing it. In *Pediatric and Adolescent Behavioural Medicine,* eds. P. MCGRATH and P. FIRESTONE. New York: Springer. pp. 132–182.

FRALICK, P. 1995. From health promotion to determinants of health: Revolution or evolution? Unpublished manuscript. Kingston: Queen's University.

FRANK, J. 1995. Why population health? *Canadian Journal of Public Health* 86 (3): 162–165.

GLANZ, M., and PICKENS, R. Eds. 1992. *Vulnerability to Drug Abuse,* 2nd ed. Washington (DC): American Psychological Association.

GOODSTADT, M. 1995. Health promotion and the bottom line: What works? Paper presented at the Seventh Annual Health Promotion Conference, Brisbane, Australia, February 12–15.

GOTTLIEB, B. 1987. Using social support to protect and promote health. *Journal of Primary Prevention* 8 (1–2): 49–70.

GREEN, L. W., and LEWIS, F. M. 1986. *Measurement and Evaluation in Health Education and Health Promotion.* Palo Alto (CA): Mayfield.

GROENEVELD, J., SHAIN, M., and SIMON, J. 1990. *Unemployment, Alcohol and Drugs: A Study.* Toronto: Addiction Research Foundation.

HAWKINS, J. D., CATALANO, R. F., and MILLER, J. Y. 1992. Risk and protective factors for alcohol and other drug problems in adolescence and early adulthood: Implications for substance abuse prevention. *Psychological Bulletin* 112(1): 64–105.

HAWKINS, J. D., CATALANO, R. and ASSOCIATES. 1993. *Communities That Care: Action for Drug Abuse Prevention.* San Francisco: Jossey-Bass.

HERTZMAN, C. 1993. The lifelong impact of childhood experiences: A population health perspective. Unpublished paper. University of British Columbia.

HILL, K. 1989. Grade retention and dropping out of school. Paper presented at the annual meeting of the American Education Research Association. Washington (DC).

HYNDMAN, B. 1996. Personal communication.

ISRAEL, B. 1985. Social networks and social support: Implications for natural helper and community-level interventions. *Health Education Quarterly* 12(1): 65–80.

JESSOR, R. 1986. Adolescent problem drinking: Psychosocial aspects and developmental outcomes. In *Development as Action in Context: Problem Behavior and Youth Development,* eds. K. SILBEREISEN, E. EYFERTH, and G. RUDINGER. New York: Springer-Verlag. pp. 241–244.

KAPLAN, S. B. 1985. Testing a general theory of drug abuse and other deviant adaptations. *Journal of Drug Issues* 14: 477–492.

KEMMIS, S., and MCTAGGART, R. Eds. 1988. *The Action Research Planner.* 3rd ed. Geelong, Australia: Deakin University Press.

KIEDROWSKI, J. AND ASSOCIATES INC. 1996. *Government Expenditures Directed at Substance Abuse in Canada: Preliminary Analysis.* Paper prepared for the Canadian Centre on Substance Abuse. Ottawa, February 1996.

KROHN, M. D., NAUGHTON, M. J., SKINNER, W. F., BECKER, S. L., and LAUER, R. M. 1986. Social disaffection, friendship patterns and adolescent cigarette use: The Muscatine study. *Journal of School Health* 56(4): 146–150.

LABONTE, R. 1993. *Making Progress: Evaluation and Accountability in Community Development.* Toronto: Department of Public Health, city of Toronto.

_____. 1995. Population health and health promotion: What do they have to say to each other. *Canadian Journal of Public Health* 86(3): 165–168.

LALONDE, M. 1974. *A New Perspective on the Health of Canadians.* Ottawa: National Health and Welfare.

LEWIN, K. 1946. Action research and minority problems. *Journal of Social Issues* 2(1): 34–46.

_____. 1952. Group decision and social change. In *Readings in Social Psychology,* eds. G. F. SWANSON, T. M. NEWCOMB, and E. L. HARTLEY. New York: Henry Holt. pp. 459–473.

LONEY, E. A., GREEN, K. L., and NANSON, J. L. 1994. A health promotion perspective on the House of Commons Report "Foetal Alcohol Syndrome: A Preventable Tragedy". *Canadian Journal of Public Health* 85(4): 248–251.

MACDONALD, S. 1989. A comparison of the psychosocial characteristics of alcoholics responsible for impaired and non-impaired collisions. *Accident Analysis and Prevention* 21(5): 493–508.

MANGA, P. 1993. Socioeconomic inequalities. In *Canada's Health Promotion Survey 1990: Technical Report,* eds. T. STEPHENS, and D. FOWLER-GRAHAM. Ottawa: Health and Welfare Canada. pp. 263–274.

MANGHAM, C., REID, G., McGRATH, P., and STEWART, M. 1995. *Resiliency: Relevance to Health Promotion.* Ottawa: Health Canada, Alcohol and Other Drugs Unit.

MARTIN, M. J., and PRITCHARD, M. E. 1991. Factors associated with alcohol use in late adolescence. *Journal of Studies on Alcohol* 52(1): 5–9.

MARTIN, S. L., RAMEY, C. T., and RAMEY, S. 1990. The prevention of intellectual impairment in children of impoverished families: Findings of a randomized trial of educational daycare. *American Journal of Public Health* 80: 844–847.

MATTAR, L. 1996. Personal communication.

McNEILL, A., JARVIS, M. J., STAPLETON, J. A., RUSSELL, M. E. H., EISNER, J. R., GRAMMAGE, P.L., and GRAY, E.M. 1988. Prospective study of factors predicting uptake of smoking in adolescents. *Journal of Epidemiology and Community Health* 43: 72–78.

McTAGGART, R. 1993. Dilemmas in cross-cultural action research. In *Health Research in Practice: Political, Ethical and Methodological Issues,* eds. P. COLQUHOUN, and A. KELLAEHEAN. London: Chapman and Hall. pp. 65–96.

MENSCH, B. S., and KANDEL, D. B. 1988. Dropping out of high school and drug involvement. *Sociology of Education* 61: 95–113.

MOSS, A. J., ALLEN, K. F., GIOVINO, G. A., and MILLS, S. L. 1992. *Recent Trends in Adolescent Smoking, Smoking Uptake Correlates, and Expectations about the Future.* Advance Data no. 221. From Vital Health Statistics of the Centers for Disease Control and Prevention/National Center for Health Statistics. Atlanta.

MUSTARD, J. F., and FRANK, J. 1991. *The Determinants of Health.* CIAR publication no. 5. Toronto: Canadian Institute for Advanced Research.

NATIONAL COUNCIL ON WELFARE. 1990. *Health, Health Care and Medicare: A Report by the National Council on Welfare.* Ottawa: Minister of Supply and Services Canada.

NEWCOMB, M. D., McCARTHY, W. J., AND BENTLER, P. M. 1989. Cigarette smoking, academic lifestyle and social impact efficacy: An eight-year study from early adolescence to young adulthood. *Journal of Applied Social Psychology* 19: 251–281.

ONTARIO GOVERNMENT. 1995. *Focus Communities Interventions Report.* Toronto: Health Communication Unit Promotion Branch, Ontario Ministry of Health.

ONTARIO HEALTH SURVEY. 1990. *Highlights Report.* Toronto: Queen's Printer for Ontario.

PARKER, D. A., and PARKER, E. S. 1980. Status and status inconsistency of parents on alcohol consumption of teenage children. *International Journal of the Addictions* 15(8): 1233–1239.

PEDERSON, L. 1993. Smoking. In *Canada's Health Promotion Survey 1990: Technical Report*, eds. T. STEPHENS and D. FOWLER-GRAHAM. Ottawa: Health and Welfare Canada. pp. 91–102.

PERRY, C. 1986. Community-wide health promotion and drug abuse prevention. *Journal of School Health* 56: 359–363.

PINDER, L. 1994. The federal role in health promotion art of the possible. In *Health Promotion in Canada*, eds. A. PEDERSON, M. O'NEILL, and I. ROOTMAN. Toronto: W. B. Saunders Canada. pp. 92–106

POSAVAC, E. J., and CAREY, R. G. 1989. *Program Evaluation: Methods and Case Studies* 3rd ed. Englewood Cliffs (NJ): Prentice-Hall.

PREMIER'S COUNCIL ON HEALTH STRATEGY. 1991. *Nurturing Health: A Framework on the Determinants of Health.* Toronto: Queen's Printer for Ontario.

RADFORD, J. L., King, A. J., and WARREN, W. K. 1989. *Street Youth and AIDS.* Ottawa: Health and Welfare Canada.

RICE, D. P. 1993. The economic cost of alcohol abuse and alcohol dependence: 1990. *Alcohol Health and Research World* 17(1): 10–11.

ROBINSON, G. C., CONRY, J. L., and CONRY, R. F. 1987. Clinical profile and prevalence of Fetal Alcohol Syndrome in an isolated community in British Columbia. *Canadian Medical Association Journal* 137: 203–207.

ROOTMAN, I. 1995. Health promotion and population health. *Centre for Health Promotion Newsletter.* February, p. 2.

SADAVA, S. W. 1987. Interactional theory. In *Psychological Theories of Drinking and Alcoholism*, eds. H. T. BLANE, and K. E. LESSARD. New York: Guilford. pp. 90–126.

SIEBER, M. F. 1979. Social background, attitudes and personality in a three-year follow-up study of alcohol consumers. *Drug and Alcohol Dependence* 4(2): 407–417.

SINGLE, E. 1995. The use and abuse of alcohol in Canada. *Canadian Profile: Alcohol, Tobacco and Other Drugs.* Ottawa: Canadian Centre on Substance Abuse.

SINGLE, E., BREWSTER, J., MACNEIL, P., HATCHER, J., and TRAINOR, C. 1995. The 1993 General Social Survey II: Alcohol Problems in Canada. *Canadian Journal of Public Health* 86(6): 402–407.

SKINNER, W. F., MASSEY, J. L., KROHN, M. D., and LAURER, R. M. 1985. Social influences and constraints on the initation and cessation of adolescent tobacco use. *Journal of Behavioral Medicine* 8(2): 353–376.

SMART, R. G. 1979. Drinking problems among employed, unemployed and shift workers. *Journal of Occupational Medicine* 21(11): 731–736.

SMART, R. G., and ADLAF, E. M. 1991. Substance abuse and problems among Toronto street youth. *British Journal of Addiction* 86: 999–1010.

SMART, R. G., and BLAIR, N. 1980. Drug use and drug problems among teenagers in a household sample. *Drug and Alcohol Dependence* 5: 171–179.

SMART, R. G., ADLAF, E. A. WALSH, G., and ZDANOWICZ, Y. 1992. *Drifting and Doing: Changes in Drug Use among Toronto Street Youth 1990–1992.* Toronto: Addiction Research Foundation.

SOKOL, R. J., and CLARREN, S. K. 1989. Guidelines for use of terminology describing the impact of prenatal alcohol on the offspring. *Alcohol Clinical Experimental Research* 13(4): 597–598.

STECKLER, A., MCLEROY, K. R., GOODMAN, R. G., BIRD, S. T., and MCCORMICK, L. 1992. Towards integrating qualitative and quantitative methods. *Health Education Quarterly* 19(1): 1–8.

STEWART-BROWN, S. L., and PROTHERO, D. L. 1988. Evaluation in community development. *Health Education Journal* 47(4): 156–161.

STREISSGUTH, A. P., AASE, J. M., and CLARREN, S. K. 1991. Fetal Alcohol Syndrome in adolescents and adults. *Journal of the American Medical Association* 265(15): 1961–1967.

THOMPSON, J. 1995. *Early Life Factors and Addictions: A Review of the Literature.* Edmonton: Alcohol and Drug Abuse Commission.

TOBLER, N. S. 1989. Drug prevention programs can work: Research findings. Paper presented at the conference What Works: An International Perspective on Drug Abuse Treatment and Prevention Research. New York, Oct. 23–25.

VAN DER EYKEN, W. 1991. Evaluating the process of empowerment. *Empowerment and Family Support* 2(2): 8–12.

VAN ROOSMALEN, E. H., and MCDANIEL, S. A. 1989. Peer group influence as a factor in smoking behavior of adolescents. *Adolescence* 24: 801–806.

VAN SANT, J. 1989. Qualitative analysis in development interventions. *Evaluation Review* 13(3): 257–272.

VOAKES, L. 1992. *A Small Town Streetworkers' Report.* Smith Falls (ON): Tri-County Addictions Program.

_____. 1995. *Town Youth Participation Strategies (TYPS).* Smith Falls (ON): Tri-County Addictions Program.

WALLERSTEIN, N. 1992. Powerlessness, empowerment and health: Implications for health promotion programs. *American Journal of Health Promotion* 6(3): 197–205.

_____. 1993. Empowerment and health: The theory and practice of community change. *Community Development Journal* 28(3): 218–227.

WEIKART, D. P. 1989. Early childhood education and primary prevention. *Prevention in Human Services* 6: 285–306.

WILKINS, R. 1988. *Special Study on the Socially and Economically Disadvantaged.* Ottawa: Minister of Supply and Services Canada.

WINDSOR, R. A., BARANSKI, T., CLARK, N., and CUTTER, G. 1984. *Evaluation of Health Promotion and Education Programs.* Palo Alto (CA): Mayfield.

WORLD HEALTH ORGANIZATION. *Ottawa Chater for Health Promotion.* 1986. International Conference on Health Promotion, November, 1986. Ottawa: World Health Organization, pp. 17–21.

STD and AIDS Prevention among Young People

GASTON GODIN, PH.D.,
AND FRANCINE MICHAUD

Research Group on Psychosocial Aspects of Health
Laval University Faculty of Nursing Sciences

SUMMARY

This document deals with the prevention of AIDS and sexually transmitted diseases (STDs) among adolescents in school and socially maladjusted youths who have been placed in rehabilitation centres or foster families.

The first section presents the situation with respect to STDs and AIDS in various age groups, while the second describes the intervention framework behind the various experimental programs. The third section gives an overview of studies examining the factors associated with risk behaviours in the two target populations, namely adolescents in school and socially maladjusted youths. In the fourth section, the types of activities and the factors that help to ensure successful intervention are reviewed.

The fifth section presents three experimental intervention programs aimed at AIDS and STD prevention. The first involves intervention with high school students by peers in a multiethnic school setting. The second is a program implemented by community educators with socially maladjusted youths who have been placed in rehabilitation centres. The objective of the third program is to train foster parents to intervene with the troubled adolescents who have been placed with them.

We conclude with a series of recommendations based on the programs tested and the difficulties encountered in order to facilitate future sexual health promotion interventions and make it possible to take action within the settings in which the various target populations live.

TABLE OF CONTENTS

LIST OF FIGURES

LIST OF TABLES

THE STD AND AIDS ISSUE

For the past ten years, AIDS and sexually transmitted diseases (STDs) have posed one of the most serious public health problems the world has known. Taking underdiagnosis and delays in reporting cases into account, the World Health Organization (WHO) estimates there have been approximately 4.5 million cases of AIDS among adults and children since the pandemic started (WHO 1995). In Canada, Ontario and Quebec are the two provinces most strongly affected by AIDS (Bureau of Communicable Disease Epidemiology 1995). Furthermore, the prospects of controlling this disease are hardly encouraging in the short term.

What is more, the prevalence of STDs has become sufficiently worrisome in several countries that for a number of years the WHO (1986) has been alerting its member countries to the seriousness of the complications these diseases can entail, both for the individuals affected and for their families and communities. Although no statistics are available for Canada as a whole, it is known that in Quebec there are over 300,000 cases a year. Although not all of these are cases in which mandatory reporting is involved, the problem is nonetheless significant, since it is estimated that one out of 20 Quebeckers contracts an STD each year (Centre québécois de coordination sur le sida 1992).

It seems entirely likely that this problem will not be resolved for some time and that as a society we will have to deal with these illnesses for many years or even decades to come.

STD and AIDS prevention as a social issue is too complex to be addressed from every angle, given the diversity of the target populations affected. A number of groups, including young people and marginalized groups such as socially maladjusted youths, intravenous drug users, persons engaged in prostitution, offenders, men who have sex with other men, young mothers experiencing difficulties and members of ethnocultural groups, form social subgroups with their own unique characteristics. This document will thus give an overview of the STD and AIDS issue, but the analysis will deal exclusively with young people in school and socially maladjusted youths.

General Public

In Canada, for women as well as men, AIDS is most prevalent among the 30 to 39 age bracket (Bureau of Communicable Disease Epidemiology 1995). The disease strikes all segments of the population, but certain groups are more strongly affected, such as men who have sex with other men, intravenous drug users and persons from countries where AIDS is endemic (Bureau of Communicable Disease Epidemiology 1995; Centre québécois de coordination sur le sida 1995). Moreover, Quebec has higher rates of heterosexual and perinatal transmission than any other Canadian province.

With regard to the various types of STDs, not only are these more frequently reported among women, but they can also lead to very serious complications, such as ectopic pregnancy, salpingitis, infertility and increased risk of cervical cancer (Centre québécois de coordination sur le sida 1992). Chlamydiosis is by far the most often reported prevalent disease and women particularly are affected (Parent and Alary 1995).

Adolescents in General

In Canada, 20 percent of known cases of AIDS occur in the 20 to 29 age bracket (Bureau of HIV/AIDS and STD). Considering that the incubation period for HIV is many years (up to 13), there is every indication that the young adults in question were infected with HIV during their teen years (DiClemente 1992). Experts maintain, moreover, that HIV can now be found in young people and that its transmission could become much more widespread by the end of the decade (Hein 1993).

As far as STDs are concerned, a number of studies carried out among high school students in Quebec (Cloutier et al. 1994; Otis 1992, 1994; Otis et al. 1994, 1995) indicate that between 1.3 and 11 percent of these young people have already been treated for an STD. For a number of STDs subject to mandatory reporting, the largest number of cases is among adolescent girls aged 15 to 19 (Parent and Alary 1995).

Socially Maladjusted Youths

In a number of studies conducted in the United States (Alexander-Rodriguez and Vermund 1987; Morris et al. 1992, 1993; Oh et al. 1993, 1994; Rotheram-Borus et al. 1991; Shafer et al. 1993), in Canada (Radford, King, and Warren 1989) and in Quebec in particular (Cloutier et al. 1994; Godin et al. 1994; Otis et al. 1994; Poulin et al. 1994), between 12 and 30 percent of socially maladjusted youths said they had already suffered from an STD. If we accept, as certain authors (Mann et al. 1992) maintain, that persons who have previously contracted an STD are more vulnerable to HIV infection, it seems entirely likely that these young people represent a very high risk group for HIV transmission.

INTERVENTION FRAMEWORK

In view of the scope of these health problems, it is essential that action be taken as quickly as possible to cut down substantially on their incidence or even eradicate them. Because the adoption of safe behaviours is the only way to prevent AIDS and STDs, activities focusing on prevention and health promotion are the most appropriate. However, for these activities to bear fruit, they must be part of a comprehensive intervention framework.

Health Determinants

More than 40 years ago, the WHO adopted a definition of health as being a state of complete physical, mental and social well-being which does not consist simply in the absence of disease or infirmity (Nutbeam 1988). More recently, a number of authors have noted that the concept of health does not apply only to the individual but also has a multidimensional character that changes depending on the social and cultural context and other individual characteristics, such as socioeconomic status and the proximity of health services. For these authors, health is determined by a variety of factors (Pineault and Daveluy 1986). These definitions thus imply that individuals in good health can fulfil their ambitions and satisfy their needs while having the capacity to evolve within their environment or adapt to it. From this perspective, health is seen to be a resource of daily life.

In short, these definitions of health call into play a series of determinants that are not confined within the parameters of the health care system. These determinants include biological factors, lifestyle and health-related behaviours, the community, the physical and sociopolitical environment, living conditions and the health care system (Department of Health and Social Services 1992). Evans and Stoddart (1994) discuss the connections between these various determinants (figure 1).

Figure 1
Model of determinants of health and well-being

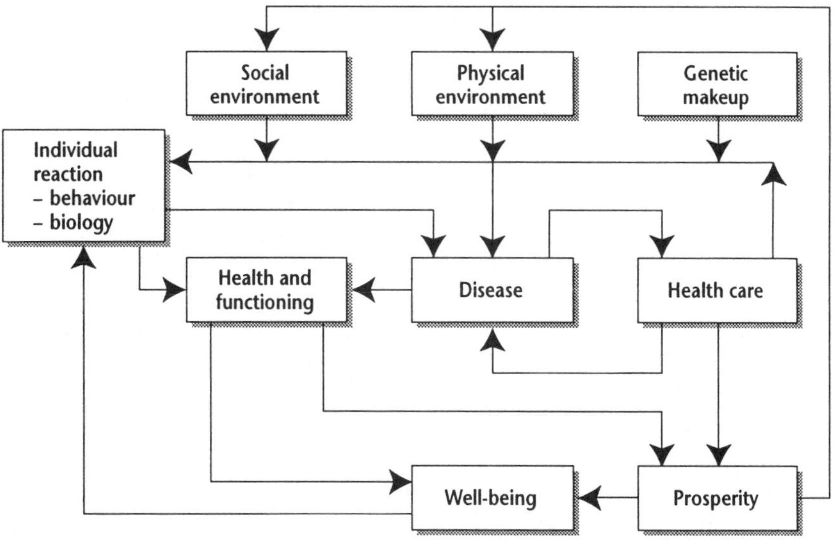

Source: Evans and Stoddart 1994.

The connections established between the various determinants of health show that the individual is not the only party that has an influence on his own health. Health is also influenced by social forces which model the choices and preferences of individuals and which may work against the adoption of desirable behaviours (for example, the inequality in the power relationship between men and women in terms of the adoption of safe sexual behaviours) (Syme 1994).

Moreover, while it may be enlightening to take into account all determinants of health when endeavouring to describe an individual's or group's state of health or assessing high-risk groups, it must also be recognized that not all the risk factors identified lend themselves equally well to intervention. That is why certain authors recommend that the effort currently being put into health promotion programs be channelled toward changing the behavioural and environmental risk factors upon which it is possible to exercise individual or collective control (Green and Kreuter 1991).

A Planning Model for Prevention and Health Promotion Activities

Health promotion is becoming increasingly recognized as an essential tool for improving the health and well-being of the population. It is part of an overall process aimed at improving the quality of life of individuals and communities and is therefore not confined to the adoption of a healthy lifestyle (ASPQ health promotion committee 1993). Health promotion is a strategy for supporting activities aimed at facilitating planned changes in individual behaviour and in the sociopolitical environment in which this behaviour takes place. This relationship between health promotion and the recommended activities is illustrated in figure 2.

Stakeholders in the field of health promotion have available to them various types of mechanisms for facilitating planned changes in individual behaviour and in the sociopolitical environment. Those mechanisms which act primarily on individual behaviour are health education, social marketing and communication. Those mechanisms that exert a marked influence on the sociopolitical environment include political action, community action and organizational change.

Among the planning models that integrate these two major determinants of health (behaviour and sociopolitical environment) is that of Green and Kreuter (1991), which is illustrated in figure 3.

For these authors, three categories of factors must be considered in the planning stage for health promotion and health education programs. First are *predisposing factors that lead to action.* These are associated with individual characteristics and with the individual's perception of his vulnerability in relation to a particular health problem. It is their beliefs, attitudes, values and so forth that determine the motivation of individuals to take action.

Figure 2
Health promotion

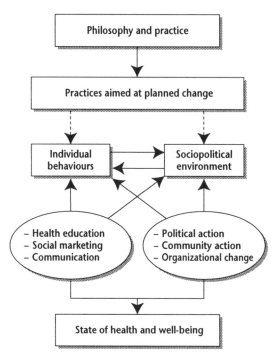

Source: Adapted from O'Neill and Cardinal 1994.

Along with these are factors that *facilitate action* and that *reinforce action*. Factors that facilitate action, which are external to the individual, are of two types. They encompass all the technical skills needed to adopt the desired behaviour and all the conditions the community must bring together (genuine access to services, genuine availability of the product, etc.) so that the behaviour can be adopted. Factors that reinforce action pertain largely to the social environment. They include members of the support network, that is, friends, family, health professionals and other persons important to the individual. Let us add that the two latter categories of factors play a different role, in that they support the individual in taking action, that is, they enable him to move from intention to the adoption of the desirable behaviour. They are conducive to the continuation or disappearance of the health-related behaviour. In addition, these two categories of factors have a direct influence on factors that lend themselves to action.

In terms of the subject at hand, the prevention of STDs and HIV infection, we focused on *factors related to the sociopolitical environment*, specifically the living environments of the young people who could be

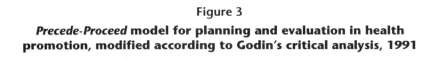

Figure 3

***Precede-Proceed* model for planning and evaluation in health
promotion, modified according to Godin's critical analysis, 1991**

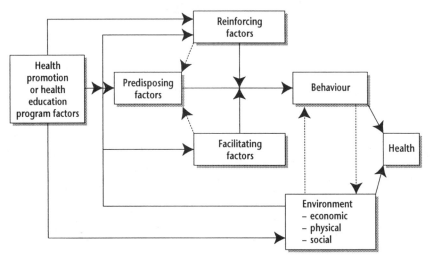

Source: Adapted from Green and Kreuter 1991.

threatened by these diseases, and on *factors related to behaviour,* that is, the
decisions young people make which may have an impact on their own
health (Health and Welfare Canada 1992).

To orchestrate effective action, it is first necessary to understand the
factors which determine a given behaviour in order to choose the most
appropriate method of intervention. The desire to change a behaviour does
not automatically suggest that an approach aimed directly at the individual
should be taken. In some cases, indirect intervention methods such as turning
to the community as a whole, regulation and the creation of a social support
network will have a greater impact on the adoption of a behaviour than
would an education program based on the dissemination of information.
The fact remains, nonetheless, that there are situations in which educational
intervention is indicated. Special attention should then be paid to the content
of the message being communicated (Godin 1991).

The Determinants of Behaviour

There is no longer any doubt that the effectiveness of the interventions
chosen depends on the determination of the psychosocial factors that
influence the adoption of a behaviour within the target population (Godin
1991). A number of theories have been developed to determine the

psychosocial factors that influence the behaviour of individuals and to explain this behaviour. These theories, which are rooted in social psychology, approach the behaviour of individuals from a social perspective, that is, by considering the interaction between the individual and his social environment. From this perspective, health-related behaviour is viewed as social behaviour in the same way as any other behaviour.

Over the past 15 years, a multitude of studies have applied various theoretical frameworks to the study of health-related behaviour. A thorough review of the research results in this area indicates it is possible to construct a synthetical model that can be used to explain and predict health-related behaviour (Godin 1996). This synthetical model, which consists of eight factors falling under three categories, is presented in figure 4, below.

Intention represents the expression of the motivation to adopt a behaviour (for example, the intention to suggest the use of a condom). While such motivation is essential to the adoption of a behaviour, intention alone is not always sufficient. There are in fact situations in which the individual has limited control over the intended behaviour (for example, a partner's refusal to use a condom); in such cases the resources and skills needed for the intention to become reality must be considered.

Figure 4
Integrative model of behaviour determinants

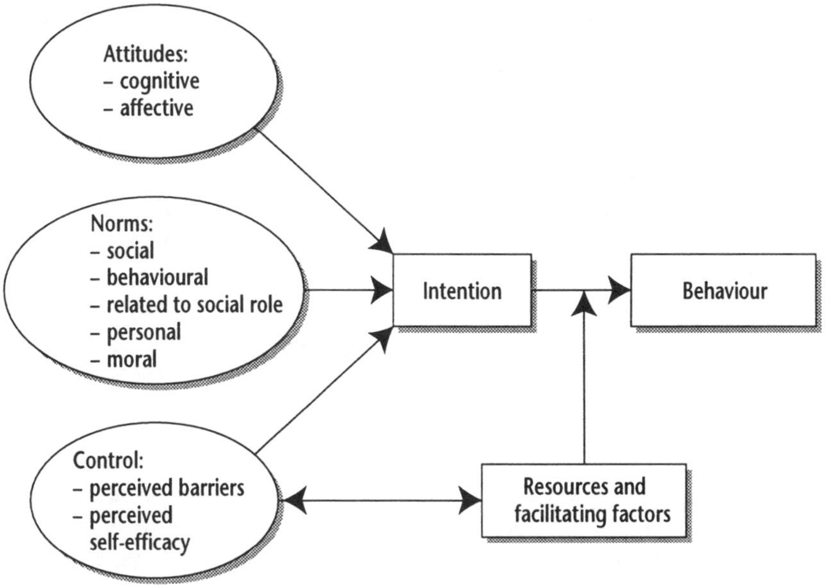

Source: G. Godin 1996.

The first category of factors conducive to the forming of intentions has to do with the attitude of the individuals concerned toward the behaviour to be adopted. Such attitudes have two components: (1) a component related to rational decision making and to cognitive evaluation of the advantages and disadvantages associated with the behaviour in question (for example, suggesting the use of a condom arouses distrust in the partner, interrupts spontaneity), and (2) a component related to the affective aspect, that is, the feeling of pleasure or displeasure that emerges at the idea of adopting this behaviour (for example, suggesting the use of a condom is stressful or embarrassing).

The second category of factors takes in the various standards that influence motivation to take action. These include social norms, which reflect our perceptions of the expectations of those around us with regard to the adoption of a given behaviour (for example, the perception that our partner or our doctor would like us to suggest a condom be used). They also reflect the standards of behaviour which prevail in our community (for example, the percentage of our friends who use condoms). Also included are the social roles taken on by a person in view of his social position (for example, a young homosexual adolescent's refusal to use a condom or a woman's suggestion that a condom be used). As to personal and moral standards, these pertain to the personal principles that govern action, and are expressed in the moral obligation we feel to adopt a given behaviour (for example, refusing to have unprotected sexual relations).

The third category represents an individual's capacity to adopt the behaviour in question, namely his perception of the degree of control over the behaviour in question. This ability stems from the impediments and degree of personal effectiveness perceived. The physical and psychological impediments that are perceived represent elements that prevent the adoption of the behaviour (for example, a partner's refusal to use a condom). With regard to personal effectiveness, this represents the ability to adopt a given behaviour despite the difficulties that may arise (for example, for a woman who would like her partner to wear a condom, to know how to suggest they use condoms and to negotiate this).

OVERVIEW OF STUDIES EXAMINING FACTORS ASSOCIATED WITH RISK BEHAVIOURS

Adolescents

According to the data derived from nearly 30 studies carried out among young people in school (Otis 1995), 12 to 23 percent of students in the early years of high school and 47 to 69 percent in the later years say they have had already had at least one sexual experience with vaginal or anal penetration. Between 13 and 38 percent of these sexually active young people say they have had sexual relations with anal penetration.

With respect to the number of partners since their first sexual relations, 21 to 41 percent of young people say they have had only one partner, 32 to 52 percent two to five partners, while 12 to 47 percent have had six or more; for the past six months, these proportions are respectively 48, 33 and 10 percent. The percentage of young people who use intravenous drugs is 0.3 to 4 percent, and the proportion of those who have had a partner who used intravenous drugs ranges between 2 and 6.4 percent. From 1 to 8 percent of young people report they have had homosexual relations, 3.1 percent say they are homosexual, and 2.6 percent have had a sexual partner who has had homosexual relations. Approximately 1 percent of young people have engaged in prostitution or have had partners who have engaged in it.

It would appear that 50 to 76 percent of young people use a condom the first time they have sexual relations. From 13 to 48 percent of young people use a condom consistently after their first sexual experience.

Over 20 percent of young people have already been screened for STDs, 14 percent have been tested for HIV, and between 2.3 and 11 percent of young people report they have received treatment for an STD. There is a much higher proportion of girls than boys among these young people.

On the whole, the studies indicate that *increased* condom use is associated with the following sociodemographic variables: younger, male, from a linguistic group other than Francophone (Quebecker) and living in a larger urban centre. It also appears from the studies that young people with a higher rate of condom use drink alcohol and use drugs less frequently and have had fewer sexual partners. In addition, fewer of them have been screened for STDs or use oral contraceptives.

In general, those young people who most strongly indicate their intention to use a condom the next time they have sexual relations are not very sexually active (fewer than 15 sexual experiences), have used a condom from the time they first started having relations, used this form of protection alone or in conjunction with oral contraceptives and have low rates of past oral contraceptive use. Moreover, young people tend to stop using condoms when they start living with their sexual partners.

Among the psychosocial variables that also influence condom use, the perception of control over this behaviour seems to play a highly important role, as do moral standards, that is, personal principles or a sense of duty. Social standards also play a significant role in that a stronger intention and more frequent condom use are associated with greater parental approval with regard to the young person's sexuality, higher levels of agreement on the part of persons whose opinions matter to the young person, the perception that friends also use condoms even when the girl is taking oral contraceptives, but primarily with the impression that using condoms is an appropriate behaviour for a young person his age.

These studies indicate that television constitutes the primary source of information for young people about STD and AIDS prevention. However, half of them indicate they have heard little specifically on risk behaviours in this regard, on how to use condoms or on safe sexual practices.

Among the impediments to condom use, embarrassment at purchasing condoms seems to be the most common one, especially among the younger adolescents. Cost and knowing where to obtain condoms are less important factors but also play a role. Moreover, there seem to be factors which, while more circumstantial, may nonetheless play a crucial role in whether or not condoms are used. These factors are forgetfulness in the heat of the moment, not having a condom when needed, and drug or alcohol use just prior to having sex.

Socially Maladjusted Youths

According to numerous studies conducted in the United States (Alexander-Rodriguez and Vermund 1987; Bell et al. 1985; Council of Scientific Affairs 1990; DiClemente 1991; DiClemente et al. 1989, 1991; DiClemente and Dunah 1989; Farrow and Schroeder 1984; Hein 1993; Lanier et al. 1991; Lanier and McMarthy 1989; Melchert and Burnett 1990; Morris et al. 1992; Nader et al. 1989; Shaffer et al. 1993), in Canada (King et al. 1988; Radford et al. 1989), and in Quebec specifically (Caron 1986; Cloutier et al. 1994; Dubois and Dulude 1986; Lévy and Dupras 1989; Otis 1995; Otis et al. 1994; Poulin et al. 1994; Van Gijseghem 1989), in many respects young people in rehabilitation centres present more risk behaviours with regard to HIV and STD transmission than do other adolescents. These young people start having sexual relations at a younger age than do other adolescents, more of them are sexually active, they are more sexually active and they have more sexual partners. A low percentage of these young people (around 20 percent) use condoms regularly even though their sexual practices place them at higher risk (DiClemente 1991; DiClemente et al. 1991; King et al. 1988; Lévy and Dupras 1989; Morris et al. 1992; Nader et al. 1989; Poulin et al. 1994; Shafer et al. 1993). They are also more reluctant to talk with their partners about the need to use condoms, although they appear to be less embarrassed about obtaining them than are young people in school (King et al. 1988).

With regard to prostitution, between 18 and 35 percent of young people in U.S. detention centres report having been involved in prostitution in the past year (Huscroft et al. 1990; Stricof et al. 1991; Temoshok et al. 1989), while in Quebec the proportion is 18 percent for girls and 10 percent for boys (Poulin et al. 1994). Drug and alcohol use is very widespread among socially maladjusted youths, not to mention the fact that some of these young people have used intravenous drugs (DiClemente 1991; Radford et al. 1989; Rotheram-Borus and Koopman 1991; Roy et al. 1992; Poulin et al. 1994; Stricof et al. 1991) and that, of this number, half have shared their needles (Poulin et al. 1994). Moreover, it would appear that a little over a third of the young people admitted to rehabilitation centres have had sexual partners who presented at least one of the risk factors referred to above, that is, they have taken intravenous drugs, have engaged in prostitution or are HIV-positive individuals (Poulin et al. 1994).

For sexually active adolescents, using condoms for all sexual relations that place them at risk is still the best way of preventing HIV and other STDs (Goldsmith 1987; Stone et al. 1986). A certain number of studies have looked at the factors associated with condom use among adolescents. Most of these studies have focused on young people in school or young people attending clinics for adolescents (DiClemente 1992), but some have dealt with young people in rehabilitation centres.

According to a U.S. study of young people in rehabilitation centres, awareness of HIV is not sufficient to motivate them to adopt preventive behaviours. Ethnicity, the ability to communicate with one's partner about AIDS and the perception that peers encourage condom use are factors associated with consistent condom use among these young people (DiClemente et al. 1991).

According to the results of a number of studies carried out in Quebec on the determinants of condom use among young people in rehabilitation centres, it would appear that a higher degree of intention to use this form of protection is primarily related to the perception that one has greater control over this behaviour, to higher personal moral standards, to a more positive attitude, to more positive social standards and to an already established habit of using condoms (Godin et al. 1994; Otis et al. 1994).

One study attempted to establish a profile of persons who use condoms consistently as compared with those who do not use them regularly or do not use them at all. Consistent users display the following characteristics: greater perception of the risk of pregnancy, STDs and AIDS and of their ability to use condoms despite certain impediments, stronger manifestations of the partner's agreement in the past, more recent entry into an active sex life, and lower rate of drug use prior to sexual relations. Consistent users also believe more strongly in the effectiveness of condoms in reducing the risks of STDs and feel secure using this form of protection (Otis et al. 1995).

The main impediments to condom use anticipated by young persons in rehabilitation centres are alcohol or drug use prior to sexual relations, the fact that the girl is using oral contraceptives, being convinced that one's partner does not have an STD and embarrassment about asking one's partner to use a condom. Not having a condom when the time comes, forgetfulness in the heat of the moment, the partner's lack of agreement and knowing one's partner well also have a negative effect on condom use (Godin et al. 1994; Otis et al. 1994).

EFFECTIVE PREVENTION STRATEGIES

Since individual behaviour is the primary cause of STD and AIDS transmission, it is not surprising that prevention depends primarily on health education as the preferred intervention strategy for combatting these diseases. It is thus appropriate to ask which prevention activities are most widely used and most effective and what makes these activities effective.

Most Common and Effective Prevention Activities

Janz et al. (1996) shed new light on these questions by analyzing the activities carried out in connection with 37 prevention programs and by evaluating their effectiveness. According to this study, the three most common strategies are small-group discussions (15 or fewer participants), large-group discussions, and training of volunteers to intervene with their peers (table 1). As to the activities considered the most effective, they indicated (1) small-group discussions; (2) intervention in the community with marginalized populations that present a high risk of infection; and (3) training of volunteers to enable them to intervene with their peers.

Small-group discussions give participants an opportunity to become involved in dynamic interventions, to speak freely, to learn from contact with others, to acquire a sense of belonging to the group, and so forth. This approach is thus considered a powerful mechanism for teaching, fostering learning and supporting the changes in behaviour needed to prevent STDs and AIDS.

Intervention in the community with populations that present a high risk of infection is particularly indicated for populations that are difficult to reach and that are marginalized from mainstream society. The effectiveness of this approach depends on the credibility of the community facilitator or streetworker with those targeted by his interventions.

Mechanisms through which volunteers intervene with their peers are effective, because they present models with whom the individuals targeted can identify. As models, these volunteers help establish a standard within the peer group, thus reinforcing the adoption of the desired behaviour.

The effectiveness of these prevention activities does vary, however, according to the target population. Certain activities seem to be more effective with certain segments of the population. Programs for women, for example, are most effective if they rely on peer training and the dissemination of materials on safer sexual practices. Programs for men, on the other hand, tend to involve intervention by community workers and individual counselling. It should also be noted that peer training and the production of videos seem to be the two most effective activities among interventions with young people.

Table 1

**Project activities rated as most effective and
their frequency of use (N = 37)**

Project activity	Number using activity	Number rated most effective	Percentage rated most effective
Small-group discussions	36	22	61
Outreach to high risk populations	25	7	28
Training peers/volunteers	30	7	23
Provide safer-sex kits	27	6	22
Large-group discussions	36	8	22
Support groups	19	4	21
Individual counselling	25	5	20

Source: Janz et al. 1996.

Factors Facilitating Intervention Effectiveness

Without describing the various interventions carried out, Janz and her colleagues (1996) identify from their analysis of 37 prevention programs a certain number of factors that contribute to the effectiveness of the activities in question. These various factors, summarized in the following paragraphs, are presented in table 2.

Design culturally relevant and language-appropriate interventions – To achieve this, it is necessary to have representatives of the target population involved throughout the planning, implementation and evaluation process. This is the best way of ensuring that the norms, values and traditions of the target population are reflected in the intervention program.

Embed STD and AIDS information into broader contexts – For example, information can be disseminated as part of a more general sex education program. With this approach, it is possible to take into account the context in which the preventive behaviour will need to be adopted.

Provide rewards and enticements to participants who play a key role in the activities' success – For example, students can be offered the opportunity to earn credit for one of their courses in recognition of their participation as volunteers with their peers. Creative rewards can be provided in order to facilitate recruitment and retention of participants in the activities offered in connection with prevention programs.

Table 2

Factors facilitating intervention effectiveness

FACTORS
• Design culturally relevant and language-appropriate interventions
• Embed STD and AIDS information into broader contexts
• Provide rewards and enticements
• Build in opportunities for program flexibility
• Promote integration into and acceptance by the community
• Repeat essential STD and AIDS prevention messages
• Create a forum for open discussion
• Solicit participant involvement

Source: Adapted from Janz et al. 1996.

Build in opportunities for program flexibility – The program should be geared to the varied circumstances and interests of the individuals it is endeavouring to help. It is the program that must adjust to these realities and not the reverse. It should be stated from the outset that a program that is overly rigid in its structure will run into serious difficulties.

Promote integration into and acceptance by the community – It is necessary to work with the target group and, to the extent possible, recruit interveners from among its members. Traditional top-down approaches whereby, for example, prevention programs intended for the community are developed by academics or health care professionals working in isolation are unacceptable and ineffective. It is necessary to work in partnership from the very beginning with the clients targeted by the program in question.

Repeat essential STD and AIDS prevention messages – "Spot" interventions, in which the message is presented one time only, are not very effective. Important messages must therefore be repeated. This is the only way to exert an appreciable amount of influence on the attitudes, values and behaviour of those targeted by the interventions.

Create a forum for open discussion – The program must not confine itself to presenting information and messages about prevention. It must also promote dialogue and give participants an opportunity to express themselves with no fear of moral judgment and to openly discuss their ideas about sexuality and safe behaviours. Such a forum can give rise to a sense of belonging to the discussion group and consequently the development of a standard which supports the adoption of safe behaviour within the group.

Solicit participant involvement – Participant involvement can take many forms. Mechanisms that allow participants to become involved in decision-making teams and with their peers are the most successful. It is important not to lose sight of the fact that we do not do things for people, but with people.

SUCCESS STORIES

The case studies presented below were carried out using the following approach. We first reviewed the documents available on these various projects, and then met at least once with the person or persons responsible for the program and the person responsible for its application within the community. Combining these two approaches enabled us to identify and explain the factors that contributed to the success of these interventions in the community in which they were implemented.

Peer Education Program in a Multiethnic School

Referred to as "Life Savers" by the young people concerned, this sex education program was introduced in a multiethnic high school in Montérégie. Volunteers in their next-to-last year of high school worked with students in the year below them to enhance their awareness of AIDS prevention. They encouraged them to delay their initial sexual experience (abstinence) and to use condoms.

Target Population and Context

This program is aimed at 14- and 15-year-old boys and girls in their second year at a high school in an urban environment in Montérégie. The setting was a Protestant school with approximately 120 students at each grade level. Students are from all denominations and over 40 ethnic backgrounds and come from middle-class families.

Various HIV prevention strategies were introduced in the school by, for example, making this issue a part of the curriculum, implementing teacher training programs, distributing teaching materials to nonteaching staff and developing local policies on HIV infection. These far-reaching initiatives notwithstanding, innovative programs based on factors that have a good chance of influencing young people are still quite rare. Prior to this initiative, it would appear that no school had implemented and evaluated an experimental peer education program based on the attitudes, perceived social norms, perceived control and intentions of young people with regard to sexual abstinence and condom use. The choice of setting proved to be particularly apt, in that it provided an opportunity for a peer education program to be tested in an ethnocultural context in which the importance of ethnic identity in the shaping of sociosexual behaviour must be taken into account.

There had previously been a number of sex education activities in this school, but with the emergence of AIDS, teachers and nonteaching professionals soon felt the need to work together on the messages, activities and courses used for intervening in terms of prevention. In addition, a great many fears, myths and prejudices about AIDS and HIV had to be addressed. The first program, developed four years ago, focused on condom use. Since a number of young people had greatly appreciated the information they had been given, the next year those in charge of the program called on volunteers recruited from among those who had already taken the program to present it to the younger students. Interestingly enough, according to a number of studies, this school has the lowest percentage of sexually active young people in the region. These results suggest that these young people are capable of speaking in terms of abstinence while accepting condom use as a proposed method of preventing STDs and AIDS.

Actors

This program was started by the nurse at the school connected with the Longueuil-Ouest local community service centre. A teacher of moral and religious instruction also played a very important role from the outset and worked together with the nurse to train peer educators. The services of a teacher of dramatic arts were also called upon during this phase. The board of education was kept up-to-date on the project from beginning to end and gave its approval throughout the process. The school's educational advisor distributed information and documentation on the project and recently applied to the Quebec Department of Education to have the program qualify as a special credit. A university researcher also participated in the project, at first on an ad hoc basis and then in a more sustained way during the fourth year of the project by supervising a research paper. This made it possible to adjust the program, which had been set up on the basis of the determinants of the desired behaviour, according to the evaluation that had been done of it.

Each year, new teachers responsible for personal and social education and biology courses as well as new peer educators can be integrated into the project, depending on staff mobility. However, the project has always been coordinated by the school nurse, despite her precarious status at the school, because of the fact that she is connected with the local community service centre.

The fact that those promoting the program are members of the community considerably facilitated its implementation in that it enabled them to mobilize individuals who had a degree of credibility with school officials (teachers, group leader, etc.).

Development of Intervention

This program is based on the idea that the influence exerted by peers on adolescent behaviour has been proven in areas such as alcohol and tobacco use. Peer education takes this tendency of young people to be easily influenced and uses it for educational purposes, endeavouring to bring teaching strategies more in line with the characteristics of students. The content is communicated in language that is age appropriate and culturally relevant.

When the program first started, third year students were asked to *volunteer* to participate in the program as peer educators. A selection committee consisting of four teachers and the school nurse selected 16 young people (12 girls and four boys) representing a variety of different ethnic backgrounds. These young people were considered by the selection committee to be reliable, responsible, dynamic and credible with their peers. They participated in a prevention-based sex education program offered after normal school hours once a week for 20 weeks, for a total of 40 hours. After taking this training, these third year peer educators worked with second year students as part of their biology and personal and social education courses.

The activities presented to the third-year students were developed by the fourth-year peer educators under the trainer's supervision and in keeping with the program objectives. In working with the peer educators, the person in charge of the program placed a great deal of emphasis on staying with the content to be presented and on consistency and uniformity in the program's implementation. However, the peer educators had a degree of latitude as to the form of the teaching activities.

Objectives and Form of Intervention

The program was developed so as to take into account the factors that influence behaviour (Greene and Kreuter's PRECEDE model 1991), the determinants of behaviour according to Ajzen's theory of planned behaviour (1985) and the results of studies dealing specifically with abstinence and condom use among young people (Otis 1992, 1993b, 1994).

The aim of this program is to reduce the incidence of sexually transmitted diseases among young people by encouraging them to delay having an active sex life (abstinence) or to use condoms systematically in all their sexual relations. A further objective is to inspire second year students to make positive changes in their attitudes, perceived control, perceived social standards and intentions with regard to abstinence and condom use.

It should be recalled that, under this program, biology and personal and social education teachers and third-year peer educators work with second-year students. All program activities take place during the same week and encourage concerted action. Activities aimed at promoting abstinence take place in personal and social education courses, while activities aimed at promoting condom use take place in biology courses. The two interventions last 50 minutes each.

The topics addressed in relation to abstinence are the advantages of sexual abstinence, the prerequisites for satisfying sexual relations, the impediments to abstinence and ways of overcoming these impediments. The topics covered in connection with the promotion of condom use are the types of condoms, the steps to be followed in putting on a condom, the impediments to condom use and the ways of overcoming these impediments, as well as the advantages and disadvantages of using this form of protection. These topics are dealt with in the context of activities such as simulation exercises followed by directed discussions aimed at clarifying values, role playing, demonstrations and discussions. Each session concludes with a summary of the content and a key message.

The 16 peer educators comprise four work teams. The objective is to have two different teams of facilitators—one team for the activities held during biology classes (condom use) and another for the activities offered during personal and social education classes (abstinence)—visit each class.

Project Funding

This program, which costs no more than a few hundred dollars a year, received funding from the board of education's Educational Development Fund (for two years), the Longueuil Ouest local community service centre and a number of individual donations for purchasing condoms and T-shirts with the *Life Savers* logo. When funding became more difficult to obtain, self-funding activities were organized. This program is inexpensive, since it can draw on community resources whose salaries are already provided for in regular budgets. However, this advantage is offset by the fact that the program's continuation depends on the availability of human resources (nurse and teachers) and the actual time investment in the project.

Results and Implications within the Community

An evaluative study of this project was carried out. The aim of the study was to examine the process used to implement the program by determining the extent to which the program that had been planned for the second year students corresponded with the program that was actually carried out and the level of appreciation for the program among the second-year students, the third-year peer educators and the teaching staff. The evaluative study also provided an opportunity to verify the impact of the intervention by the third-year peer educators on attitudes, perceived control and perceived social standards and the intentions of the second-year students with regard to abstinence and condom use.

The program was taken by 123 second-year students. The evaluation, however, covered a sampling of the 70 students who had completed the impact assessment (pretest and posttest) and formative assessment.

The results of the formative assessment show that the content that had been planned for both the biology courses (condoms) and the personal and social education courses (abstinence) were presented by the peer educators in a fairly satisfactory manner on the whole, since the level of satisfaction ranged from 62 to 89 percent. The overall level of satisfaction with the program among students, peer educators and teachers was very high, particularly for the biology courses (condoms). The level of satisfaction with the peer educators was very high or fairly high; they were perceived by the students as respectful, well prepared, trustworthy, likable, convincing, dynamic and as having a sense of humour. The teachers felt they had grown in maturity. The activities presented by the peer educators were considered educational, not boring in the least, moderately amusing and moderately successful. On the whole, the peer educators and the students the program was aimed at agreed their attention and interest had been very high during the biology class and moderately high during the personal and social education classes.

For the peer educators, the program had the following positive effects: it strengthened their self-confidence, enhanced their personal growth, enabled them to acquire certain skills in terms of facilitating groups, gave them a sense of having met a major personal challenge and, overall, gave them a great deal of pride, joy and satisfaction. These young people felt this experience changed things in their lives and they said they were more comfortable talking about sexuality with their friends. They are perceived by their peers as being more knowledgeable than other young people, and as people one can talk to if one has a problem, and being a "life saver" has become a source of prestige. In some cases, their parents would even have given them the responsibility for intervening with their younger sister or brother. What is more, the school rewards them for their participation as peer educators by giving them a plaque or a trophy along with two additional credits for their personal and social development course.

The results of the evaluation indicate that the program had a positive effect on the second-year students in terms of abstinence and condom use, particularly with regard to the cognitive aspect of attitude. It also strengthened their intention to use condoms even when the girl is using oral contraceptives. The perception of impediments among young people who use condoms was also higher after the intervention. With regard to abstinence, the perception of peer approval decreased; this is a positive result in that there was greater distancing in relation to peer influence.

The benefits of the training program for peer educators have been recognized by the Quebec Department of Education. Beginning with September 1996 it is part of the local school's curriculum. The young people who participate in it receive two additional credits for their personal and social development course.

This project was widely publicized. It was the subject of official presentations (Caron 1993c, 1995; Caron et al. 1990; Karunananthan 1995) and unofficial presentations and publications (Caron 1992, 1993a, 1993b, 1996). Moreover, the board of education frequently receives requests from other organizations that would like to set up the program. Further presentations are anticipated, as are publications on the evaluation of this intervention.

Replicability

The strength of this type of intervention stems from the fact that it enlists young facilitators from the peer group. It does, however, rely on the support of teachers and the quality of the communication with the person in charge of the project. In order for the intervention to go smoothly and for the messages about STD and AIDS prevention to be heard, it is essential that the interactive teaching strategies that call on peers be geared to the students. The teachers are in the best position to determine whether such is in fact the case.

This form of intervention can easily be reproduced at minimal cost. In order to do so, the organization must assign responsibility for the program to a person who can devote a great deal of time and energy to building relationships of close cooperation between the various partners: the local community service centre, the board of education, the school, the teachers and the young people. Furthermore, implementation would be greatly facilitated if the program were integrated into the board of education's curriculum instead of being offered as an extracurricular activity.

Intervention Program on Sexuality and STD and AIDS Prevention for Young People in Rehabilitation Centres for Troubled Youths and Young Mothers

This is a sex education and STD and AIDS prevention program for maladjusted youths. The program, which endeavours to modify their risk behaviour, has been implemented in rehabilitation centres for troubled youths and young mothers.

Target Population and Context

This program is aimed at all young people aged 12 to 18 who have been placed in rehabilitation centres for troubled youths and young mothers. The target population thus consists of young people who have been placed in such centres by order of the Youth Court or as a result of voluntary placement measures. The length of such placements varies from one day to six months and in exceptional circumstances is renewed for a period of three to six months.

Although a certain number of rehabilitation centres in Quebec had introduced sex education activities starting in the 1980s, very few of them have been subject to systematic evaluation. Where AIDS and STD prevention are concerned, no programs from Quebec have been reported in the literature on the research that has been done in this area. Furthermore, a consultation carried out with the institutions concerned showed that most of the rehabilitation centres involved in the project in question did not have any kind of structured sex education program, even if informal and ad hoc interventions had been carried out on certain aspects of sexuality. STD and AIDS prevention were not covered anywhere in the curriculum covered by the young people. What is more, the interveners felt they did not have the tools needed to carry out an effective educational intervention on this subject with a group of young people. They did say, however, that they were very motivated to address this problem with their young people if adequate support could be provided to them (Carbonneau 1989).

A number of measures intended to mobilize the community had, however, been taken previously, including support for the development and application of a policy on AIDS in these institutions, promoting awareness among staff members of the primary aspects of HIV and AIDS, and training sex education teachers. But above all, the program met a need that had been identified and a working group on social maladjustment had even officially expressed a desire to see a sex education and STD and AIDS prevention program for socially maladjusted youths set up (Bédard et al. 1991).

Actors

This program is an initiative carried out by university and public health researchers. It was carried out in collaboration with all rehabilitation centres for troubled youths and young mothers that accept young people aged 12 to 18 from eastern Quebec, that is, the Quebec metropolitan area, la Chaudière-Appalaches, Saguenay–Lac-St-Jean–Chibougamau, North Shore, Lower St. Lawrence and Gaspésie–Îles-de-la-Madeleine regions.

The program facilitators are educators who work with young people from each living unit (or group home) in the institutions in which the program is offered. These persons were chosen because they were interested in the program and wanted to deal with the issue of sexuality with the adolescents in their charge. Those responsible for the project provided them with training during the weeks prior to delivery of the program.

Development of Intervention

The educational intervention that is the subject of this case study came about as a result of a research program. A review of the epidemiological data on the sexual experiences of these young people and their risk behaviour initially indicated that using a condom during sexual relations with a new partner was an aspect of behaviour that required further study. A study was therefore carried out to identify the psychosocial determinants that could predict and explain this behaviour in the case of young people in rehabilitation centres for troubled youths and young mothers. The program was subsequently developed taking into account all the important factors highlighted by the study (Godin et al. 1994).

This program was developed in partnership. Each group was asked to delegate an educator with a good knowledge of the target population, the dynamic in effect within these groups of young people, and the constraints within the group. A senior researcher from the university community and a sexologist representing the public health network also participated. The committee adopted an approach based on the following: meetings to facilitate the sharing of ideas, production of written documents, work sessions, discussions, feedback on documents, revision of documents, and consensus on the final product to be offered to the young people. Six work sessions with the advisory committee were held over a seven-month period to develop the program. In short, the program is the result of a consensus based on the research data and the data that came out of direct knowledge of the target populations and the constraints within the group (Godin et al. 1994).

Objectives and Form of Intervention

The aim of the intervention program on sexuality and STD and AIDS prevention is to promote the adoption of safe sexual practices by maladjusted boys and girls in order to reduce their risk of contracting an STD or of being infected by HIV. This is an innovative and original program since it focuses on the determinants of safe behaviour. During 10 sessions (a total of 765 minutes), the following topics are covered: the reality of AIDS, knowledge about AIDS and STDs, the significance of sexual relations, high-risk and low-risk sexual activities, condoms, the advantages and disadvantages of using condoms, values and sexuality, communicating about sexuality and risk-free sex. The latter includes negotiating safe sexual practices, assertiveness, initiating conversation and taking a stand in relation to the impediments to adopting safe sexual practices.

These topics are dealt with in the context of various activities: formal and informal presentations, sharing of ideas, discussions, debates, personal reflection, group work, quizzes, role playing, problem solving, handling condoms, improvisational games, and songs and audiovisual documents.

This program was integrated into the programming for the living units or group homes along with all the other activities in which young people in rehabilitation centres must participate. It is offered to groups of between 8 and 12 young people, the number generally found in these units (or homes).

Project Funding

The preparatory research aimed at identifying the needs of the young people and the determinants of the adoption of safe behaviour was supported by the research program of the senior researcher, whose funding came from the Social Sciences and Humanities Research Council of Canada (SSHRC). This research was also supported by its research infrastructure, which was funded by the Government of Quebec's Fonds pour la formation de chercheurs et l'aide à la recherche (FCAR) (Fund for researcher training and research assistance).

Development of the program on sexuality and STD and AIDS prevention was funded by the Centre de santé publique de Québec (Quebec City public health centre). The evaluation project for the intervention program is currently being funded by the Conseil québécois de la recherche sociale (CQRS) (Quebec council for social research).

The rehabilitation centres showed a great deal of interest in the program. However, while the quality of the development was crucial to the program's success in the community, it was the seven-month period allocated to this phase which was the most difficult to obtain funding for. There does not seem to be any agency or program whose mandate is to fund the development of interventions.

Results and Implications within the Community

The results of the study on behaviour and the determinants of risk behaviour among these young people have been published (Godin et al. 1994; Godin et al., soon to be published) and presented at various scientific congresses (Godin et al. 1994a, 1994b). The program was also the subject of a publication (Godin et al. 1994).

This program, which is still at the experimental stage, has thus far been presented by 53 educators to 42 groups of young people consisting of a total of 500 boys and girls who have taken it either in whole or in part. It is expected that the program will be offered on an experimental basis to 15 new groups—nearly 200 young people—by some twenty new facilitators. In each of the rehabilitation centres involved, almost all the groups (living units, group homes, etc.) will have taken the program at least once by the time its implementation ends. Moreover, at least one facilitator from each unit will have presented the program for the first time and will therefore be able to offer it again to other young people.

Once they are known, the results of the evaluation will lead to greater understanding of the sexual and preventive behaviour of this target group, and above all will help to identify those strategies with a genuine impact on the adoption by these young people of behaviour aimed at preventing STDs and AIDS. With these results it will also be possible to improve the effectiveness of interventions. If the results are positive, this type of program could become more widely available to other young people in rehabilitation centres in other parts of Quebec.

It has been noted thus far that the simple fact of presenting this new program has had an impact on those working in this area in the sense that it has already changed their intervention approaches and the way they view the problem of STDs and AIDS and of dealing with sexuality with their target population. These workers say they feel more comfortable intervening in a greater number of situations by pursuing objectives pertaining to sex education and STD and AIDS prevention. This program stimulated discussion within the various groups and required the institutions to take a clear position on making condoms truly accessible to their target population and on screening tests.

Furthermore, by calling on the educators who work with these young people, those concerned clearly showed their desire to assume responsibility in the medium and long term for the prevention activities and services they wish to offer their clients on an ongoing basis. Providing training to at least one educator from each living unit or group home helped ensure sustainable implementation within the community.

Replicability

This program has already aroused a great deal of interest in the community. We have even had to rein in the extreme enthusiasm of rehabilitation centres in other parts of Quebec at this point of the evaluative research. This intervention can certainly be implemented in other settings, since it has been planned in such a way as to use tools that are readily obtainable and inexpensive. What is more, it is geared to the realities of these settings. Thanks to its flexibility, the program enables young people to join in at any time. This is an invaluable asset in settings in which young people come and go all throughout the year.

Foster Parents and STD and AIDS Prevention

This STD and AIDS prevention program offers training to foster parents taking care of teenagers. The program's objective is to equip them for their roles as educators in STD and AIDS prevention with the teens placed in their care by Centres jeunesse de Québec (Quebec City youth centres).

Target Population and Context

Quebec City youth centres are agencies whose mandate is to ensure the protection and rehabilitation of troubled youth whose health and well-being are in jeopardy and to stop them from committing delinquent acts. They are also responsible for placing the young people entrusted with them and offer them rehabilitation services. From the perspective of the overall development of the individual, the health of these young people is of concern to the youth centres.

As of January 1, 1994, Quebec City youth centres were responsible for 430 adolescents who had been placed in foster families. The average length of placement with these families is approximately two years. The foster families are accredited by the youth centres' resources unit. By way of guidance in their roles as educators with the young people they take in, these families receive support and advice from the social workers responsible for providing supervision. For region 03, most of the families are native Quebeckers, are from middle-class backgrounds and live in semi-urban settings on the outskirts of Quebec City.

By virtue of their daily contact with them, these foster parents play a socializing and educational role with the young people placed with them which complements that of their families of origin. In their daily contact with these young people, the foster families feel the need for support in various areas, such as their love relationships, contraception, and STD and AIDS prevention. They frequently call upon the social workers from the youth centres regarding the young people's sexuality, because they must deal with troubled teens whose behaviour is sometimes very different from that of their own children. Like other Quebec families, foster families are not immune from the fears and taboos that surround sexuality, STDs and AIDS. As a result, these parents need assistance and ask for the tools they need to more effectively support the young people.

This training program is intended for the Quebec City youth centres' foster parents. It was implemented on a trial basis in the greater Quebec, Portneuf and Charlevoix region, because these subregions fall within the jurisdiction of Quebec City youth centres. Groups of no more than 15 parents were recruited in each of these subregions, for a total of 46 persons (twice as many women as men). This intervention project was based on a number of criteria in order to recruit as volunteers parents who were motivated and who wished to learn more about sexuality and STD and AIDS prevention. First, the foster family had to be responsible for at least one teen aged 12 or older. The other criteria involved the level of interest in and the ability to think critically about sex education for young people, strong analytical ability (with regard to potential improvements to the program) and the ability to deal with the subject of young people's emotional and sexual experiences in a group setting.

Actors

The Quebec City youth centres were the promoters for this project through their resources unit, in conjunction with the research and education directorate and the rehabilitation centres' health services. L'Association régionale des familles d'accueil (Regional association of foster families) is a special partner. A professor from Laval University school of social services also acted as a consultant on the evaluation of this project.

There was a great deal of collaboration between institutions. This collaboration was facilitated by the fact that each partner was convinced of the importance of taking action to prevent STDs and AIDS and that these institutions report to the Quebec City youth centres, thus eliminating any potential competition with regard to recognition of participation and ownership of the program.

Development of Intervention

This project came about because of the realization that there was a shortcoming in the system: the social worker responsible for the foster families had noticed that there were no specific STD and AIDS prevention programs in place for young people placed in foster families associated with Quebec City youth centres. Given this situation, the youth centres' representative on the regional STD and AIDS committee and the coordinator of the resources unit applied for funding in order to develop a pilot project for foster families.

The project is based on the thesis that foster parents can become invaluable guides with regard to STD and AIDS prevention with the young people in their care. Increasing their level of awareness puts them in a better position to help these young people. This contention is based on a number of factors: (1) foster parents are the adult resource persons who have the most direct contact with the young people placed with them; (2) foster parents are selected on the basis of their ability to establish good relations with young people and they are likely to represent models with whom they can identify; (3) in most cases, no educator has been assigned to follow up with the young people placed in foster families; (4) these young people do not have daily contact with the social worker responsible for following up their case; and (5) the personal and social development courses offered in high schools deal with the question of STD and AIDS prevention, but only briefly, and they are intended for groups, which makes it difficult for them to take into account the special needs of young people in foster families.

The intervention is based on the principles of adult education and social group work and focuses on the participants' interaction on the basis of their experience as parents. The tools and activities were designed so as to build on the foster parents' assets, such as their training and contact with their own children and their knowledge of contemporary society.

This program mobilized a multidisciplinary team made up of a social worker responsible for the foster families of children from the resources unit, a social worker from the adoption unit, two nurses and an educator working in a rehabilitation centre. Also consulted were a social worker with expertise in social group work and a professor from Laval University for the program evaluation. The design work was done individually and in groups, in close collaboration with the project's promoters. A few modifications were made as the sessions progressed in order to more adequately meet the needs expressed by the participating parents.

One of the factors behind the project's success was the fact that the multidisciplinary team participated in every phase of the project, from the design phase through to the presentation of the program to the foster parents. It was the members of this team who were truly responsible for making this project a reality, and their contribution was all the more valuable since it was directly related to the expertise they had acquired by working with parents and young people. In addition, the enthusiasm generated by the project and the keen interest of those concerned in the issue of STDs and AIDS helped the project come about.

Objectives and Form of Intervention

The objective of this program was to ensure that foster parents have the means to play an educational role with regard to STD and AIDS prevention with the adolescents placed in their care by Quebec City youth centres.

The topics covered with the foster families were the adolescent experience of love and sexuality, knowledge about STDs and AIDS, and preventive measures. The approach used, of the "structured group" type, included periods of reflection, listening and sharing, role playing, self-assessment exercises to evaluate knowledge and attitudes, presentations, testimony, games and audiovisual materials. Print materials were also distributed. The program was offered in five consecutive weekly sessions of three hours each. There were no more than 15 people in each group.

In general, participants were offered numerous opportunities to share all throughout the program and it was they who had the floor at the last meeting. In addition to reviewing the topics dealt with in the previous sessions, they had an opportunity at that time to express their needs in terms of follow-up as well as to make suggestions for modifying or improving the program.

Project Funding

This project was made possible through grants obtained from the public health branch of the Régie régionale de Québec (Quebec City regional board) and contributions from Quebec City youth centres and from Laval University. The grant was used to free up a professional from a portion of her normal workload to allow her to concentrate on the design, promotion and coordination of the program's activities. With this funding, it was also possible to retain the services of a consultant in group dynamics and to obtain teaching materials.

The funding provided by the youth centres more or less paid for the salaries of the staff freed up to facilitate the sessions, the secretarial services and the travel costs for the interveners as well as travel and child care costs for the foster families. Quebec City youth centres and Laval University also contributed to the project by each providing a consultant to work on the project. This project could not have taken place without the grant, since Quebec City youth centres would not have been able to free up a staff member to develop and test the program without adversely affecting client services.

Results and Implications within the Community

The program evaluation made it possible to ensure the objectives had been met. Data pertaining to preestablished indicators were collected at each session by a resource person who had not participated in the facilitation. In addition, at the end of the session the participants filled out a questionnaire designed to evaluate their level of satisfaction. With the project's completion, the evaluators consider on the basis of the comments regarding the evaluation indicators that there was an increase in the participants' awareness concerning STD and AIDS prevention—particularly with regard to knowledge and positive behaviours and attitudes—that will be useful to them in their roles as educators.

At the beginning and end of the program, the parents filled out a questionnaire to assess their knowledge, the purpose of which was not to evaluate the program but to give participants an opportunity to update their knowledge about AIDS and STDs. For most of the questions, the results were better on the posttest than on the pretest.

The formative and summative evaluation of the project showed that the foster parents were interested in talking about the young people's affective lives and that they were motivated to play a role in STD and AIDS prevention. After taking the program, they felt better equipped to play an educational role in this regard and they wished that other parents and foster parents and even young people could receive this training. They also said they were very satisfied with the training, the organization in general, the way the sessions were facilitated, the length of the session and what they had learned. One parent expressed his satisfaction in the following terms: "It's like a toolbox. You don't necessarily need it every day, but it's comforting to know that you can use it when you need it." A follow-up session held a year later at each of the target sites provided an opportunity to validate the various topics covered by the training and confirmed that the foster parents felt more comfortable dealing with these issues. Over the course of the year, they also became aware of the limitations of their intervention, in that they could not adopt the preventive behaviour in the young people's place.

The first outcome of this program is undoubtedly the fact that the foster parents now feel more comfortable intervening and that they say they are in fact intervening with regard to sexuality and STD and AIDS prevention. The foster parents had an opportunity to review the documentation made available to them and to then use it to work on prevention with the young people entrusted to their care. There is no doubt that the program helped build up their self-confidence and gave them a feeling of being "better equipped" to intervene.

In addition, as a result of the recommendations made by the parents at the end of the program and at the request of a number of young people placed in these foster families, a new funding application was submitted in order to carry out a second phase of the project. While still working towards the same objective, that of STD and AIDS prevention among adolescents in foster families, this second phase will involve interventions with both foster families and young people.

However, this project has a number of limitations that must be pointed out. First, although the program had a great deal of success with the foster families, it cannot be assumed it had a genuine impact on STD and AIDS prevention with the young people for whom they were responsible, which was the real objective. The modest funding received for the development and implementation of this initial project was not sufficient to evaluate the true impact on the young people. Another limitation stemmed from the fact that the team of facilitators for the program consisted solely of women. The foster parents invited to participate in the program included men as well as women. It would have been interesting to have had both male and female facilitators, which would have allowed the fathers to identify with another man and to confide in him the difficulties they sometimes face in their interventions.

This program has been written about in publications (Berlinguet et al. 1995; Quebec City youth centres 1996), has been the subject of official and unofficial presentations (Beaupré et al. 1994; Berlinguet et al. 1995;

Brochu and Brousseau 1994) at conferences, and has been covered in social work courses at Laval University. Other presentations on the evaluation of this program are also in the works.

Replicability

Now that the program has been developed and subsequently modified after being offered at three test sites, it would be less costly to offer it again. Moreover, with the facilitation guide that will soon be available (Quebec City youth centres 1996), it will be very easy for other trainers to offer it elsewhere in future. In addition, if the second phase is in fact carried out, agencies will be better equipped to intervene, since they will have access to two programs: one for parents and one for parents and young people.

RECOMMENDATIONS FOR STD AND AIDS PREVENTION

A careful review of the literature on this subject and of the three case studies presented here shows that most of the initiatives are based on knowledge of the living environment while focusing on individual behaviour. The description of these prevention activities also indicates that they posed certain difficulties which appeared sufficiently serious at times to jeopardize the implementation of these interventions. The assessment of health determinants as well as factors facilitating effective interventions gave rise to a number of observations on the basis of which we have been able to make certain recommendations for future STD and AIDS prevention interventions.

Since STDs and HIV are still transmitted largely through sexual contact, any preventive measures to be set up or expanded must focus on the development of healthy and responsible sexuality in young people. Educational efforts to that end can be effective only to the extent that they go beyond the mere acquisition of knowledge and promote the adoption of attitudes and the acquisition of skills and values with regard to sexuality. Moreover, information on AIDS must be offered as part of a more general framework of sex education.

Furthermore, it is well known that, after the family, the school setting constitutes the primary place of socialization and education for young people (Desaulniers 1990; Moore and Rosenthal 1993). This fact must be taken as a point of departure and there must be an end to the continual questioning of the appropriateness of sex education in the schools so that young people's interests can be served. Education on AIDS and STD prevention should begin as soon as possible, starting in the later years of primary school, for a number of reasons. First, trends over the past few decades show that young people are having sexual relations at an earlier age (Carballo et al. 1991; Moore and Rosenthal 1993; Otis 1995). In addition, young people who wait to have an active sex life generally adopt safer sexual practices. As well, young people who use condoms when they have sexual relations for the first time are more apt to use them afterwards (Otis 1995).

Of course, the data from the research that has been done indicates that there has been a marked decrease among young people aged 15 to 19 in certain STDs, such as chlamydiosis and gonorrhea, over the past ten years. There are a number of possible reasons for this decrease, including the prevention efforts that have been made during this period. However, it must be emphasized that HIV infection does not seem to have reached the schools yet and that measures must be taken to ensure that this does not in fact take place. We therefore recommend:

- *That prevention and education efforts in the schools be continued and even intensified;*
- *That sex education courses be offered to all young people starting in the second level of primary school to promote healthy sexuality and to help them understand the importance of delaying their first sexual experience;*
- *That young people have easy access to condoms in the schools.*

Among the variables associated with condom use by adolescents in their sexual experiences, alcohol and drug use and the use of oral contraceptives warrant special attention. It is becoming increasingly recognized that alcohol and drug use, which alter the ability to make decisions, are associated with unprotected sexual relations in young people. Moreover, according to a number of studies that addressed the antagonism between "pill and condom", the use of oral contraceptives by teenage girls is the best predictor of *decreased* condom use (Otis 1995). This shows the importance of addressing these questions before young people start having an active sex life. Pregnancy, STDs and AIDS, despite their various impacts (in terms of meaning and consequences), must be dealt with together. Sexual health should also be linked with more general health-related values, particularly with regard to substance abuse. We therefore recommend:

- *That programs on sexuality, STDs and AIDS make connections with the prevention of teenage pregnancy and the prevention of substance abuse.*

One of the primary difficulties inherent in the development of effective promotion interventions pertains to the amount of time and money that must be invested. Not only must the needs of the target population be clearly identified, but the intervention must be carefully developed. This crucial step must be carried out in partnership. Thus, contents validated by research results must be negotiated along with elements that are more incidental but attractive for the target population. Moreover, no program, no matter how attractive, is sufficient in itself. It must be part of a general framework and be sustained by resource persons for a sufficient period of time to ensure its continuity; otherwise, it will be doomed to failure. It thus becomes essential to create a structure to support the implementation of new prevention programs. Health professionals in the schools (such as the school nurse), who play a very important role in carrying out prevention activities and objectives, all seem to be designated as the pillars of this structure. Through the energy of these interveners, organizations are able to conduct prevention activities for little cost and, in conjunction with teachers, nonteaching staff and young people, carry out programs in the schools. These health professionals in fact serve as a liaison between the schools and the health community. We therefore recommend:

- *That schools have a person responsible for initiating dynamic prevention activities that are in keeping with the realities of the school setting.*

The appropriateness of relying on interveners who are already in place in the school, including educators in youth centres and foster parents of socially maladjusted young people, has been demonstrated. In our opinion, this intervention model should be adopted with other target populations, because these interveners represent the most significant persons for these various groups. Furthermore, interveners are likely to come in contact with a sufficient number of persons to make it cost effective to call upon them. In addition, counting on them also means counting on the fact that the community will take ownership of the intervention, a major advantage. Finally, using this approach is consistent with one of the criteria for successful interventions: genuine understanding of the living environment.

To promote STD and AIDS prevention among the various target groups, whether they be in schools, youth centres, community agencies, etc., the issue of sexual practices must be addressed along with other facets of the sexuality of individuals. It is thus important that the basic training of the professionals (interveners) working in these various settings enable them to intervene in STD and AIDS prevention programs. We therefore recommend:

- *That a policy of continuous training in the various intervention communities be established to ensure that* all *interveners called to work directly with the target populations have the skills needed with regard to sex education and STD and AIDS prevention;*
- *That training for parents and key players in the natural support system (such as peers and foster parents) be offered so that prevention interventions can be developed in interaction with the living environment.*

The media are now a part of the Canadian people's cultural universe. Television in particular has acquired a stunning level of popularity over the years. For example, young people spend an average of 24 hours a week in front of the television set (Duquet 1991). Grégoire notes that, as the pre-eminent medium for contemporary culture, television obviously plays a key role in the emergence, development and incarnation of values surrounding the things that interest young people: love, work, the beautiful and the good, recreation, relationships with others, the family, knowledge, religion and so forth (Grégoire 1982). Consequently, the fact that almost all television series deal with sexuality and show sexual relations with no consideration of the risks of STDs or unwanted pregnancy tends to promote a lack of responsibility among television viewers with regard to these problems in their own sex lives.

One major benefit of using the media stems from the fact that it makes it easy to reach people in remote areas and other groups that are hard to reach through our normal work methods. Highly rated television series and miniseries could thus be used to at least put forth messages about prevention and preferably to present models of persons who are assuming their responsibility with regard to sexuality and STD and AIDS prevention when they have sexual relations with a new partner. Artists who are popular and credible with the public should be approached to deliver these messages. We therefore recommend:

- *That broadcasters (particularly public broadcasters) and those who work with them (producers, writers and artists) be made aware of the importance of presenting television viewers with responsible role models in terms of sexuality and STD and AIDS prevention.*

It is estimated that an average of five to six years must be spent on the development and implementation of an intervention program, including evaluation of the program (Bouchard 1991). In view of how essential evaluation is to program quality, it is obvious that ad hoc or piecemeal funding will not only make programs vulnerable and precarious from the outset but can also have an adverse effect on the level of motivation within the community in which the prevention project is being implemented. Consequently, in order for new programs to be implemented, there is a need for reliable funding that is at least sufficient to enable all the phases of a project's implementation to be carried out, including the training of staff able to offer this program and to ensure continuity after the evaluation. When there is insufficient funding the partners give up, the program must be interrupted or it becomes necessary to work with understaff resources. In general, funding agencies are very receptive to applications for funding for needs analyses, but they become more stringent when it comes to establishing protocols for program evaluation, and funding for the intermediate (implementation) phase does not seem to fall within the mandate of any specific organization. This state of affairs can have unfortunate consequences on the mobilization of partners and renders worthless all the effort put into the needs analysis. We therefore recommend:

- *That funding be allocated to needs analyses as long as such analyses are part of a comprehensive research program leading to the probable implementation of an intervention followed by evaluation of the intervention.*

Another factor that can have an impact on effectiveness is the use of a multidisciplinary approach, that is, the harmonization of the programs implemented by various interveners from the realms of health, education, justice and so forth. Prevention interventions often target populations for which other agencies are responsible, agencies whose primary mission does not pertain to physical health. The support of the organizations to which these agencies report must nonetheless be enlisted for the implementation of prevention activities as well as for providing funding. We therefore recommend:

- *That the various levels of government facilitate the use of a multidisciplinary approach and collaboration when interventions fall within the jurisdiction of more than one department.*

Gaston Godin, *Ph.D., is a full professor in the Faculty of Nursing Sciences at Laval University. He graduated in community health from the University of Toronto, specializing in behavioral sciences. He coordinates the activities of two research groups: one on the study of the adoption and maintenance of health-related behaviours and one relating to AIDS prevention. He has published close to a hundred articles in both national and international scientific journals.*

BIBLIOGRAPHY

AJZEN, I. 1985. From intention to action: A theory of planned behavior. In *Action Control: From Cognition to Behavior*, eds. KUHL, and J. BECKMANN. Berlin: Springer-Verlag. pp. 11–39.

ALEXANDER-RODRIGUEZ, T. and VERMUND, S. H. 1987. Gonorrhea and syphilis in incarcerated urban adolescents: Prevalence and physical signs. *Pediatrics* 80 (4): 561–564.

BEAUPRÉ, P., LaVIGUEUR R., and GAGNÉ, N. 1994. Les familles d'accueil pour adolescents: agents multiplicateurs dans la prévention des MTS/SIDA (Foster families for adolescents: Educators in STD/AIDS prevention) Workshop held during the meeting of the Conseil multidisciplinaire des Centres jeunesse de Québec (Multidisciplinary council of Quebec City youth centres) under the theme "Intégrer les approches et connaissances nouvelles à nos pratiques" (Integrating new approaches and knowledge into our practice), held in Quebec City on November 25, 1994.

BÉDARD, D., FORTIER, P., LAROUCHE, Y., LETARTE, G., and DUVAL, B. 1991. La problématique de l'hépatite B en centres de réadaptation pour jeunes et mères en difficulté d'adaptation (CRJDA et CRMDA) (Hepatitis B in rehabilitation centres for troubled youths and young mothers). Proposal adopted by the Commission régionale sur la mésadaptation sociale (Regional board on social maladjustment), Conseil de la santé et des services sociaux de la région de Québec (Quebec City regional council on health and social services) (03–12).

BELL, T. A., FARROW, J. A., STAMM, W. E., CRITCHLOW, C. W., and HOLMES, K. K. 1985. Sexually transmitted diseases in females in a juvenile detention center. *Sexually Transmitted Diseases* 12: 140–144.

BERLINGUET, M., CHAGNON, G., and TROTTIER, G. 1995. *Parents d'accueil et prévention des MTS et du sida chez les adolescents à risque (Foster parents and STD and AIDS prevention among adolescents at risk)*. Evaluation report on intervention program. Quebec: Centres jeunesse de Québec.

BERLINGUET, M., BROCHU, C., BROUSSEAU, J., and GAGNÉ, N. 1995. *Parents d'accueil et prévention des MTS et du sida chez les adolescents qui leur sont confiés par les Centres jeunesse (Foster parents and STD and AIDS prevention among adolescents placed with them by youth centres)*. Presentation submitted during the meeting of the provincial association of resource directors for Quebec youth centres, held in Quebec City on May 18, 1995.

BOUCHARD, C. 1991. *Un Québec fou de ses enfants (Quebec is crazy about its children)—Report of the working group on youth*. Quebec: Government of Quebec, Department of Health and Social Services, Direction des communications (Communications branch).

BROCHU, C., and BROUSSEAU, J. 1994. Parents et jeunes en difficulté. Presentation made at provincial HIV/AIDS symposium "La prévention plus que jamais" (Prevention: Now more than ever), held in Sherbrooke on November 24 and 25, 1994.

BUREAU OF COMMUNICABLE DISEASE EPIDEMIOLOGY. 1995. *Quarterly Surveillance Update: AIDS in Canada*, Health Canada, Laboratory Centre for Disease Control, Division of HIV/AIDS Surveillance.

CARBALLO, M., TAWIL, O. and HOLMES, K. 1991. Sexual behaviors: Temporal and cross-cultural trends. In *Research Issues in Human Behavior and Sexually Transmitted Diseases in the AIDS Era*, eds. J. N. WASSERHEIT, S. O. ARAL, K. K. HOLMES, and P. J.HITCHCOCK. Washington(DC): American Society for Microbiology.

CARBONNEAU, D. 1989. *Rapport de consultation auprès des organismes jeunesse (Report on consultation with youth agencies)—Region 03*, Sainte-Foy, Département de santé communautaire du Centre hospitalier de l'Université Laval (Laval University hospital community health department), Équipe de prévention et dépistage—Infection à VIH et sida (Prevention and screening team—HIV and AIDS infection)—Region 03 and Eastern Quebec.

CARON, D. 1986. De l'information à l'intervention (From information to intervention). In *Jeunesse et sexualité (Youth and sexuality)*, eds. A. DUPRAS, J. J. LÉVY, and H. COHEN. Longueuil: les Éditions Iris. pp. 567–587.

CARON, F. 1992. High school youth trained as peer educators. *Canadian AIDS News: The New Facts of Life* 5(2): 3.

_____. 1993a. *Formation des jeunes agents multiplicateurs en prévention des MTS et du sida en milieu scolaire: les Life Savers (Training of peer educators on STD and AIDS prevention in a school setting: The Life Savers)*. South Shore Regional Board of Education, Saint-Lambert, Quebec.

_____. 1993b. Programme de formation de jeunes agents multiplicateurs en prévention des MTS/ sida en milieu scolaire (Training program for peer educators on STD/AIDS prevention in a school setting). *Canadian Journal of Infectious Diseases* 4 (suppl. D): 13.

_____. 1993c. Programme de formation de jeunes agents multiplicateurs en prévention des MTS/ SIDA en milieu scolaire (Training program for peer educators on STD and AIDS prevention in a school setting). Presentation at "Continence ou condom: quel choix laissons-nous aux adolescents?" (Abstinence or condom: What choices are we leaving to our teenagers?). Workshop at the AIDS and STD conference "L'impact de nos actions" (The impact of our actions), held in Quebec City, December 1–3, 1993.

_____. 1995. L'expérience des Life-Savers (The Life Savers experiment). Presentation at the 5th regional conference of ACSA, "Affectivité et sexualité à l'adolescence, développer les compétences des intervenants et des adolescents" (Affectivity and sexuality in adolescence, developing skills in interveners and adolescents), May 1995.

_____. 1996. Évaluation d'un programme d'éducation à la sexualité orienté sur la prévention du sida présenté par des jeunes dans une école secondaire multi-ethnique de la Montérégie (Evaluation of a sexuality education program focusing on AIDS prevention presented by young people in a multi-ethnic high school in Montérégie). Activity report (brief) submitted to l'Université du Québec à Montréal, Sexology department.

CARON, F., NEWELL, M., OTIS, J., and LAMBERT, J. 1990. The AIDS travelling road show: Evaluation of a peer education program on AIDS awareness and prevention in the high school. Sixth International Conference on AIDS, San Francisco, summary 3083.

CENTRE QUÉBÉCOIS DE COORDINATION SUR LE SIDA (Quebec centre for coordination on AIDS). 1992. *Stratégie québécoise de lutte contre le sida et de prévention des maladies transmissibles sexuellement (Quebec strategy for combatting AIDS and preventing sexually transmitted diseases), Phase 3, 1992-1995 action plan*, Quebec City, Government of Quebec, Department of Health and Social Services, Centre québécois de coordination sur le sida.

_____. 1995. *Surveillance des cas de syndrome d'immunodéficience acquise (sida) (Surveillance of cases of acquired immuno-deficiency syndrome), Quebec City, cumulative cases 1979–1995—Update no. 95–3*, Quebec City, Centre québécois de coordination sur le sida, STD/AIDS prevention and control module.

CENTRES JEUNESSE DE QUÉBEC. 1996. *Facilitation Guide for Training Program "Parents d'accueil et prévention des MTS et du SIDA chez les adolescents à risque" (Foster parents and STD and AIDS prevention among adolescents at risk)*. Quebec City, Centres jeunesse de Québec and Department of Health and Social Services, Centre québécois de coordination sur le sida.

CLOUTIER, R., CHAMPOUX, L., and JACQUES, C. 1994. *"Ados, familles et milieu de vie—La parole aux ados" (Teens, families and living environments: Giving teens the floor)*, Quebec City, Université Laval, Centre de recherche sur les services communautaires (Centre for research on community services).

CLOUTIER, R., CHAMPOUX, L., JACQUES, C., and LANCOP, C. 1994. *"Nos ados et les autres" (Our teens and others: Comparative study of adolescents in Quebec youth centres and high school students)*. Quebec City, Université Laval, Centre de recherche sur les services communautaires (Centre for research on community services).

COMITÉ DE PROMOTION DE LA SANTÉ DE l'ASPQ. 1993. *Document de consensus sur les principes, stratégies et méthodes en promotion de santé (Consensus document on health promotion principles, strategies and methods)—Supporting document for the Déclaration québécoise sur la promotion de la santé et du bien-être (Quebec declaration on the promotion of health and well-being).* Montreal, Association pour la santé publique du Québec (Quebec Public Health Association).

COUNCIL OF SCIENTIFIC AFFAIRS. 1990. Health status of detained and incarcerated youths. *Journal of the American Medical Association* 263: 987–991.

DEPARTMENT OF HEALTH AND SOCIAL SERVICES. 1992. *Policy on Health and Well-Being,* Quebec City, Government of Quebec.

DESAULNIERS, M. P. 1990. *L'éducation sexuelle: définition (Sex education: A definition),* Montréal: Éditions Agence d'ARC Inc.

DICLEMENTE, R. J. 1992. Epidemiology of AIDS, HIV prevalence, and HIV incidence among adolescents. *Journal of School Health* 62(7): pp. 325–330.

———— 1991. Predictors of HIV-preventive sexual behavior in a high-risk adolescent population: The influence of perceived peer norms and sexual communication on incarcerated adolescents' consistent use of condoms. *Journal of Adolescent Health* 12: 385–390.

DICLEMENTE, R. J., and DUNAH, R. 1989. A Comparative Analysis of Risk Behaviors among a School-Based and Juvenile Detention Facility Sample of Adolescents in San Francisco. 5th International Conference on AIDS, Montreal, abstract D.508.

DICLEMENTE, R. J., LANIER, M. M., HORAN, P. F., and LODICO, M. 1991. Comparison of AIDS knowledge, attitudes, and behaviors among incarcerated adolescents and a public school sample in San Francisco. *American Journal of Public Health* 81(5): 628–630.

DUBOIS, R., and DULUDE, D., 1986. La perception de la relation sexuelle par des adolescentes dites mésadaptées socio-affectives (Perceptions of sexual relationships by "socio-affectively maladjusted" teenage girls). *Revue québécoise de psychologie* 7(3): 21–32.

DUQUET, F. 1991. *La violence et le sexisme dans les vidéoclips—Guide de participation à la session de perfectionnement (Violence and sexism in music videos—Guide to participation in development session).* Quebec City, Government of Quebec, Department of Education.

EVANS, R. G., and STODDART, G. L. 1994. Producing health, consuming health care. In *Why Are Some People Healthy and Others Not? The Determinants of Health of Populations,* eds. R. G. EVANS, M. L. BARER, and T. R. MARMOR. New York: Aldine De Gruyter.

FARROW, J. A., and SCHROEDER, E, 1984. Sexuality education in juvenile detention. *Adolescence* 19(76): 817–826.

GODIN, G. 1991, L'éducation pour la santé: les fondements psychosociaux de la définition des messages éducatifs (Health education: Psychosocial basis of the definition of educational messages). *Sciences sociales et Santé* IX(1): 67–94.

————. 1996. L'application des théories sociales cognitives à l'étude des comportements liés à la santé: une application au non-usage du tabac (Application of social cognitive theories to the study of health-related behaviours: An application to the non-use of tobacco). *Alcoologie* 18(3): 237–242.

GODIN, G., MICHAUD, F., and FORTIN, C. 1994. *Programme d'intervention sur la sexualité et la prévention des MTS et du sida pour les jeunes en CRJDA et CRJMDA (Intervention program on sexuality and STD and AIDS prevention for young people in rehabilitation centres for troubled youths and young mothers).* Sainte-Foy, Université Laval, École des sciences infirmières, Groupe de recherche sur les aspects psychosociaux de la santé (Research group on the psychosocial aspects of health, University Laval Faculty of Nursing Science).

GODIN, G., FORTIN, C., MICHAUD, F., and BRADET, R. 1994a. Self-efficacy and outcomes expectations as determinants of condom use among adolescents living in juvenile detention centers. Fourth Annual Canadian Conference on HIV/AIDS Research, Toronto, June 1994.

————. 1994b. Use of condoms: Intention and behavior of adolescents living in juvenile detention centers. 15th annual meeting, The Society of Behavioral Medicine, Boston, April 1994.

GODIN, G., MICHAUD, F., FORTIN, C., and DESRUISSEAUX, D. 1994. *Étude sur les comportements associés à la transmission des MTS et du sida chez les jeunes et les jeunes mères en difficulté d'adaptation en CRJDA et CRJMDA—Rapport de recherche (Study on behaviours associated with STD and AIDS transmission among young people in rehabilitation centres for troubled youths and young mothers—Research report).* Sainte-Foy, Université Laval, École des sciences infirmières, Groupe de recherche sur les aspects psychosociaux de la santé (Research group on the psychosocial aspects of health, University Laval Faculty of Nursing Science).

GODIN, G., FORTIN, C., MICHAUD, F., BRADET, R., and KOK, G. (soon to be published). Use of condoms: Intention and behaviour of adolescents living in juvenile rehabilitation centres. *Health Education Research.*

GOLDSMITH, M. 1987. Sex in the age of AIDS calls for common sense and condom sense. *Journal of the American Medical Association* 257: 2261–2266.

GREEN, L. W., and KREUTER, M. W. 1991. *Health Education Planning: An Educational and Environmental Approach.* 2nd ed. Palo Alto (CA): Mayfield.

GRÉGOIRE, R. 1982. *Grandir avec la télévision (Growing up with television).* Quebec City, Government of Quebec, Superior Council on Education.

HEALTH AND WELFARE CANADA. 1992. *User's Guide to 40 Community Health Indicators.* Ottawa: Health and Welfare Canada, Health Services and Promotion Branch, Community Health Division.

HEIN, K. 1993. "Getting real" about HIV in adolescents. *American Journal of Public Health* 83 (4): 492–494.

HUSCROFT, S., MORRIS, R., RE, O., BAKER, C., AQUINO, K., and ROSEMAN, J. 1990. *Survey of Sexual Behavior Risk Factors for HIV Infection in Incarcerated Adolescents,* Sixth International Conference on AIDS, San Francisco, summary 3018.

JANZ, N. K., ZIMMERMAN, M. A., WREN, P. A., ISRAEL, B. A., FREUDENBERG, N., and CARTER, R. J. 1996. Evaluation of 37 AIDS prevention projects: Successful approaches and barriers to program effectiveness. *Health Education Quarterly* 23(1): 80–97.

KARUNANANTHAN, M. 1995. Presentation in connection with the "Youth for Youth". Conference sponsored by the Canadian AIDS Society, April 1995.

KING, A. J. C., BEAZLEY, R. P., WARREN, W. K., HANKING, C. A., ROBERTSON, A. S., and RADFORD, J. L. 1988. *Canada Youth and AIDS Study.* Kingston: Queen's University.

LANIER, M., and MCMARTHY, B. R. 1989. AIDS awareness and the impact of AIDS education in juvenile corrections. *Criminal Justice* 16: 395–411.

LANIER, M., DICLEMENTE, R. J., and HORAN, P. F. 1991. The impact of ecological factors and cultural diversity: Incarcerated adolescents' AIDS awareness and precautionary measures. *Criminal Justice* 16: 257–262.

LÉVY, J. J., and DUPRAS, A. 1989. Les comportements sexuels et contraceptifs au Québec: aspects contemporains (Sexual and contraceptive behaviours in Quebec: Contemporary aspects). In *La sexologie au Québec (Sexology in Quebec),* ed. A. DUPRAS. Longueuil: les Éditions Iris. pp. 129–164.

MANN, J. M., TARANTOLA, D. J. M., and NETTER, T. W. Ed. 1992. *AIDS in the World,* Cambridge: Harvard University Press.

MELCHERT, T., and BURNETT, K. F. 1990. Attitudes, knowledge, and sexual behavior of high-risk adolescents: Implications for counseling and sexuality education. *Journal of Counseling and Development* 68(3): 293–298.

MOORE, S. M. and ROSENTHAL, D. A. 1993. *Sexuality in Adolescence.* New York: Routledge.

MORRIS, R. E., BAKER, C. J., and HUSCROFT, S. 1992. Incarcerated youth at risk for HIV infection. In *Adolescents and AIDS: A Generation of Jeopardy,* ed. R. J. DICLEMENTE. Newbury Park: Sage Publications Inc. pp. 52–70.

MORRIS, R., LEGAULT, J., and BAKER, C. 1993. Prevalence of isolated urethral asymptomatic chlamydia trachomatis infection in the absence of cervical infection in incarcerated adolescent girls. *Sexually Transmitted Diseases* 20(4): 198–200.

MORRIS, R., BAKER, C., HUSCROFT, S., EVANS, C. A. and FIRPO, R. 1992. Three years variations in HIV risk behaviors in detained minors. 8th International Conference on AIDS, Amsterdam, PoD 5063.

NADER, P. R., WEXLER, D. B., PATTERSON, T. L., MCKUSICK, L., and COATES, T. 1989. Comparison of beliefs about AIDS among urban, suburban, incarcerated, and gay adolescents. *Journal of Adolescent Health Care.* 10(5): 413–418.

NUTBEAM, D. 1988. Glossaire de la promotion de la santé (Health promotion glossary). In *La promotion de la santé: une perspective, une pratique,* eds. H. ANCTIL, and C. MARTIN. Santé et Société, Collection promotion de la santé (Health promotion: perspective and practice, Health and Society, Health promotion collection), Government of Quebec, Department of Health and Social Services.

OH, K. M., BERMAN, S., PASS, R. F., CLOUD, G. A., and FLEENOR, M. 1993. Sexual behavior and prevalence of STDs among detained adolescent females in U.S. 9th International Conference on AIDS/HIV STD World Congress, Berlin, summary WS-D11-5.

OH, M. K., CLOUD, G. A., WALLACE, L. S., REYNOLDS, J., STURDEVANT, M., and FEINSTEIN, R.A. 1994. Sexual behavior and sexually transmitted diseases among male adolescents in detention. *Sexually Transmitted Diseases* 21(3): 127–132.

O'NEILL, M., and CARDINAL, L. 1994. Health Promotion in Quebec: Did it ever catch on? In *Health Promotion in Canada,* eds. A. PADERSON, M. O'NEILL and I. ROOTMAN. Toronto, W. B. Saunders.

OTIS, J. 1992. La théorie du comportement planifié appliquée à l'utilisation du condom chez les adolescents et adolescentes de cinquième secondaire (Theory of planned behaviour applied to condom use among fifth year high school students). Doctoral thesis. Montréal: Université de Montréal.

———. 1993a. Connaissances, attitudes et comportements d'élèves de la région montréalaise en matière de prévention des MTS et du sida (Knowledge, attitudes and behaviours of students from the Montreal area with regard to STD and AIDS prevention). *Bulletin de Nouvelles,* Association canadienne pour la santé des adolescents (*Newsletter,* Canadian association for adolescent health) 2(4): 10–13.

———. 1993b. *Connaissances, attitudes et comportements des élèves en matière de prévention des MTS et du sida: étude en milieu scolaire—Résultats préliminaires (Knowledge, attitudes and behaviours of students with regard to STD and AIDS prevention—preliminary results).* Summary document for school interveners, Montreal, Université du Québec à Montréal, Sexology department.

———. 1994. Connaissances, attitudes et comportements des élèves en matière de prévention des MTS et du sida (Knowledge, attitudes and behaviours of students with regard to STD and AIDS prevention)—Study conducted in May 1993 with second to fifth year high school students. Summary document for school interveners, unpublished document, Université du Québec à Montréal, Sexology department.

———. 1995. *Comportements et déterminants des comportements liés à la prévention des MTS et de l'infection par le VIH chez les jeunes québécois(e)s: état des connaissances (Behaviours and behaviour determinants associated with STD and HIV prevention among young people in Quebec: Level of awareness).* Document submitted to the evaluation branch of the Department of Health and Social Services, Montreal, Université du Québec à Montréal, Sexology department.

OTIS, J., ROY, E., and FRAPPIER, J. Y. 1995. *Determinants of Condom Use among Adolescents in Custodial Facilities.* 27th annual meeting of the Society for Adolescent Medicine, Vancouver.

OTIS, J., GODIN, G., LAMBERT, J., and SAMSON, J. M. 1995. Étude longitudinale des facteurs associés à l'adoption et au maintien de comportements sexuels sains chez les adolescents: temps 3 (Longitudinal study of factors associated with the adoption and retention of healthy sexual behaviours among adolescents: Phase 3). Working document, Université du Québec à Montréal, Sexology department.

OTIS, J., LONGPRÉ, D., GOMEZ, B., and THOMAS, R. 1994. L'infection par le VIH et les adolescents: profil comportemental et cognitif de jeunes de milieux communautaires différents (HIV infection and adolescents: Behavioural and cognitive profile of young people from various backgrounds). In *Éduquer pour prévenir le sida (Education for AIDS prevention)*, eds. N. CHEVALIER, J. OTIS, and M. P. DESAULNIERS. Beauport: Publications MNH Enr. pp. 37–56.

PARENT, R., and ALARY, M. 1995. *Analyse des cas de chlamydiose, de gonorrhée, d'infection par le virus de l'hépatite B et de syphilis déclarés au Québec par année civile, 1990-1994 (Analysis of cases of chlamydiosis, gonorrhea, hepatitis B infection and syphilis reported in Quebec by calendar year, 1990-1994)*. Quebec City, Centre de santé publique de Québec (Quebec City public health centre).

PINEAULT, R., and DAVELUY, C. 1986. *La planification de la santé, concepts, méthodes, stratégies (Health planning, concepts, methods, strategies)*. Montreal: Éditions Agence d'ARC Inc.

POULIN, C., ALARY, M., RINGUET, J., FRAPPIER, J. Y., and ROY, E. 1994. *Prévalence de l'infection chlamydienne et comportements à risque de MTS et d'infection par le VIH chez les jeunes en difficulté du Québec (Prevalence of chlamydiosis infection and STD and HIV risk behaviours among troubled youths in Quebec)*. Sainte-Foy, Centre de santé publique de Québec (Quebec City public health centre).

RADFORD, J. L., KING, A. J. C., and WARREN, W. K. 1989. *Street Youth and AIDS*. Kingston: Queen's University

ROTHERAM-BORUS, M., and KOOPMAN, C. 1991. AIDS and adolescents. *Encyclopedia of Adolescence* 1, A-L, pp. 29–36.

ROTHERAM-BORUS, M. J., KOOPMAN, C., and EHRHARDT, A. A. 1991. Homeless youths and HIV infection. *American Psychologist* 46(11): 1188–1197.

ROY, E., FRAPPIER, J. Y., NADEAU, D., GIRARD, M., MORIN, D. A., MORIN, D. H. and O'SHAUGHNESSY, M. 1992. Demographic characteristics and HIV risk behaviours of detained adolescents in metropolitan Montreal. 8th International Conference on AIDS. Amsterdam, summary PoD. 5068.

SHAFER, M. A., HILTON, J. F., EKSTRAND, M., KEOGH J., GEE, L., DIGIORGIO-HAAG, L., SHALWITZ, J., and SCHACHTER, J. 1993. Relationship between drug use and sexual behaviors and the occurence of sexually transmitted diseases among high-risk male youth. *Sexually Transmitted Diseases* 20(6): 307–313.

STONE, K. M., GRIMES, D. A., and MAGDER, L. S. 1986. Primary prevention of sexually transmitted diseases. *Journal of the American Medical Association* 255: 1763–1766.

STRICOF, R. L., KENNEDY, J. T., NATTELL, T. C., WEISFUSE, I. B., and NOVICK, L. F., 1991. HIV seroprevalence in a facility for runaway and homeless adolescents. *American Journal of Public Health* 81 (suppl.): 50–53.

SYME, S.L. 1994. The social environment of health. *Daedelus, Journal of the American Academy of Arts and Sciences* 123(4): 79–86.

TEMOSHOK, L., MOULTON, J. M., ELLMER, R. M., SWEET, D. M., BAXTER, M., and SHALWITZ, J. 1989. Youth in detention at high risk for HIV: Knowledge, attitudes, and behaviors regarding condom usage. 5th International Conference on AIDS, Montreal, summary T.D.P.13.

VAN GIJSEGHEM, H. 1989. *Commission d'enquête portant sur des allégations d'abus sexuels impliquant des enfants résidant dans un centre d'accueil de la région de Montréal (Commission of inquiry into allegations of sexual abuse involving children living in a reception centre in the Montreal area). Report of the Commission*. Jean Denis Gagnon, president of the Commission, Montreal, June 1989.

WORLD HEALTH ORGANIZATION. 1995. Global Situation of the HIV/AIDS pandemic. *Weekly Epidemiological Record* 70, July 7, pp. 195–96

————. 1985. *Control of Sexually Transmitted Diseases*. Geneva: World Health Organization.

Improving the Health of Street/Homeless Youth

TULLIO CAPUTO, PH.D., AND KATHARINE KELLY

*Department of Sociology and Anthropology
Carleton University*

SUMMARY

*During the last decade, young people were the fastest growing segment of the homeless population, with runaways and street youth accounting for a significant proportion of this group (*Children Today *1989; Price 1989; Ward 1989). This paper examines various aspects of homeless youth through a detailed review of relevant literature and an examination of the results of two case studies. Specific attention is given to runaways and street youth, since these two groups make up the bulk of the homeless youth population. However, other young people who are associated with the street lifestyle, such as curbsiders and wannabees, are also considered.*

Estimates of the number of homeless youth in Canada vary widely. For example, the RCMP Missing Children's Registry 1991 annual report stated that the rate of missing children in Canada was 13 per 100,000 in 1986. Of the 61,248 missing children reports filed in Canada in 1990, 44,800 were identified as runaways (Fisher 1992). Estimates of the number of homeless youth also vary for individual cities. In Toronto, they range from 5,000 to 10,000 or even 12,000 street youth (McCullagh and Greco 1990, 24; Appathurai 1988).

A more restrictive definition than "runaways and missing children" is proposed based on a model developed by Brannigan and Caputo (1993). It identifies street/homeless youth according to the amount of time spent on the street and the extent of their involvement in the street lifestyle. Applying this definition dramatically lowers estimates of the size of the population of interest. Estimates in several Canadian cities of the number of entrenched street/homeless youth range from 200 or 300 hundred in winter to 500 or 600 in summer. While estimates based on this definition are much smaller than the estimates of the number of runaways and missing children, they still represent a significant number of young people who are living in marginal and precarious situations and engaging in the dangerous practices associated with surviving on the street.

The street youth population has been described as between 12 and 24 years in age (Regional Municipality of Ottawa-Carleton 1992). There are slightly more males than females on the street, particularly at the upper end of the age range (Social Planning Council of Winnipeg 1991; Kufeldt et al. 1988; Smart et al. 1990; Janus et al. 1986). They experience a variety of challenges to their well-being while living on the street. For example, street/homeless youth have been found to be especially vulnerable to mental health problems, with many experiencing depression or attempting suicide (Stiffman 1989a; Yates et al. 1988; Denoff 1987). Molnar et al. (1990) stated that homeless children experience physical, psychological and emotional damage. Luna (1987) reported that these young people lead emotionally damaging, unstable and hazardous lives.

Young people living on the street are also exposed to the violence that is a common feature of street life. A needs assessment of street/homeless youth in Ottawa reported that 40 (62 percent) of the 64 street youth in the study had been hurt while on the street (Regional Municipality of Ottawa-Carleton 1992). Of these, 72.5 percent said they had been beaten up or assaulted. Many street youth engage in high-risk sexual activities (McCullagh and Greco 1990; Social Planning Council of Winnipeg 1990; Webber 1991; Michaud 1988; Brannigan and Caputo 1993). Another major health risk is the extent of drug use. Canadian research suggests that "substance abuse amongst street youth is almost universal, and usually takes the form of dual drug and alcohol use (McCullagh and Greco 1990, 34). Radford et al. (1989, 124) found that "two thirds of all street youth were using drugs and/or alcohol weekly or daily."

The involvement of street/homeless youth in delinquent or criminal activities also places them at risk. Numerous studies report on their participation in various delinquent acts, such as theft, prostitution and drug dealing (McCarthy 1990; Powers et al. 1990; Janus et al. 1986, 1987b; Janus et al. 1987a). McCullagh and Greco (1990, 39–45) described the involvement of Toronto street youth in prostitution, theft, robbery and shoplifting, drug dealing and panhandling. In Winnipeg, the Social Planning Council study (1990, 40) found extensive street youth involvement in delinquent or criminal activities including prostitution, drug dealing, theft, robbery, joy riding, shoplifting, forgery and fraud.

The correlates of running away from home are well documented in the research literature (Rotheram-Borus 1991). These include individual problems (Nye and Edelbrock 1980; Stiffman 1989a; Yates et al. 1988; Denoff 1987), problems related to conflictual or dysfunctional families (Kufeldt and Nimmo 1987; Shane 1989; Kufeldt and Perry 1989; Price 1989) school-related difficulties (Brennan 1980; Windle 1989), problems with substance abuse (Radford et al. 1989; Smart et al. 1990; Social Planning Council of Winnipeg 1990) and participation in delinquent or criminal activities (Kufeldt and Nimmo 1987; Social Planning Council of Winnipeg 1990; McCullagh and Greco 1990; McCarthy 1990; McCarthy and Hagan 1991).

This research on the correlates to running away outlines the crucial factors that influence a young person's decision to leave home prematurely. They also identify instances where service providers might intervene to prevent these young people from going to the street in the first place, thereby avoiding the risks found there.

Various studies have also examined the health needs of street/homeless youth once they are on the street. In addition to meeting basic requirements, the following needs have been identified:

- *access to various types of personal counselling;*
- *contact with caring adults or peers;*
- *family counselling;*
- *appropriate social and recreational opportunities;*
- *specialized educational or employment training programs;*
- *consistent and integrated services;*
- *access to socially and culturally relevant services; and*
- *services delivered at times and places appropriate to this population.*

Many Canadian communities have recognized that the problem of youthful homelessness extends far beyond the needs of individual homeless youth. These problems are part of a complex pattern of behaviour that places the health of a significant number of young people at risk. Increasingly, interagency networks are being recognized as the most effective and efficient way of addressing such complex problems as youthful homelessness, juvenile delinquency and youth violence (Regional Municipality of Federation of Canadian Municipalities 1994). Many communities have developed comprehensive, interagency, multi-disciplinary, community-based networks to respond to this problem.

Two case studies were examined as the source of "stories" that illustrate both the successes and failures of interagency networks in two Canadian communities: Saskatoon and Ottawa. These interagency networks were designed, in part, to meet a broad range of social, economic, health and personal needs of the street/homeless youth population in these communities.

Data from these case studies are presented to highlight the views of street youth in these two communities regarding the services available to them. In general, street youth in both communities reported using available services. The exception was the low use of shelter services in Saskatoon and the avoidance of social services by Aboriginal youth in that community. Otherwise, use of health, educational and maintenance services in both communities was high. Moreover, most of the street youth evaluated the services they used quite favourably.

Socially and culturally relevant services, provided in an appropriate manner by sensitive staff were highly used and well respected by the street youth. The difficulties they noted had to do with access and availability and the fragmented nature of existing services. In many cases, street youth could not gain access to the mainstream services they required. For others, the services they most needed were unavailable.

These views were assessed in light of the interagency efforts in place in both communities. In both instances, extensive youth services were available. And both had developed specific interagency responses to this population. In Saskatoon, E'Gadz represents a unique interagency approach. It was formed by a committee of youth-serving agencies as a focal point for the community's response to street/homeless youth. Its counterpart in Ottawa, the Youth Services Bureau (YSB), provides a range of services to street/homeless youth, including outreach, drop-in centres, counselling, housing and referral services. Unlike E'Gadz, YSB does not house the services of member agencies in its buildings. Rather it acts as a broker for services needed by street youth in the community.

The street youth in Saskatoon spoke favourably of E'Gadz and made extensive use of its services. They trusted the staff and maintained contact with staff members. The challenges facing E'Gadz revolve around its location and relationship with member agencies. The fact that E'Gadz has a large building means that many agencies serving high-risk youth can offer programs there as is the case for the health, education and criminal justice system. Their location, however, means that they do not attract street youth from congregation areas in other parts of the city. In response, E'Gadz has started an outreach program. But this, too, is somewhat contradictory since it places E'Gadz in competition with service providers who are members of its board of directors.

Interagency cooperation and "turf" related issues are a challenge facing Saskatoon's interagency effort. While E'Gadz was intended as a place where all service providers could offer programs, only a few do so. Some have tested program ideas in E'Gadz and then located successful programs in their home agencies.

Similar successes and challenges were found in Ottawa. The efforts of YSB have been well received by the local street youth, and agency staff are trusted and respected. The challenge in Ottawa is that many street youth find it difficult to gain access to the mainstream services they need. Conversely, some of these services are not available. YSB has an excellent working relationship with other youth-serving agencies in the community. In its role as broker, YSB refers street youth to the services they require. For the most part this works quite well. However, many needs are not being met and, like Saskatoon, "turf" issues are always a concern.

A number of creative community responses were being developed in Ottawa while the case study there was under way. For example, a youth employment initiative which involved the downtown business community supported the efforts of street/homeless youth to establish and operate their own business. The Rideau Street Youth Initiative provides street youth with employment training, experience and contacts with members of the business community.

Recommendations

Key conclusions drawn from the relevant literature and the case studies point to a number of policy implications.

1. *Numerous opportunities exist for implementing preventive measures. These should be directed at the correlates of running away in order to forestall going to the street in the first place.*
2. *A range of services should be available to young people once they are on the street. These should include prevention, crisis intervention, maintenance, transition and incapacitation services. These services should be socially and culturally relevant, and delivered at times and places accessible to the target population.*
3. *Interagency initiatives are the most efficient and effective way of responding to the problem of youthful homelessness. They provide an opportunity to maximize limited resources by reducing or eliminating duplication, and filling service gaps.*
4. *If interagency initiatives are used, efforts must be taken to minimize "turf" issues among the participants. Services should be consistent and continuity must be maintained.*

TABLE OF CONTENTS

INTRODUCTION

The problem of homelessness has received increasing attention in both Canada and the United States over the last decade. Numerous media reports, books, films as well as government-sponsored studies and academic research have documented the issue of youth homelessness (Kufeldt and Burrows 1994; Caputo et al. 1994a, b; Brannigan and Caputo 1993; McDonald and Peressini 1992; Rossi 1989). During this period, young people were the fastest growing segment of the homeless population, with runaways and street youth accounting for a significant proportion of this group (*Children Today* 1989; Price 1989; Ward 1989).

    This paper examines various aspects of the issue of youthful home-lessness. A detailed review of relevant literature is provided with specific attention to runaways and street youth, since these two groups comprise the bulk of the homeless youth population. However, other young people, such as curbsiders and wannabees, who are associated with the street lifestyle are also considered. A description of the target population is presented, with some consideration of who should be included in a definition of homeless youth. This is followed by a discussion of the health risks associated with living in marginal and precarious situations on the street. In particular, the potential consequences of engaging in the risky and often dangerous activities associated with the street lifestyle are discussed. These activities include substance abuse, high-risk sex and involvement in illegal activities in order to survive.

    Many observers have noted that interagency, multidisciplinary, community-based approaches offer the best opportunities for addressing the problem of street/homeless youth. Two case studies are used as the source of "stories" that illustrate both the successes and failures of interagency networks in two Canadian communities: Saskatoon and Ottawa. These interagency networks were designed, in part, to meet a broad range of social, economic, health and personal needs of the street/homeless youth population in these communities. Various issues are also discussed, including the antecedents and consequences of young people going to the street.

    Key conclusions drawn from the relevant literature are then considered in a final section which includes a discussion of the policy implications of this work. This discussion is couched in terms of the broad determinants of population health. Relevant principles are identified to help guide the actions of governments, youth-serving agencies, communities and others providing services to homeless youth.

ESTIMATING THE SIZE OF THE HOMELESS YOUTH PROBLEM

Estimates reported in the research literature of the size of the homeless youth population vary widely. For example, American estimates of the number of missing children range from two hundred thousand to several million cases per year (*Society* 1988). This is consistent with other American research, such as Rotheram-Borus (1991) who reported that in 1979 there were approximately 1.5 million runaways and homeless youth in the United States, and Shane (1989) who put this figure at two million runaways per year in the early 1980s. A study by Finkelhor et al. (1990) estimated a rate of 205 runaways per 100,000 in the United States.

In Canada, the RCMP Missing Children's Registry 1991 annual report stated that the rate of missing children in Canada was 13 per 100,000 in 1986. In 1990, 61,248 missing children reports were filed in Canada. Of these, 44,800 were identified as runaways, the majority of whom were children who ran away multiple times over the course of the year (Fisher 1992). Additional Canadian estimates are provided by Radford et al. (1989, 9) who cited Covenant House statistics which estimated that there are 150,000 runaways in Canada each year. They also noted a suggestion by the Select Committee On Youth that the number of children who run away from home each year in Canada is unknown.

Estimates of the number of homeless youth in particular Canadian cities also vary widely. For example, the Coalition of Youth Work Professionals in Toronto stated that there are about 5,000 street youth in the city. By contrast, the Evergreen Drop-In Centre estimated that approximately 12,000 young people are living on the street in Toronto (McCullagh and Greco 1990, 24). Appathurai (1988) put this figure at 10,000. Anderson (1993, 3) summarized the difficulty in estimating the size of the homeless youth population by noting the following:

> As reported by Smart et al. (1990), the actual number of street youth in Toronto is unknown. This information gap applies to all urban centres across the country. In fact, there are not even rough approximations, as illustrated by Toronto media reports that have put forward various estimates ranging from 1,500 to 10,000 persons. Apparently, no one has even hazarded a guess as to how many curb youth there might be.

Some of the difficulties involved in estimating the size of the homeless youth population, and in interpreting the statistical data, are based on the definitions used. While some studies provide estimates of the number of missing children, others refer to runaways. The method used in counting these populations also has an effect. For example, should a young person who runs away from home several times during the year be considered a missing child or a runaway? Should each episode be reported to the authorities and counted as a case of a missing child or should this young person be considered a repeat runner and counted as a runaway only once?

Who Do We Include in a Definition of Homeless Youth?

One of the challenges facing researchers and policymakers is identifying who should be included in a definition of homeless youth. A variety of terms have been used to describe the various subgroups present on the street. These include runaways, curbsiders, throwaways, societal rejects, missing children, homeless youth, street youth and youth at risk (Finkelhor et al. 1990; Burgess 1986; Adams et al. 1985). These categories are problematic since they are not mutually exclusive. Moreover, they do not refer to discrete groups. For example, a young person who was forced by parents or guardians to leave home prematurely, could be described as a throwaway. This same young person could also be identified as a street youth, a homeless youth or a youth at risk by police officers or service providers, depending on the situation.

The problem of defining homeless youth arises, in part, because there are few young people on the street who are homeless in the strict sense of the term. Most have some place to stay, at least for limited periods of time. For example, some may crash with friends or other young people they meet on the street. In some cases, resources are pooled and a room or apartment is rented by one young person which then becomes home for the entire group. Other youth may find a place to sleep in emergency shelters, flop houses or other forms of temporary or marginal shelter. A few, however, actually live on the street—in city parks, under bridges, in stairwells or in abandoned buildings—depending on the time of year and availability of suitable alternatives.

The question of definition is further complicated by the methodological problems encountered in counting such an illusive and suspicious population. As McDonald and Peressini (1992, 11) pointed out, "the size of the homeless population has serious implications for policy formation, the cost of housing, health and social services, and the requisite manpower to deal with the problem." The larger the estimates of the size of the street youth population, the greater the claims for resources. As noted above, the definition of homelessness that is used is important because a more inclusive definition can result in higher estimates of the size of the homeless youth population. Similarly, the methodology employed in counting this population is important because it can be more or less effective in identifying and including members of the target population. This can have a significant effect on the resulting size estimates. As McDonald and Peressini (1992, 3,11) noted:

> ...the pressure "to do something about the problem" has promoted the outpouring of articles that exaggerate the problem and its characteristics in order to gain attention and attract dollars to ameliorate the situation... Different constituencies use different definitions to manipulate the size of the problem according to their own vested interests.

Another problem complicating the definition is that the young people on the street are not a homogeneous group. There are many subgroups which reflect the different reasons young people have for going there. For some, the street is the only viable alternative they see to an abusive and conflict-ridden home situation (Caputo et al. 1996). For others, the street provides freedom and excitement while they are still living at home and going to school.

Many young people on the street are in a state of transition: old identities are being discarded and new ones created (Caputo et al. 1996). While some become entrenched in the street lifestyle, others struggle to leave the street. This constant state of flux makes it difficult for researchers and policymakers to determine who is on the street, who is in need of assistance and what type of help they need. Various authors have devised typologies that attempt to categorize the different youth present on the street. Several are considered below.

Typologies of Street and Homeless Youth

McCullagh and Greco (1990, 9–18) identified five kinds of street youth: runners from intolerable homes, runners to adventure, throwaways who are pushed out by parents, absconders from care who are on the run from the Children's Aid Society or young offender facilities, and curb-kids (curbsiders) who live at home but spend considerable time on the street and participate extensively in the street lifestyle. The young people in each of these categories are on the street for different reasons. They arrive with a variety of skills and abilities, and have a range of needs and service requirements.

Another typology is provided by Kufeldt and Nimmo (1987) who distinguished between two different groups on the street: the runners who leave home for extended periods of time and who have little or no intention of returning home, and the in and outers for whom running to the street is a temporary and short-term coping mechanism. These two categories were expanded by Kufeldt and Perry (1989) to include runaways, throwaways, runners and run-arounds.

Brannigan and Caputo (1993) developed a model for addressing these definitional problems. They focused on two key criteria which are characteristic of the homeless youth population: the amount of time young people actually spend on the street and the extent to which they are involved in the street lifestyle. These are conceptualized as separate continua. The first—time spent on the street—distinguishes between entrenched street youth and others on the street. Thus, while some young people, such as curbsiders, may spend a considerable amount of time on the street, they are usually still living at home and going to school. This contrasts with entrenched street youth who are more likely to be homeless and on the street all the time.

Participation in practices associated with the street lifestyle is the second continuum identified by Brannigan and Caputo (1993). This allows for a distinction between those young people who come to the street to dabble vicariously in the street lifestyle and those who are entrenched in it. In this case, wannabees and curbsiders can be distinguished from entrenched street youth according to the extent of their participation in the risky and dangerous activities associated with life on the street. For example, many entrenched street youth are engaged in prostitution in order to meet their needs for food, shelter and drugs. By contrast, few wannabees become extensively involved in the sex trade. Similarly, while many youth on the street engage in illegal activities such as theft and selling drugs, entrenched street youth are much more likely to be systematically involved in these types of activities than wannabees or curbsiders.

Brannigan and Caputo (1993) also pointed out that there is a great deal of movement along these continua. For example, a young person who lives at home but spends a considerable amount of time on the street (a curbsider) may leave home and go to the street for a period of time. While living on the street the young person becomes increasingly entrenched in the street lifestyle. This young person may then receive help getting off the street, return home and reenroll in school. All may be stable for a while until a crisis occurs and the cycle of going to the street is repeated. This pattern is quite common for some youth, and may continue for several years (Caputo et al. 1994a).

Following Brannigan and Caputo (1993), the terms street youth, homeless youth and street/homeless youth are used interchangeably, in this paper, to refer to those young people who spend considerable amounts of time on the street, who live in marginal or precarious situations and who participate extensively in street lifestyle practices. Street/homeless youth is preferred over other terms since it reflects both the lack of a stable living situation and involvement in the street lifestyle. The young people included in this definition can range from entrenched street youth to curbsiders, depending on the amount of time they spend on the street and their involvement in the street lifestyle.

The Street/Homeless Youth Population

Using the above definition of street/homeless youth results in much lower estimates of the number of street/homeless youth in Canada than are provided for the number of runaways and missing children. For example, research in several large Canadian cities reveals that there are limited shelter resources available for street/homeless youth (Regional Municipality of Ottawa-Carleton 1992; Brannigan and Caputo 1993). Even in the largest centres, the number of shelter beds rarely exceeds several hundred. Claims that there are thousands of street/homeless youth in a city must be assessed in this context. While some street/homeless youth do not avail themselves of existing services, those providing food and shelter are able to give some estimates of the entrenched street/homeless youth population they serve.

In Ottawa, for example, estimates by service providers of the number of "entrenched" street youth range from 200 to 300 in winter up to 500 to 600 in summer (Regional Municipality of Ottawa-Carleton 1992; Caputo et al. 1994b). There are less than 100 shelter beds in the city, although there are more than 500 youth on student welfare in the region. Moreover, the number of youth on the street can fluctuate dramatically since Ottawa forms part of a triangle with Montreal and Toronto that is popular with street youth. Many entrenched street/homeless youth migrate from city to city to evade parents and authorities, and to seek better circumstances and opportunities.

A similar situation exists in Saskatoon (Caputo et al. 1994a). As a catchment area for smaller surrounding communities, Saskatoon has a street youth population that reaches several hundred during the winter. However, this figure can double or even triple during summer months. The street/homeless youth population in Saskatoon differs from that in Ottawa in several important respects. First, a large proportion is made up of Aboriginal youth whose running patterns differ markedly from those of non-Aboriginal street/homeless youth. Unlike most non-Aboriginal street youth, many of the Aboriginal street youth in Saskatoon retain close ties with family members. They often leave small northern reserves to stay with relatives in the city. Not wanting to be a burden on relatives, many of these young people spend a considerable amount of time on the street and are extensively involved in street life practices in order to survive. Nevertheless, they are not, strictly speaking, homeless. They do stay with relatives from time to time and retain contact with parents or guardians.

In western Canada, Calgary, Edmonton and Vancouver play the same role as Ottawa, Toronto and Montreal with respect to street youth migration. There is considerable movement by street youth among these cities throughout the year, with many favouring Vancouver during the winter months. Smaller centres, such as Saskatoon, form part of localized networks that feed into the tri-city migration pattern (Caputo et al. 1994b; Brannigan and Caputo 1993).

The Demographic Characteristics of Entrenched Street/Homeless Youth

The demographic characteristics of street/homeless youth are described in numerous Canadian studies. Street/homeless youth are typically 12 to 24 years of age, with more females at the younger end and more males at the older end of this age range. Brannigan and Caputo (1993) discussed some of the difficulties in precisely defining the age range for the target group. Among other considerations are the constraints imposed by legislation relevant to this population such as provincial child welfare laws or the federal *Young Offenders Act.* For the latter, youth are defined as being between 12 and 17 years of age. Some service providers, however, include young people up to age 24 or older in their mandates. At the lower end of this age range, there is a great deal of pressure by police and child protection authorities to identify and take these young people into care if they appear on the street. As a result, they are often "invisible" to service providers and other authorities, staying away from popular youth congregation areas and other public places. Young females, in particular, may be hidden from view by older males who initially befriend and care for them and later force them into the sex trade (Regional Municipality of Ottawa-Carleton 1992).

Various studies have also reported on the gender ratio of street/homeless youth. For example, of the 127 youths interviewed in the Social Planning Council of Winnipeg study (1990, 13), 60 percent (76) were females while 40 percent (51) were males. Similar results were reported by Kufeldt et al. (1988) whose exploratory study of homeless youth in Calgary included 52 percent females and 48 percent males. Different findings were presented by Smart et al. (1990) in a study of drug use among street youth in Toronto which indicated that 64 percent (93) of the respondents were male while 36 percent (52) were female. These results were echoed in a report by Janus et al. (1986) whose sample of street youth consisted of 63 percent males and 37 percent females.

The Nature of the Problem

If the definition of street/homeless youth provided above is used, the target population, and the nature and extent of the problem can be more accurately described. The number of street/homeless youth does not reach the hundreds of thousands as do estimates of the number of runaways or missing children. They do, however, represent a significant number of young people. Moreover, the definition of street/homeless youth being proposed identifies these young people as entrenched in the street lifestyle and living in very precarious circumstances. They face a variety of challenges to their physical and emotional well-being. As noted in Kufeldt and Burrows:

> Homeless teenagers must hustle and scavenge to eke out an existence, worrying about where they will next sleep or eat. They often must contend with the problems of drug and alcohol abuse, disease and conflict with the law. They are at high-risk of falling victim to violent crime, being abused on the street and victimizing others through such activities as theft, assault or drug dealing (Krammer and Schmidt cited in Kufeldt and Burrows 1994).

For many young people, life on the street is fraught with danger. The consequences of street life can reverberate throughout a person's life. For some, it leads to a lifetime of homelessness and economic marginalization. For others, the street becomes part of their identity, remaining with them for the rest of their lives (Social Planning Council of Winnipeg 1990).

Exploring the health risks of street/homeless youth sheds light on a number of factors related to being homeless. For example, homelessness is not defined as a "medical" problem, per se, although the homeless suffer from a variety of afflictions related to their lifestyles. The health-related consequences of inadequate access to sanitary facilities are considerable. Uncertain sleeping arrangements mean exposure to cold, wet sleeping conditions and to the risk of being robbed or beaten. Insufficient funds mean street youth cannot afford medicines if they do seek help. A lack of a place to store medical supplies may mean they may not take prescriptions, even when these are provided free of charge. The lack of a residence also means being unable to get a health card. This, in turn, leads to a denial of access to medical clinics and health services. Fear of being picked up by the police or social service agencies makes street youth wary of mainstream services which also results in not seeking assistance. All of these factors compound the health risks of street youth. It is important to note that these factors go beyond the control or choice of individuals reflecting, instead, the challenges endemic to life on the street.

The way these young people meet their existing needs also places them at risk. Lacking ongoing care and nurturing relationships, street youth form ties to other youth on the street. These connections, loosely described as street families, provide emotional support while simultaneously entrenching these young people further in the street lifestyle. Greater entrenchment and participation in the street lifestyle increases the risks to one's health. For example, those street youth who need to "turn tricks" to survive are not likely to refuse to perform sexual acts without protection when the alternative is to lose a customer. In this case, the risk of contracting AIDS or other sexually transmitted diseases is overshadowed by the immediate need for cash. The decision to engage in unprotected sex is not shaped simply by the choices of youth engaged in the sex trade but by their need for money and the demands made by their customers.

Some of the specific health-related risks experienced by street/homeless youth have been described in many Canadian studies (Webber 1991; Social Planning Council of Winnipeg 1990; Brannigan and Caputo 1993; Kufeldt and Burrows 1994). A needs assessment conducted by a community task force sponsored by the Regional Municipality of Ottawa-Carleton (1992) outlined the health-related risks associated with youthful homelessness in detail. This study found that life on the street can result in many serious consequences for an individual's general health and physical well-being. Psychological problems were also noted, including suicide attempts and self-mutilation. Other dangers included exposure to the violence that characterizes the street scene; the participation of street/homeless youth in high-risk sexual activities; health risks associated with substance abuse, especially intravenous drug use; and problems related to participation in delinquent or criminal activities. Each of these is described in greater detail below.

The General Health of Street/Homeless Youth

Health problems of street/homeless youth are directly related to the street environment and lifestyle. This includes the physical challenges that homelessness presents, such as having a safe and healthy place to live, sufficient food and clothing, and access to sanitary facilities. The lack of these fundamental necessities results in many health-related consequences. For example, many of the respiratory and skin problems reported by street youth are the direct result of poor living conditions, poor nutrition and poor personal hygiene related to the lack of access to sanitary facilities (Regional Municipality of Ottawa-Carleton 1992). These findings are consistent with American research which has also noted that runaways do not receive adequate medical care (JAMA 1989).

The Psychological Health of Street/Homeless Youth

A variety of psychological factors can play an important role in determining the health status of street/homeless youth. Many feel marginal, lonely and rejected while living at home (Caputo et al. 1996). They suffer from low self-esteem and have negative self-images. This often contributes to their participation in dangerous or risky behaviour, including intravenous drug use and high-risk sex. Many have an extremely fatalistic view of life, feeling that no one cares whether they live or die.

Street/homeless youth have been found to be especially vulnerable to mental health problems, with many experiencing depression or attempting suicide (Stiffman 1989a; Yates et al. 1988; Denoff 1987). Molnar et al. (1990) noted that homeless children experience physical, psychological and emotional damage. Luna (1987) reported on a study of the content of the graffiti of homeless youth. The findings from this research suggest that these young people lead emotionally damaging, unstable and hazardous lives. Runaways have been found to have low general intelligence, low self-sufficiency, hostility and a sense of isolation, and they are at risk of becoming psychotic (Speck et al. 1988; Hier et al. 1990).

The emotional problems young people bring to the street also contribute to their remaining there. Many street youth are lonely and seek acceptance and emotional support. Once on the street, they meet and gain acceptance from other youth in similar circumstances (Regional Municipality of Ottawa-Carleton 1992; Caputo et al. 1994a, b; Caputo et al. 1996). These new "friends" help the young person make it by providing information, food, shelter and other necessities in exchange for sexual favours and support. Many street youth refer to the acceptance of street families as a primary attraction of the street. They say that their new family members understand and accept them in ways they have never experienced before (Caputo et al. 1996). This attachment comes with high costs, including physical and sexual abuse, and pressure to engage in illegal and dangerous activities. Paradoxically, street families provide both needed support and care while tying youth to the street and to dangerous practices.

Violence and the Experiences of Street/Homeless Youth

Whether it is over drugs or "turf" or identity, violence is a common feature of life on the street. The Regional Municipality of Ottawa-Carleton (1992) needs assessment stated that 40 (62 percent) of the 64 street youth participating in the study reported "being hurt" while on the street. Of these 29 (69 percent) said they had been beaten up or assaulted, six (14 percent) had been sexually assaulted/raped and five (12 percent) had been stabbed or shot, or both. In answer to a related question, 42 (65 percent) said they had been the victim of a crime while living on the street. Theft, physical assault and sexual assault/rape were the crimes identified.

The Participation of Street/Homeless Youth in High-Risk Sexual Activities

Participation in high-risk sexual activity is an integral part of the street lifestyle. For many, sex is the currency of exchange since they have few other resources. In the Regional Municipality of Ottawa-Carleton (1992, 10) needs assessment, "one-third of the young people interviewed had traded sex for a place to sleep since living on the street." Moreover, numerous Canadian studies have noted the participation of street/homeless youth in the sex trade (McCullagh and Greco 1990; Social Planning Council of Winnipeg 1990; Webber 1991; Michaud 1988; Brannigan and Caputo 1993). Research also indicates that this transient and hard-to-service population is at high risk for contracting AIDS (Kaliski et al. 1990; Radford et al. 1989; Woodruff et al. 1989). Some studies have attempted to determine how much runaways and street youth know about AIDS and to develop educational programs for this population (Rotheram-Borus and Koopman 1991a, b; Luna 1989).

Drug Use by Street/Homeless Youth

Another major area of concern is the extent of drug use by runaways and street youth (Smart et al. 1990; Windle 1989). Canadian research has suggested that "substance abuse amongst street youth is almost universal, and usually takes the form of dual drug and alcohol use" (McCullagh and Greco 1990, 34). In a study by the Social Planning Council of Winnipeg (1990, 34), 22 percent of the 100 respondents reported intravenous drug use. Radford et al. (1989, 120) found that 12 percent of the 712 street youth in their sample said they had used intravenous drugs. Radford et al. (1989, 124) also found that "two thirds of all street youth were using drugs and/or alcohol weekly or daily." In the Regional Municipality of Ottawa-Carleton (1992, 15) needs assessment, the respondents ranked drug/alcohol abuse as the most important problem facing street/homeless youth.

The Participation of Street/Homeless Youth in Delinquent or Criminal Activities

The involvement of street/homeless youth in delinquent or criminal activities is a common theme in the literature. Numerous studies report on their participation in various delinquent acts, such as theft, prostitution and drug dealing (McCarthy 1990; Powers et al. 1990; Janus et al. 1986, 1987b; Janus et al. 1987a). For example, in a study of 84 respondents from various agencies providing services to runaways and street youth, Whitbeck and Simons (1990) found a positive relationship between running away from home and involvement in delinquent activities. McCullagh and Greco (1990, 39–45) described the involvement of Toronto street youth in prostitution, theft, robbery and shoplifting, drug dealing and panhandling. The Social Planning Council of Winnipeg (1990, 40) study found extensive involvement of street youth in delinquent or criminal activities including prostitution, drug dealing, theft, robbery, joyriding, shoplifting, forgery and fraud.

McCarthy (1990) provided the most systematic study in the Canadian literature of the involvement of street youth in delinquency. His year-long study included 390 interviews with homeless youth in Toronto. The respondents were asked about their involvement in delinquent acts both before and after leaving home. McCarthy found a strong relationship between experiences on the street and the propensity to participate in delinquent and criminal behaviour.

In a follow-up study, McCarthy and Hagan (1991) elaborated on these results by comparing findings from the street sample with a sample of 563 young people still living at home. The results indicated a pattern that is consistent with the bulk of the research on runaways, street and homeless youth. For example, McCarthy and Hagan found that homeless youth were more likely to come from unstable families characterized by conflict and abuse. Having problems at school was another important theme, with homeless youth experiencing more conflict with teachers and greater school failure. Finally, street/homeless youth were found to have engaged in both more serious and minor property crimes than young people still living at home.

Nonmedical Factors and the Health of Street/Homeless Youth

As the discussion above demonstrates, participation in the high-risk activities associated with the street lifestyle contributes, in significant ways, to the health problems of street youth. The activities themselves, however, fall outside the medical model. Furthermore, participation in these activities is unlikely to be changed through appeals to the young people involved to live in healthier ways or to make healthier choices. Street/homeless youth who engage in such activities are seeking more than a thrill. They are often trying to anesthetize themselves against the psychological pain of their current and past circumstances (Caputo et al. 1996; Caputo et al. 1994a, b). The returns, momentary and transitory, of being high are likely to outweigh the appeals to these young people by mainstream service providers to adopt a healthier way of life. This, in turn, influences their participation in these unhealthy activities. If this analysis is correct, the underlying causes of homelessness and emotional trauma must be addressed before these individuals can be expected to stop engaging in risky behaviour.

This discussion also highlights the nonmedical correlates of being homeless. In addition to the immediate physical consequences of living on the street, the literature identifies the psychological needs of these young people and their feelings of alienation and marginalization. The impact of living in conflictual or dysfunctional families has also been discussed. Economic marginalization has been mentioned briefly in this paper, as it relates to the need to engage in risky or delinquent activities in order to survive. Economic marginalization, however, affects the health of these young people in several other ways. Research indicates that while there are youth from all social classes on the street, increasingly, economic marginalization is resulting in more marginalized youth becoming homeless (Fuchs and Reklis 1992). Moreover, the lack of employment opportunities is a serious obstacle to youth trying to get off the street and into stable living situations.

These types of nonmedical factors clearly have a direct impact on the health of street/homeless youth. As such, they must be considered in any effort to improve the health status of this segment of the population. Seen in this way, the problem of homelessness is a public issue whose basis lies in the structure of a society. Such an approach displaces the tendency to view homelessness in terms of the specific ailments of homeless individuals. It calls, instead, for solutions that transcend a narrow focus on technical, medical interventions. Broader social policy responses are required that address both the causes and the consequences of homelessness and the particular needs of those who are on the street.

Meeting the needs of such high-risk individuals and improving their overall health requires the proper identification of their problems (Hill and Piper 1995). It also necessitates their having access to a range of appropriate services. These requirements are not simply matters of choice for street youth. Quite the contrary. They reflect the way the health care and social service systems design and deliver services (Hill and Piper 1995; Kaskutas et al. 1992).

Having recognized the problem of homelessness as a public issue, many Canadian communities have come together to develop comprehensive, multidisciplinary, interagency, community-based networks to respond to the problem. This is the case for both of the communities that participated in the case studies examined here. Interagency networks are increasingly being recognized as the most effective and efficient way of addressing such complex problems as youthful homelessness, juvenile delinquency and youth violence (Federation of Canadian Municipalities 1994).

While meeting the immediate medical needs of these young people is part of most community-based efforts, these interagency networks usually go far beyond narrowly defined medical needs. They often involve young people, families, community groups and youth-serving agencies, as well as representatives from education, health, social services and the youth justice system, in the design and delivery of a wide array of services. Health is defined very broadly to include the whole individual and his environment. The determinants of health are understood to encompass the physical, psychological, social, economic and cultural dimensions of people's lives.

In the next section, a more detailed description is provided of the antecedents to running away and ending up on the street This information is crucial for designing appropriate response strategies. In particular, it allows emphasis to be placed on preventive measures which may keep young people from going to the street in the first place. Many of these responses speak to the nonmedical correlates of running away and becoming homeless. They provide a context which will be used later in the paper to examine the effectiveness of interagency approaches to street/homeless youth issues used by the two communities that participated in the case studies being examined.

THE CORRELATES OF RUNNING AWAY

The correlates of running away from home are well documented in the research literature (Rotheram-Borus 1991). These include individual problems (Nye and Edelbrock 1980; Stiffman 1989a; Yates et al. 1988; Denoff 1987), problems related to conflictual or dysfunctional families (Kufeldt and Nimmo 1987; Shane 1989; Kufeldt and Perry 1989; Price 1989), school-related difficulties (Brennan 1980; Windle 1989), problems with substance abuse (Radford et al. 1989; Smart et al. 1990; Social Planning Council of Winnipeg 1990) and participation in delinquent or criminal activities (Kufeldt and Nimmo 1987; Social Planning Council of Winnipeg 1990; McCullagh and Greco 1990; McCarthy 1990; McCarthy and Hagan 1991).

The correlates to running away from home were examined in detail in a recent study by Caputo et al. (1996). The findings from this study are particularly pertinent to the current paper since they identify potential factors which might be important in preventing some young people from leaving home prematurely, thereby forestalling the consequences of participation in street life. This study also examined the experiences of these young people once on the street and the process involved in their making the transition off the street.

Caputo et al. (1996) conducted in-depth interviews with 70 former street youth in five Canadian cities. The findings revealed four distinct patterns which lead young people to the street: those who had come from conflictual home situations, those rebelling against parental/guardian authority, those who were forced from their homes prematurely (throwaways) and those who ended up on the street inadvertently, after seeking employment or adventure in a new city. In general, these patterns coincide with the categories identified by McCullagh and Greco (1990). They do, however, differ in some respects and these differences are elaborated on below.

The most common pattern reported by Caputo et al. (1996) involved young people who experienced conflictual situations at home before going to the street. This included young people who had been victims of psychological, emotional, physical or sexual abuse. In many instances, the conflict was compounded by the substance abuse problems of either the young people, their parents or both. Many respondents also reported having parents or siblings who had a history of conflict with the law.

In the conflictual home situation category, youth reported two very distinct sets of experiences. The first consisted of those involved in repeated incidents of conflict over an extended period of time. These episodes usually culminated in the young person running away from home. After numerous running episodes, these youth came to believe that returning home was no longer possible and the street was the only viable option open to them.

Some young people who had lived in a conflictual home situation had a different experience. Unlike the previous pattern, these young people did not engage in repeated running episodes. Instead, they went through a slow build-up after ongoing episodes of conflict. They reported leaving home when they could no longer tolerate the existing situation or when the street appeared as a more palpable alternative. These young people did not engage in repeated episodes of running away. Instead, once they left, they were usually gone for an extended period, with some never returning home.

The importance of family background cannot be overstated. Family instability and conflict are closely associated with running away from home in many studies (Price 1989; Stiffman 1989a, b; Comer 1988; Caputo et al. 1996). Many young people report experiencing physical, sexual and emotional abuse at home before going to the street. This, in turn, can have an impact on their subsequent involvement in delinquent or criminal activities while on the street. For example, McCormack and Wolbert-Burgess (1986) found that females with previous experiences of sexual abuse were significantly more likely to engage in delinquent activities than female runners who had not had these experiences. Similarly, early sexual abuse has been found to be related to increased victimization and a greater likelihood of involvement in prostitution (Whitbeck and Simons 1990; Seng 1989).

The second pattern described by Caputo et al. (1996) also involved young people who lived in conflictual home situations. In this case the conflict was based on the rebellion of the young person against parental/guardian authority. While arguing and fighting were reported by young people in this category, it did not involve the type of abuse reported by those in the previous category. Youthful rebellion is a common feature of adolescent life. For these young people, however, the rebellion reached an extreme and they chose to leave home. It should be noted that conflict over youthful rebellion is not restricted to individual families. Indeed, many Canadian studies of street youth have noted the preponderance of young people on the street who are running from group homes, young offender facilities or other forms of institutional care (Brannigan and Caputo 1993).

Young people in the rebellion category are in conflict with parents or guardians over rules, curfews and other decisions affecting their freedom. A common basis of the conflict experienced by these young people involved the attempt by parents/guardians to restrict their ability to "hang out" on the street and participate in street lifestyle activities. Curfews were identified as a major source of conflict and many of the respondents rebelled against such restrictions by running away.

The third group of youth identified by Caputo et al. (1996) found their way to the street after being forced to leave home prematurely. Some of the common experiences of these youth included being asked to leave home once they reached a certain age (e.g., 16 or 18). In other cases, the appearance of a new partner after a marriage breakdown led to the young person being asked to leave the home. These young people fit into the throwaway category described by McCullagh and Greco (1990). Their lack of resources leads them to the street where they learn that they have to participate in the street lifestyle in order to meet basic needs.

The final pattern identified by Caputo et al. (1996) consisted of those young people who ended up on the street inadvertently. Many in this category left small towns in search of jobs or excitement. A poor labour market coupled with a lack of experience or job skills forced many to the street. Once there, they had few options available to meet their needs. While not originally intending to be there, these young people engaged in street life activities in order to survive.

McCullagh and Greco (1990) also identified a curb-kid category consisting of young people who spent a considerable amount of time on the street while still living at home. These young people are often referred to as curbsiders. They have similar experiences to those in the conflict and rebellion patterns reported by Caputo et al. (1996). For some curbsiders, being on the street is a way of avoiding conflict at home. For others, spending significant amounts of time on the street is a reflection of their rebelliousness and the source of conflict with parents/guardians. In both cases, curbsiders learn about life on the street while still living at home. Making the transition to the street is much easier since they know what to expect. They know that they can "make it" on the street and they have contacts with peers who are already in the street scene. Curbsiders need support and assistance if they are to be prevented from moving to the street. They represent an important target group for policymakers attempting to deal with health issues related to homeless youth since they are not yet entrenched in the street lifestyle.

As these categorizations and patterns of going to the street show, street youth and their experiences are quite heterogeneous. One of the important implications of these findings is that youth who appear on the street come for different reasons and with different resources. Consider, for example, the difference between a young person fleeing an intolerable home situation characterized by long-term abuse and one leaving a small town seeking excitement or employment in a distant city. These individuals come to the street with very different backgrounds which may influence how each sees the possibilities available and the decisions they make. They may also bring very different personal repertoires—the sets of skills and abilities they use to deal with life's challenges (Caputo and Ryan 1991). Someone growing up in a conflictual/intolerant home situation may have quite a different repertoire than someone who left a supportive home voluntarily and often with parental blessings.

In addition to different paths to the street, Caputo et al. (1996) found considerable variation in the experiences of young people once they got to the street. Briefly, the respondents indicated that the first two or three weeks were a crucial decision-making period for newcomers to the street. Many reported an initial feeling of relief, at finding others in similar circumstances who shared common experiences and empathized with them. The initial foray into the street lifestyle was exciting and pleasurable, often encouraging these young people to become further involved. As this occurred, some newcomers became frightened or unsure about their participation in the risky or dangerous practices associated with life on the street. At this point, some decided that street life was not for them and they looked for alternatives. Some returned home while others found their way into programs or agencies available to this segment of the youth population. Others continued to participate getting increasingly entrenched in the street lifestyle. For these young people, leaving the street became less and less an option as their time on the street increased. Some never left the street and became part of the adult homeless population. Others stayed on the street for an extended period of time, ranging from one year to six or seven years or more. Data collected by Caputo et al. (1996) indicated that their departure from the street became possible only after they had "bottomed out" or experienced some type of crisis. For example, many noted that the death of a friend or the threat of arrest and imprisonment jarred them into taking stock of their lives. During these moments, leaving the street was more possible, especially if the appropriate help was available.

As can be expected, the experiences of youth on the street can vary dramatically. Some are able to engage at the margins of the street scene, dabbling in street life activities without becoming overly committed. This is largely restricted to the social aspects of the street lifestyle, including substance use, partying and engaging in high-risk sex. Youth in this group often engage in criminal activities to meet immediate needs. This can include selling sex to pay for drugs, food and a place to sleep. The length of time people are able to maintain this type of marginal connection to the street scene depends on the resources available to them and the absence of pressure from pimps or drug dealers to engage more systematically in organized criminal activities such as prostitution, breaking and entering or the drug trade.

The more entrenched the young person becomes, the more difficult it is to leave the street. The pull of the street includes such things as having a feeling of belonging, of being part of a group of friends. Many of the respondents in the Caputo et al. (1996) study reported that they had become part of a "family" on the street and had friends they could count on. The street was also described by these young people as a place where they could exercise some power and control over their lives. They could come and go as they pleased and do what they wanted. Many valued the freedom and independence the street provided. Another factor pulling people to the street was knowing what was expected of them and knowing they could make it on the street. Many reported not fitting in and feeling marginal before going to the street.

Experiences of young people in getting off the street reflected both the factors that had pushed them to the street in the first place and those that kept them there once they arrived. Some of the respondents in the Caputo et al. (1996) study saw few alternatives to the street available to them. Many either could not or would not return home. In some cases, there was no home to which they could return and going back to an institution or group home was not a viable alternative.

The services available to assist these young people to leave the street were another important factor influencing their decisions to leave. A noteworthy finding was that the young people wanted service providers to "hang in there" with them and be ready when they asked for help. Many mentioned how important nonjudgmental and accessible services were in this regard.

One of the more significant factors for the young people who made a successful transition off the street was "fitting in." This included having appropriate educational, employment, social and recreational opportunities. Leaving the street meant leaving a social support network behind. Service agencies were crucial in assisting these young people in rebuilding their support base.

RESPONDING TO HOMELESS YOUTH: "STORIES" FROM TWO CASE STUDIES

The findings discussed in the previous section outline some of the key patterns regarding the experience of running away and ending up on the street. The needs of the young people living on the street were also discussed. In this section, case studies of the way two Canadian communities responded to the needs of street youth are examined. Data gathered in the case studies are presented to highlight the perceptions held by the street/homeless youth of the services available to them.

The case studies were conducted in Saskatoon, Saskatchewan and Ottawa, Ontario during 1993-1994 (Caputo 1994a, b). Multifaceted and detailed methodological strategies were used in both sites, including in-depth interviews with runaways and street youth, surveys of average high school youth and in-depth interviews with youth-serving professionals from health, criminal justice, education and social service agencies. Community consultations were also held in both cities. These involved the participation of representatives of the youth-serving agencies that had been involved in the study as well as representatives of various segments of the youth population. During these case studies, in-depth interviews were conducted with over 150 runaways and street youth, and an equal number of youth-serving professionals.

This work represented Phase II of the Runaways and Street Youth Project sponsored by an interdepartmental working group of the federal government. Phase I of this project consisted of a literature review and research design exercise. Phase II was in-depth case studies of the initiatives taken in two communities in response to the challenges facing runaways and street youth. Information was gathered from both service providers and service recipients (i.e., street youth in these communities) regarding services being provided as well as services that were most needed. This led to a detailed assessment of the youth services system in both communities and recommendations for addressing current and future concerns.

A list of criteria was developed to assist in the identification of suitable research sites. For example, potential sites had to have a sufficiently large street youth population to make such a study viable. Other considerations included geographical location and the presence of Aboriginal street youth in at least one of the study sites. Eventually, Saskatoon and Ottawa were selected among a number of potential sites on the basis of these criteria. Discussions were held with key actors in both communities and, after some negotiation, both agreed to take part in the study.

In Saskatoon, considerable concern existed over the plight of inner-city neighbourhoods and the large numbers of Aboriginal youth who were on the street. A great deal of interagency activity was already under way at the time the Saskatoon case study got started. The research team tapped into this energy by calling a community meeting of key stakeholders to discuss their participation in the study. One of the potential benefits of the case study to the community was that it could contribute to a simultaneous, systemwide review of what was going on with respect to this high-risk population. Such a review was attractive to the key stakeholders since they were experiencing systemwide change as a result of several major initiatives by their provincial government. Better information about the operation of the overall youth services system would be helpful in light of the wholesale changes already under way or in the planning stage. Though some of these changes were directed at the health care system itself, the broader changes to the youth services system could have a considerable impact on nonmedical determinants of the health of this population.

In Ottawa, community concern focused on the issue of youth violence, including the role of street youth in this problem. As with Saskatoon, Ottawa has a long history of interagency cooperation. The research team once again worked with existing groups and called a community meeting to discuss their participation in the study. A needs assessment of homeless/street youth had been conducted in Ottawa the previous year. This had to be taken into account. In addition, a community-wide youth and violence initiative was being developed. Negotiations were started with the Youth and Violence Steering Committee to determine if its interests were compatible with those of the case study. This was discussed at a community meeting where an agreement to collaborate was reached. The research team agreed to collect specific data on youth and violence issues in exchange for access to the information required for the case study.

The "Needs" of Street/Homeless Youth

Some of the more pressing needs of street/homeless youth identified in the literature are discussed in this section. This information is derived from the Regional Municipality of Ottawa-Carleton (1992) needs assessment and builds on the findings of the Caputo et al. (1996) study already discussed. The key findings from the Saskatoon and Ottawa case studies are then assessed to determine how well each of these communities met the identified needs. While no formal evaluations were conducted in either community, both service providers and service consumers were interviewed regarding the availability and quality of services for street/homeless youth. The reliability of the findings from these interviews was tested at a community meeting. As noted in the findings of each case study, there was general consensus among both service providers and consumers at the community meeting, about the operation of the youth service system in each community.

A number of specific needs of street/homeless youth were outlined in the Regional Municipality of Ottawa Carleton (1992) study. The 64 street youth who participated were asked to identify the services needed most by street youth. Multiple responses were coded resulting in 101 answers to this question. The largest response category was shelter and permanent housing. This was mentioned by 37 respondents. A drop-in centre was identified by 23 of the respondents while 11 thought that emotional support and counselling was needed most. Food services for youth was noted by nine respondents and nine also reported a need for financial resources. Six of the respondents felt that outreach/advocacy was needed most while another six respondents didn't know what was needed.

These findings should be considered in light of what these young people identified as the most serious problems facing street youth. As noted earlier, 18 (28.1 percent) reported that drugs/alcohol abuse was the most important problem while 16 (25 percent) identified shelter/day and night. Safety/survival was mentioned by 10 (15.6 percent) of the respondents and money was identified by five (7.8 percent) of them. Finally, counselling was noted by four (6.3 percent) street youth. Other services were identified as most important by 12 (18.8 percent) respondents.

In the Caputo et al. (1996) study, 70 interviews were conducted with former street youth. The study explored a range of factors related to going to the street. These included self-image, family experience, school problems and involvement in delinquency. The findings indicated that 50 of the 70 (71 percent) former street youth had had a very negative self-image before going to the street. Some said they hated themselves while others said they had contemplated committing suicide. Many also reported a negative family experience. For 27 (39 percent) respondents, this consisted of conflict over family rules such as curfews, which resulted in arguments and fighting but no physical abuse. More serious family conflict was reported by 21 (31 percent) respondents. This included harmful verbal abuse, as well as physical and sexual abuse. Many of these young people described their family situations as intolerable.

The respondents were asked about their association with delinquent peers as well as their own contact with the police. The interview data revealed that 45 (64 percent) of the 70 respondents were involved with delinquent peers and 32 (46 percent) of the 69 had had personal contact with the police. The reasons for police involvement included 19 (59 percent) for property crimes, such as shoplifting or break and enter; seven (22 percent) were involved in assaults; and six (19 percent) for other reasons.

The former street youth were asked if anything could have prevented them from going to the street in the first place. In response, 44 (63 percent) of the 70 said that some support would have helped. This included having access to appropriate counselling services as well as personal support from a caring adult or peer. Specifically, 21 (48 percent) of the 44 stated that they would have benefitted from counselling for personal problems, substance abuse, anger management or life skills training. An additional 19 (43 percent) stated that family counselling may also have been helpful in preventing them from going to the street.

The respondents were asked about the factors that kept them on the street. Responses included 27 (39 percent) of the 70 who said freedom, 18 (26 percent) who mentioned friendships and 17 (24 percent) who were attracted to the money they could get on the street. These were the three largest response categories for this question. The remaining eight (11 percent) respondents gave other answers. The former street youth were then asked to identify the hardest thing about leaving the street. In response to this question, 43 (67.2 percent) of the 64 who responded, identified breaking with the way of life on the street while 12 (19 percent) mentioned taking control of one's life and nine (13 percent) stated that obtaining and accepting help was the hardest thing about leaving the street.

The findings reported here from the Regional Municipality of Ottawa-Carleton (1992) needs assessment and the Caputo et al. (1996) study identify the need for a number of important services for street/homeless youth. These include meeting basic needs for food, shelter, clothing and access to financial resources. A series of personal needs was also identified, including professional counselling for substance abuse and mental health concerns. Both studies also noted the need for social, employment/educational and recreational opportunities. The Caputo et al. (1996) study, in particular, emphasized the need for "fitting in." This was reflected in the important role street families play in attracting and keeping young people on the street. Meeting these needs satisfactorily is a considerable challenge for service providers.

In general, a similar range of services aimed at high-risk youth are found in most midsize Canadian communities. These usually include some element of prevention, crisis intervention, maintenance, transition and incapacitation services (Brannigan and Caputo 1993; Kufeldt and Burrows 1994). Some services deal with immediate problems while others address longer-term needs. For example, prevention programs are designed to identify youth at risk and help them deal with the circumstances that are pushing and/or pulling them to the streets. This may include identifying youth when they first "hit" the street and intervening quickly to get them off.

Crisis intervention normally consists of emergency care and includes an immediate response to medical, housing, food and clothing needs. Most crisis intervention services are short term and aimed at specific problems. These types of programs usually provide referral services. Maintenance services meet the day-to-day needs of clients for things like food and shelter while transition services are designed to get youth off the street. Incapacitation services protect society and the individual clients from any harm they might cause if they were not placed in a restricted setting.

In the following section, the Saskatoon and Ottawa case studies are examined to consider how these two Canadian communities have attempted to meet some of the needs discussed above. The section begins with a discussion of the interagency initiatives undertaken in each community to meet the needs of street/homeless youth. Next, the views of the service system held by street youth in each of the communities are presented. Finally, the successes and failures experienced by each community in meeting the needs of its street/homeless youth are discussed.

The Saskatoon Case Study

The case study undertaken in Saskatoon provides a detailed overview of the workings of the youth services system in that community, the experiences of street youth and the way the community responded to their needs. The most salient of these findings are outlined below. They are organized around issues related to youth needs and the system's response to these needs. Of particular interest is how the system itself, despite many well-intentioned actors, contributed to the problems facing homeless youth.

At the time the case study in Saskatoon began, a well-developed interagency initiative was in place. Like most Canadian communities of its size, Saskatoon provides a variety of services for youth ranging from prevention and crisis intervention to transition and incapacitation. The unique aspect of the interagency initiative in Saskatoon, however, is the existence of one particular agency, E'Gadz, which was created by the youth-serving community, specifically to meet the needs of its street/homeless youth.

This agency was designed as a central clearinghouse of services for the city's street youth population. Most youth services in the community participate in E'Gadz by having a representative on its board of directors. In addition, they are encouraged to offer programs and services in space provided on-site at E'Gadz. Thus, while the E'Gadz building serves as a drop-in and social and recreational centre for the community's street youth, many other services are also available on-site provided by the medical, educational or youth justice systems. For example, the educational system offers specialized courses at E'Gadz while a public health nurse provides medical services and the justice system operates a community-based corrections program in the centre.

In addition to E'Gadz, a number of services are extensively involved with the street/homeless youth population. These include outreach services provided by Mobile Crisis; the Community Health unit which operates a needle exchange program and clinics for sexually transmitted diseases; the MacNeill Clinic which provides mental health counselling; the Hands On drop-in centre; the YM/YWCA which offers a range of services and programs; the educational system which provides specialized schooling programs; and the social services system which has responsibility for general welfare as well as youth justice in the province.

As this short description demonstrates, Saskatoon has an extensive and well-developed set of services in place for street/homeless youth. The existence of E'Gadz reflects the considerable attention and resources the community has devoted to these young people. The results of the community case study revealed that the community has experienced both considerable success and some setbacks in responding to the needs of street/homeless youth. This is expanded on below, after an examination of how the street youth themselves viewed and assessed the services available to them.

The research in Saskatoon included in-depth interviews with 61 street youth from different congregation areas in the city. Of these, 30 were female and 31 were male. Their ages ranged from 12 to 20 years, with 16 being the median age of the sample. When asked why they had gone to the street, 25 percent gave family conflict as their first reason while 18 percent said they had been abused in some way. Parental substance abuse was mentioned by 12 percent as the reason for leaving home while 3 percent indicated they left because of their own substance abuse.

Street youth in Saskatoon were asked a series of questions about the services they were familiar with or had used. These young people were both knowledgeable and had used the youth services system extensively. For example, 76 percent said they had received some form of counselling, including 20 percent for substance abuse, 42 percent for personal adjustment and 15 percent for other reasons. Food services had been used by 55 percent of the respondents. However, when asked if they had used shelter services in the city during the last year, only two people said they had. This indicates that these young people were staying with relatives, friends or on the street.

While welfare or social assistance was used by 33 percent of the Saskatoon street youth, some youth said it was unavailable to them. The respondents were asked to identify other social services besides food and shelter that were needed. In response, 43 percent identified counselling, 15 percent said clothing, 13 percent said recreation and 6 percent answered education. (Multiple answers were coded for these questions so they may total more than 61.)

Next, the street youth were asked to assess the availability and quality of the services they used. This drew a mixed response. For example, only 5 percent thought social services were very available while 39 percent said they were somewhat available. The majority of respondents, (56 percent) reported that these services were not very available or not at all available. Responses about the quality of the social services, were more positive with

49 percent stating they were very good or good, and 16 percent rating them as fair. The remaining 35 percent rated them as poor or very poor.

Extensive use of health care services was reported by the street youth. Many had seen either their family doctor or a doctor in a clinic or emergency room during the last year. When asked what health care services were needed by street youth, 37 percent stated storefront health clinics, 33 percent identified birth control services and 37 percent said STD testing. Access to medical services without having to provide personal identification was mentioned by 57 percent of the respondents as needed. Drug rehabilitation, emergency care and free medical supplies were also identified as needs.

When asked about the accessibility of health care, responses varied. Health care services were seen as very or somewhat accessible by 55 percent of the respondents while 45 percent said they were not very or not at all accessible. However, 71 percent of the street youth rated the health care services they received as very good or good.

Respondents were asked to identify the educational needs of street youth. High school equivalency, upgrading or correspondence programs were mentioned by 9 percent of those interviewed. An additional 15 percent identified job/skills training while 20 percent mentioned flexible, individually tailored programs. Sex and drug educational programs were identified by 15 percent of the respondents while 9 percent said that educational programs oriented toward Aboriginal youth were needed.

Almost half the respondents indicated that they were in contact with the educational system. Their assessment of these programs was positive with 50 percent rating them as good or very good and 32 percent saying they were fair. The remaining 18 percent said they were poor or very poor. However, accessibility was poor with 74 percent of the street youth stating that these types of programs were not very or not at all available.

The Saskatoon data suggest that where services are appropriate and accessible, various needs of street/homeless youth can be met. This can occur despite an environment of funding cutbacks and scare resources. However, the research also indicates that targeting key, nonmedical determinants of health is insufficient if the delivery system is not socially and culturally relevant to the target population. For example, some agencies in Saskatoon put considerable effort into making their services sensitive to the needs of Aboriginal youth. Notably, the Joe Duquette School met a wide range of needs of Aboriginal youth in the community—including street youth—by providing a culturally sensitive environment and programming. This led to youth participation in a wide range of activities. Educational programs that can attract and keep high-risk youth involved have positive, long-term consequences for population health.

A wider range of educational opportunities aimed at high-risk youth were being developed in Saskatoon at the time of the case study. For example, some programs were experimenting with compressed course schedules. This would allow students to work on and complete one course at a time during a short but intensive period. Students are more likely to complete credits in such a system compared to the regular schedule because of their pattern of dropping out and then returning to school. This way, they could make some progress and build on past successes. This type of flexibility reduces frustration and increases the likelihood that these students will return to the school system and complete their education. It demonstrates how success can be achieved with young people living chaotic and unpredictable lives.

Despite the creativity and flexibility of the educational programs described above, the street youth interviewed indicated that more could be done. For example, almost 75 percent stated that access to education was limited even though half of the street youth interviewed were in contact with the educational system in one way or another. Additionally, 50 percent of respondents rated these services as very good or good. These results suggest that educational programs have to be tailored to this particular high-risk population.

Similar results were found for the medical and social services provided for the target population. Thus, while use of medical services was high and they received high ratings, more than half of those interviewed reported poor accessibility to needed medical services. Access was also a problem with social services such as welfare. Here, again, more than half of the sample said they were not available.

The assessment of E'Gadz highlights some of the paradoxical elements of the Saskatoon interagency initiative. E'Gadz provides a range of services in a safe, youth-friendly environment. The supportive staff and environment, the format of delivery and the ability of youth to walk in and gain access to services, underlie the success enjoyed by E'Gadz. Unlike many other agencies, E'Gadz has ongoing contact with youth. This gives them a level of credibility that makes it possible for them to work with this high-risk population. The results of the interviews with street/homeless youth indicated that they felt safe using the services provided at E'Gadz and saw them as being of high quality.

While E'Gadz enjoyed considerable success providing culturally and socially appropriate services to street/homeless youth, it was less successful in other ways. For example, the centre had been established as a place for all youth services in the community to deliver their programs to the target population. In a number of cases, this worked very well. For example, on-site medical services designed with street/homeless youth needs in mind were used extensively and were highly regarded by the street/homeless youth. On the other hand, some of the partners in E'Gadz offered services for street/homeless youth in their own locations. Some had even tested their programs at E'Gadz and once found to be successful, had moved the programs back to their home locations. These activities reflect the ongoing tensions over "turf" that are characteristic of most interagency initiatives. And while Saskatoon had gone a considerable distance in averting them through the creation of E'Gadz, some elements of the "turf" issue were still apparent.

Another challenge facing E'Gadz was its physical location: it did not reach large segments of the street youth population in Saskatoon from its location quite a distance from one of the major street youth congregation areas in the city. To respond to this problem, E'Gadz established an outreach program shortly after the case study was completed. Using a large van, E'Gadz workers visit various street youth congregation areas each night. They provide a range of services, including hot drinks, food and counselling. This put E'Gadz in direct competition with other service providers who were on the board of directors at E'Gadz. Moreover, while having a large building meant that E'Gadz could provide a wide range of services and programs, access to these programs was difficult for youth outside of the area. In this way, one of the strengths of E'Gadz was also one of its limitations.

An important success noted in Saskatoon's interagency effort was the willingness of formal youth-serving agencies to work with community representatives. This was visible in one initiative that got started while the case study was under way. In this instance, social service dollars were re-allocated for a much needed shelter for female youth. The need for such a shelter was emphasized during the case study and particularly at the community meeting. Community representatives were involved from the outset in the design and delivery of this service. This initiative signalled an opportunity for more cooperative relations between the community and the traditional social service system. It represented an attempt to make social services more open and accessible as well as more culturally relevant to those using the services. This was extremely important since even though many social services exist in the community, only 33 percent of the youth interviewed said they used these services and over half identified them as not at all available.

The Ottawa Case Study

As can be expected in a major urban centre, Ottawa has an extensive array of services available for street/homeless youth. The community has a long history of interagency activity directed at high-risk youth. Over the years, it has addressed numerous issues related to this group. At the time the Ottawa case study began, an interagency initiative aimed at the youth violence problem was receiving attention in the community.

Earlier interagency efforts in Ottawa had resulted in the establishment of the Youth Services Bureau (YSB) as a main service provider for high-risk youth. YSB operates drop-in centres across the region and offers a range of services, such as outreach, housing, various types of counselling, employment referrals and a needle exchange program. YSB also plays a pivotal role as an intermediary between street/homeless youth and mainstream services in the region.

In addition to YSB, a number of services formed part of a loosely connected interagency network. For example, the task force that conducted the needs assessment supported by the regional municipality's social services department, included the participation of some 30 community agencies. The youth and violence initiative attracted over 450 participants from over 35 agencies to a one-day conference at a downtown hotel. Many agencies went on to take part in various committees and activities developed at this conference.

Interviews with street youth regarding the operation of the youth services system in Ottawa revealed that while they were very knowledgeable about existing services, their use of these services varied. For example, 89 percent said they had used food services, while only 58 percent said they had used shelter services. Besides food and shelter, the respondents identified the need for other services including 62 percent who said recreation, 42 percent clothing, 23 percent financial aid and 12 percent who identified counselling.

Social services were rated as very available by 17 percent of the respondents while 44 percent said they were somewhat available, By contrast, 39 percent said they were not very available or not at all available. The quality of the social services was rated high by 71 percent of the respondents while 30 percent rated them as fair, poor or very poor.

The use of health care was high, although a varied response was given when street youth were asked what health care or medical services they thought were most needed. The responses revealed that 53 percent thought clinics were needed, 20 percent identified the need for needle exchange services and 9 percent saw a need for AIDS/STD testing. Perceptions of the accessibility of health care also varied. In this case, 50 percent of respondents said that health care services were very or somewhat accessible, while the other 50 percent said they were not very or not at all accessible. These services were rated as good and very good by 71 percent of the street youth.

The assessment of the educational system was also mixed. Participation was low with 58 percent of those interviewed indicating they had no contact with the educational system. This was reflected in their responses to questions about the availability of educational programs. In this case, 9 percent said these programs were very available and 39 percent said they were somewhat available. However, 58 percent said they were not very or not at all available. The street youth indicated that a number of educational programs were needed, including, 46 percent who identified high school upgrading, correspondence programs or a drop-in high school program. Job/skills training was identified by 17 percent while 21 percent wanted some other kind of education, including sex education, drug education or programs aimed at keeping/getting people off the street. The quality of the educational programs they were in contact with was rated as good or very good by 90 percent of those interviewed.

When asked to identify the most important problem facing street youth, 15 percent noted a lack of money, a further 15 percent said drug and alcohol addiction and 15 percent mentioned violence. When asked to identify what services street youth needed most, 50 percent of the respondents identified recreation centres, 42 percent mentioned clothing, 23 percent said financial aid and 15 percent indicated education programs were needed.

The research in Ottawa revealed that while the community had sought to provide culturally and socially relevant services to street youth, these programs had not been successful in reaching various segments of this population. In response, new and innovative programs and services were being developed in Ottawa as the case study began. The educational system had developed several programs for identifying youth at risk of dropping out of school—often a prelude to going to the street. As with any preventive program, it is often difficult to measure success. The program provided youth with recreational activities designed to improve self-esteem and coping skills. One of the encouraging signs was that a majority of the youth involved in the program stayed in touch with program staff long after completing the program. Many have been hired as mentors for the next generation of youth entering the program. Most have maintained school ties and are doing better within the system. These successes have reduced their exposure to the risks of life on the street and have helped to ensure a better future.

Despite the interagency approach, the Ottawa research indicated a need for more integrated and consistent services. Service providers reported difficulty organizing services to connect youth with the right workers. Also, once contact has been made, it is difficult for a worker to "stick" with a young person through the entire service delivery process because of the way services are organized. Instead, each agency provides a new worker which often results in inconsistency and the fragmentation of services. This is particularly problematic because schools, courts and other youth-serving agencies often rely on the existence of such a support network to achieve objectives. In the absence of the network, street youth are forced to rely on themselves. The difficulty of negotiating the system means that they frequently do not make it. The failure appears to be individual but it also reflects, at least in part, a failure of the service system.

Recognition of this shortcoming led many of the youth-serving professionals to consider an advocate system which would give each youth a contact person and a say in assessing whether agencies had been helpful. This would include having someone remind these young people about appointments, encourage them to attend school or other programs, and motivate them to accomplish their goals. Support workers could also act as advocates. The likelihood of accessing needed services is far greater for these young people when they are involved with an adult, in a supportive and consistent relationship. It would also address some of the problems with fragmentation.

There was considerable consensus that the service delivery system in Ottawa was becoming more rigid. Respondents indicated that stricter rules and regulations were appearing in more and more mainstream services. This was due, in part, to growing public concern over youth violence. It may also be indicative of a wider social concern over eligibility and access to publicly funded services. The increasing rigidity of the system makes it more difficult for street youth to connect with mainstream services. Their lifestyles and behaviour patterns often conflict with strict rules, including attendance and eligibility criteria for programs. Rules limit the access of these young people without dealing with the underlying problems.

The results of the Ottawa study suggest that while the job market is tight for all young people, street youth face particular difficulties. Their lack of marketable skills and their lifestyle restrict an already limited employment situation. This is especially important in the current period of economic restraint, in which minimum qualifications have increased for most jobs. Under these circumstances, education becomes even more vital for securing a job than it was in the past. The lack of education that is characteristic of most street youth is a considerable barrier to their obtaining employment.

The regular process of getting jobs does not work for street youth. Moreover, employment programs that do exist have been designed to prepare young people for traditional employment opportunities. They are not really geared to deal with the challenges confronting street youth who have few marketable skills and even fewer employment prospects.

Less traditional approaches to securing youth employment have been developed in Ottawa, based on the involvement of young people and the business community in partnership with community agencies. The Rideau Street Youth Initiative, one of these less traditional approaches, has helped street youth in Ottawa develop their own business. Funded in part through donations by local merchants, the program provides space, support, craft materials and equipment so the youth can make and sell crafts. It also provides a key contact point to other agencies.

Here again, the existence of a loose interagency network enhances the integration of services, and improves accessibility and the potential for success. In the case of the Rideau Street Youth Initiative, this includes bringing the local business community into the picture in a more integrated response to the employment needs of the target population.

As these examples indicate, much has been accomplished in Ottawa as a result of a loosely knit interagency network. The various agencies know each other and work well to integrate programs and avoid duplication. Agencies such as the Youth Services Bureau have proven quite effective in meeting many of the needs of the street/homeless youth population. However, as the case study findings indicate, availability and accessibility to services remain challenges. While multiagency educational and employment programs have been quite successful, there is still considerable fragmentation in the youth service system. Attempts to respond to this problem will have to address the same type of "turf" issues noted in the Saskatoon case study and present in most communities.

POLICY IMPLICATIONS: IMPROVING THE HEALTH STATUS OF STREET/HOMELESS YOUTH

The research on street/homeless youth presented above demonstrates that many nonmedical factors contribute to the challenges these young people face to their overall health and well-being. Before going to the street, these revolve around experiences at home and at school. The extent to which conflict in the family was a factor that led many young people to the street suggests that response strategies should target this area for intervention. This might include programs for young people and their parents that provide counselling, parenting skills and assistance with specific problems such as substance abuse. It might also include ensuring that young people have access to adults who are approachable and willing to listen and help them with their problems.

Other ideas are more traditional. They focus on enhancing parenting skills to address the need young people expressed for freedom and independence. In many cases, family conflicts occurred over curfews or rules about going out and participating in various social or recreational activities. Programs aimed at enhancing parenting skills may assist some parents in dealing more effectively with their children's demands for freedom and independence. At the same time, the availability of appropriate social and recreational opportunities for young people may lessen parental concern over their children engaging in less acceptable activities, thereby reducing family conflict.

The school represents another excellent site for intervention, since early signs of problems can be identified and an integrated approach developed. As well, educational programs provide an opportunity for reintegrating youth who have had difficulties. Many excellent alternative educational programs exist, some of which were described above. The positive evaluation given to educational programs by the street youth interviewed in the studies discussed here demonstrates that properly constructed programs delivered in an appropriate manner and setting can have a positive impact on these young people.

Building on the points made above, the literature provides a remarkably consistent picture that family conflict, school difficulties, substance abuse and conflict with the law are all factors that contribute to the decisions many young people make about going to the street. Each of these factors affords an opportunity for intervention. In most cases, the interventions should encompass more than one factor. A more holistic approach can be developed that moves beyond focusing on one particular problem to address the entire situation of a young person.

The different sectors in the youth services system should each have a way of picking up early indications that a young person may be at risk. This includes public health agencies, the school and the criminal justice system. Once identified, resources devoted to these individuals should be maximized to ensure that they receive the assistance they need at this stage and do not proceed to more risky or dangerous situations. Such an approach requires that the primary contact agencies work closely together.

Another important policy implication is the need for a variety of flexible services. The design and delivery of services for street youth must take into account the situational factors affecting them, their individual needs and changing funding conditions. Each of these is discussed briefly below. The main point here is that, to be useful, services must be tailored to the particular client group they serve. This may mean very different approaches in different communities, depending on the service needs of the street youth population. Certainly, a core of essential services is needed in most areas (food, shelter, clothing, counselling, life skills training, education and addiction treatment programs). The specific service mix, however, must reflect local realities such as the existence of a large populations of minority or Aboriginal youth on the street.

Situational Factors

For homeless youth, situational factors include the reality of street life and the limits it imposes on opportunities, service use and well-being. The research repeatedly emphasized accessibility. Services for street youth have to be provided in a user-friendly way, at times and locations that make them accessible to street youth and in ways that ensure they are socially and culturally relevant. When the environment is factored in, the need for outreach and storefront services becomes obvious. The potential for success is increased by going to street youth and by making programs accessible and responsive to their needs.

Individual Needs

Homeless youth are not a heterogeneous population. Their reasons for being on the street, their levels of entrenchment and their personal circumstances vary considerably. If, for example, the system responds only to entrenched street youth, there will be a continual flow of youth onto the streets and through the system. If it responds only in a preventive manner, then youth currently living on the street will face increased problems and greater difficulties getting off the street. Thus, responses must be available to different segments of the street youth population—from curbsiders to newcomers to entrenched street youth and to those trying to get off the street.

Further, youth vary in the kinds of personal problems they experience. A "one size fits all" approach to serving this population is inappropriate. For example, awareness of the long-term and far-reaching consequences of surviving severe abuse is critical for some young people and not relevant to others. Cultural factors are more important to some street youth and less so for others. Some have extensive repertoires they can draw on while others lack basic life skills. These kinds of individual difference must be taken into account if the services are to be relevant for the clients for whom they are intended.

Changing Funding Environments

Both case studies indicated that funding cutbacks were creating tensions within the system and limiting services provided to street youth. Paradoxically, the decline in funds has created some momentum toward developing a more streamlined and efficient service system. Interagency cooperation and nonduplication of services were prominent themes among service providers in both communities. While such interagency relations existed in the past, they have been given greater urgency during this period of financial shortages and disappearing services.

The accompanying returns of working together go beyond simply saving money. They provide the basis for a more comprehensive service response based on a better understanding of the complex problems associated with life on the street. For example, the tendency in the past had been for each agency to identify a particular issue or problem for attention. Young people with multiple problems had to deal with numerous agencies to receive assistance. In Saskatoon, E'Gadz was established as a type of service centre for street/homeless youth. In Ottawa, YSB is responsible for this population and acts as a referral source for other mainstream services. Many of the challenges being discussed here reflect both the successes and challenges encountered in implementing effective interagency initiatives.

The case studies indicated that street youth require continuity in the delivery of consistent, caring and long-term support. The existing system was often described as fragmented and lacking in continuity. In fact, many agencies have regulations that actually inhibit consistency in the provision of services. For example, some agencies limit the length of time a staff member can work with a particular client. The rationale is that the agencies want to avoid the development of a dependent relationship by their clients. Unfortunately, it takes time to develop a trusting relationship with clients such as street youth. They are suspicious of the system and reluctant to get involved with it. Making contact with someone in the system they can trust is an important first step. Having to deal with multiple workers who are constantly changing is frustrating. It discourages these young people from seeking the services they need. After a while, many simply give up trying.

A number of respondents mentioned that continuity can best be obtained through a more client-driven approach to care. A useful suggestion that emerged during the research was to have a single person act as an advocate or broker for the street youth. This person could work with the client, assess needs, discuss preferences and so on. The young person would be informed about the services available and helped in making decisions about which services to seek and in gaining access to these services. Such an approach would help in tailoring the service response to the specific needs of each client and ensure continuity in service delivery.

A final point here concerns the participation of service consumers in the design and delivery of services. A client-driven approach was described as having a built-in mechanism for ensuring that the types of services offered and the way they were presented matched the needs of the target population. Services that do not meet the needs of the target group would not be selected. This would send a strong message to service providers that they should reassess what they are doing and how they are doing it. This takes us back to the need to include the clients (i.e., the street youth) in the design and delivery of services. Interestingly, the young people participating in the study indicated the need for services that closely resembled what was currently available. The difference, however, was in how these services were packaged and delivered.

The Saskatoon and Ottawa case studies also indicated that involving local community groups is highly productive. For example, involving local businesses in providing employment opportunities and funds for developing youth-run enterprises helps to build bridges for these young people to future jobs. It also reduces the need for police intervention by minimizing the conflicts between youth and local businesses and others.

Local communities can also provide a range of resources that are helpful to the youth-serving community. For example, these can include access to recreational facilities, information, support to service agencies on culturally appropriate responses and a forum where street youth and local residents can come together to discuss mutual concerns.

The evidence reviewed above supports the notion that interagency, community-based approaches are required to meet the various needs of street/homeless youth. The complexity of the problems these young people have cannot be adequately dealt with by one or two agencies alone. Moreover, the problems are not restricted to the ailments or shortcomings of particular individuals but reflect broader social concerns. These implicate families, schools and communities as the sources and solutions to the problem. The nonmedical determinants of the health of street/homeless youth must clearly be addressed if we are to begin to meet the needs of this high-risk youth population.

Tullio Caputo *is an associate professor in sociology at Carleton University. He earned his doctorate in 1984 from Michigan State University. Since then he has taught at several Canadian universities including the University of Manitoba and the University of Calgary. His research areas include criminology, sociology of law, juvenile justice and youth at risk. He is currently working on a project examining the effectiveness of current responses to high-risk youth.*

BIBLIOGRAPHY

ADAMS, G. R., GULLOTTA, T. and CLANCY, M. A. 1985. Homeless adolescents: A descriptive study of similarities and differences between runaways and throwaways. *Adolescence* 20 (79): 715–724.

ANDERSON, J. 1993. *A Study of Out-of-the-Mainstream Youth in Halifax Nova Scotia.* Ottawa: Minister of Supply and Services.

APPATHURAI, C. 1988. *Runaway Behaviour: A Background Paper.* Toronto: Ministry of Community and Social Services.

BRANNIGAN, A., and CAPUTO, T. 1993. *Studying Runaways and Street Youth in Canada: Conceptual and Research Design Issues.* Ottawa: Minister of Supply and Services.

BRENNAN, T. 1980. Mapping the diversity among runaways: A descriptive multivariate analysis of selected social psychological background conditions. *Journal of Family Issues* 22(9): 189–209.

BURGESS, A. W. 1986. *Youth at Risk: Understanding Runaway and Exploited Youth.* Washington (DC): National Center for Missing and Exploited Children.

CAPUTO, T., and RYAN, C. 1991. *The Police Response to Youth at Risk.* Ottawa: Solicitor General.

CAPUTO, T, WEILER, R., and ANDERSON, J. 1996. *The Street Lifestyles Project: Final Report.* Ottawa: Health Canada (forthcoming).

CAPUTO, T., WEILER, R., and KELLY. K. 1994a. *Phase II of the Runaways and Street Youth Project: The Saskatoon Case Study.* Ottawa: Minister of Supply and Services.

_____. 1994b. *Phase II of the Runaways and Street Youth Project: The Ottawa Case Study.* Ottawa: Minister of Supply and Services.

*Children Today.*1989. The dynamics of homelessness. 18 (3): 2–3.

COMER, J. P. 1988. Kids on the run. *Parents* 63 (1): 146.

DENOFF, M. S. 1987. Irrational beliefs as predictors of adolescent drug abuse and running away. *Journal of Clinical Psychology* 43 (3): 412–423.

FEDERATION OF CANADIAN MUNICIPALITIES. 1994. *Youth Violence and Youth Gangs: Responding to Community Concerns.* Ottawa: The Federation of Canadian Municipalities.

FINKELHOR, D., HOTALING, D., and SEDLAK, S. 1990. *Missing, Abducted, Runaway and Thrownaway Children in America. First Report: Numbers and Characteristics.* Washington (DC): Office of Juvenile Justice and Delinquency Prevention.

FISHER, J. 1992. Personal correspondence. Ottawa: Ministry of the Solicitor General of Canada.

FUCHS, V., and REKLIS, D. 1992. America's children: Economic perspectives and policy options. *Science* 255 (3): 41–46.

HIER, S. J., KORBOOT, P. J., and SCHWEITZER, R. D. 1990. Social adjustment and symptomatology in two types of homeless adolescents: Runaways and throwaways. *Adolescence* 25 (100): 761–771.

HILL, H., and PIPER, D. 1995. "Us Planning For Them": The social construction of community prevention for youth. *International Quarterly of Community Health Education* 15 (1): 65–89.

JAMA. 1989. Health care needs of homeless and runaway youths. *Journal of the American Medical Association* 262 (10): 1358–1361.

JANUS, M.-D., McCORMACK, A., WOLBERT-BURGESS, A., and HARTMAN, C. 1987a. *Adolescent Runaways.* Lexington (DC): Heath.

JANUS, M.-D., WOLBERT-BURGESS, A., and McCORMACK, A. 1987b. Histories of sexual abuse in adolescent male runaways. *Adolescence* 22 (86): 405–417.

JANUS, M.-D., WOLBERT-BURGESS, A., and McCORMACK, A. 1986. Runaway youths and sexual victimization: Gender differences in an adolescent runaway population. *Child Abuse and Neglect* 10 (3): 387–395.

KALISKI, E., RUBINSON, L., LAWRANCE, L., and LEVY, S. 1990. AIDS, runaways and self-sufficiency. *Family and Community Health* 13 (1).

KASKUTAS, L., MORGAN, P., and VAETH, P. 1992. Structural impediments in the development of a community-based drug prevention program for youth: Preliminary analysis from qualitative formative evaluation study. *International Quarterly of Community Health Education* 12 (3): 169–182.

KUFELDT, K. 1987. Youth on the street: Abuse and neglect in the eighties. *Child Abuse and Neglect* 11 (4): 531–543.

KUFELDT, K. 1991. Social policy and runaways. *Journal of Health and Social Policy* 2 (4): 37–49.

KUFELDT, K. and BURROWS, B. A.1994. *Issues Affecting Public Policies and Services for Homeless Youth.* Ottawa: Human Resources Development Canada.

KUFELDT, K., and NIMMO, M. 1987. Kids on the street they have something to say: Survey of runaway and homeless youth. *Journal of Child Care* 3 (2): 53–61.

KUFELDT, K. and PERRY, P. 1989. Running around with runaways. *Community Alternatives* 1 (1): 85–97.

KUFELDT, K., McDONALD, M., DURIEUX, M., and NIMMO, M. 1988. Providing shelter for street youth: Are we reaching those in need? Paper presented at the Seventh International Congress on Child Abuse and Neglect, Rio de Janeiro, September 25–28, 1988.

LUNA, C. C. 1987. Welcome to my nightmare: The graffiti of homeless youth. *Society* 24, 6 (170): 73–78.

———. 1989. Youth: Adaptation and survival in the AIDS decade. Paper presented at the Annual International Conference on Acquired Immunodeficiency Syndrome, Montreal, Canada, June 4–6, 1989.

McCARTHY, W. D. 1990. Life on the street: Serious theft, drug selling and prostitution among homeless youth. *Dissertation Abstracts International* 51 (4): 1397 A.

McCARTHY, W. D., and HAGAN, J. 1991. Mean streets: The theoretical significance of desperation and delinquency among homeless youth. *American Journal of Sociology.*

McCORMACK, A., and WOLBERT-BURGESS, A. 1986. Influence of family structure and financial stability on physical and sexual abuse of a runaway population. *International Journal of Sociology of the Family* 16 (2): 251–262.

McCULLAGH, J., and GRECO, M. (1990). *Servicing Street Youth: A Feasibility Study.* Toronto: Children's Aid Society.

McDONALD, L. P., and PERESSINI, T. L. 1992. *The East Village Community Study: Final Report.* Calgary: The City of Calgary Task Force on Housing in the Downtown.

MICHAUD, M. 1988. *Dead End: Homeless Teenagers, A Multi-Service Approach.* Calgary: Detselig.

MOLNAR, J. M., RATH, W. R., and KLEIN, T. P. 1990. Constantly compromised: The impact of homelessness on children. *Journal of Social Issues* 6 (4): 109–124.

NYE, F. I., and EDELBROCK, C. 1980. Some social characteristics of runaways. *Journal of Family Issues* 1 (2): 147–150.

POWERS, J. L., ECKENRODE, J., and JAKLITSCH, B. 1990. Maltreatment among runaway and homeless youth. *Child Abuse and Neglect* 14 (1): 87–98.

PRICE, V. A. 1989. Characteristics and needs of Boston street youth: One agency's response. *Children and Youth Services Review* 11 (1): 75–90.

RADFORD, J. L., J. C. K. ALAN and WARREN, W. K. 1989. *Street Youth and AIDS.* Ottawa: Health and Welfare Canada.

REGIONAL MUNICIPALITY OF OTTAWA-CARLETON. 1992. *Support Services to Homeless/Street Youth in Ottawa-Carleton: A Needs Assessment and Plan for Action.* Ottawa: Regional Municipality of Ottawa-Carleton.

ROTHERAM-BORUS, M. J. 1991. Serving runaway and homeless youth. *Family and Community Health* 14 (3): 23–32.

ROTHERAM-BORUS, M. J., and KOOPMAN, C. 1991a. Reducing HIV sexual risk behaviors among runaway adolescents. *JAMA, Journal of the American Medical Association* 266 (9): 1237–1241.

———. 1991b. Sexual risk behaviours, AIDS knowledge, and beliefs about AIDS among runaways. *American Journal of Public Health* 81 (2): 208–210.

ROSSI, P. 1989. *Down and Out in America: The Origins of Homelessness.* Chicago: University of Chicago Press.

SENG, M. J. 1989. Child sexual abuse and adolescent prostitution: A comparative analysis. *Adolescence* 24 (95): 665–675.

SHANE, P. G. 1989. Changing patterns among homeless and runaway youth. *American Journal of Orthopsychiatry* 59 (2): 208–214.

SMART, R. G., ADLAF, E. M., and PORTERFIELD, K. M. 1990. *Drugs, Youth and the Street.* Toronto: Addiction Research Foundation.

SOCIAL PLANNING COUNCIL OF WINNIPEG. 1990. *Needs Assessment on Homeless Children and Youth.* Winnipeg: Social Planning Council.

Society. 1988. Profile of a runaway child. 25 (3): 4.

SPECK, N. B., GINTHER, D. W., and HELTON, J.-R. 1988. Runaways: Who will run away again? *Adolescence* 23 (92): 881–888.

STIFFMAN, A. R. 1989a. Suicide attempts in runaway youth. *Suicide and Life Threatening Behaviour* 19 (2): 147–159.

_____. 1989b. Physical and sexual abuse in runaway youths. *Child Abuse and Neglect* 13 (3): 417–426.

WARD, J. 1989. *Organizing for the Homeless.* Ottawa: Canadian Council on Social Development.

WEBBER, M. 1991. *Street Kids: The Tragedy of Canada's Runaways.* Toronto: University of Toronto Press.

WHITBECK, L. B., and SIMONS, R. L. 1990. Life on the streets: The victimization of runaway and homeless adolescents. *Youth and Society* 22 (1): 10–125.

WINDLE, M. 1989. Substance use and abuse among adolescent runaways: A four-year follow up study. *Journal of Youth and Adolescence* 18 (4): 331–344.

WOODRUFF, J. D., et al. 1989. *Troubled Adolescents and HIV Infection.* Washington (DC): Child Development Center.

YATES, G.L., MACKENZIE, R., and PENRIDGE, J. 1988. A risk profile comparison of runaway and non-runaway youth. *American Journal of Public Health* 28 (37): 820–821.

Series
Canada Health Action: Building on the Legacy
Papers Commissioned by the National Forum on Health

Volume 1

Determinants of Health

Children and Youth

Series

Canada Health Action: Building on the Legacy
Papers Commissioned by the National Forum on Health

Volume 2

Determinants of Health

Adults and Seniors

William R. Avison
The Health Consequences of Unemployment

Mary J. Breen
Promoting Literacy, Improving Health

Neena L. Chappell
Maintaining and Enhancing Independence and Well-Being in Old Age

Sandra O'Brien Cousins
Promoting Active Living and Healthy Eating among Older Canadians

Victor W. Marshall and Philippa J. Clarke
Facilitating the Transition from Employment to Retirement

Dr. Robyn Tamblyn and Dr. Robert Perreault
Encouraging the Wise Use of Prescription Medication by Older Adults

Daphne Nahmiash
*Preventing, Reducing and Stopping the Abuse and Neglect of Older Canadian
Adults in Canadian Communities*

Series
Canada Health Action: Building on the Legacy
Papers Commissioned by the National Forum on Health

Volume 3
Determinants of Health
Settings and Issues

Series
Canada Health Action: Building on the Legacy
Papers Commissioned by the National Forum on Health

Volume 4
Striking a Balance
Health Care Systems in Canada and Elsewhere

Series
Canada Health Action: Building on the Legacy
Papers Commissioned by the National Forum on Health

Volume 5
Making Decisions

Evidence and Information

Joan E. Tranmer, S. Squires, K. Brazil, J. Gerlach, J. Johnson, D. Muisner,
B. Swan, Dr. R. Wilson
Using Evidence-Based Decision Making: What Works, What Doesn't

Paul Fisher, Marcus J. Hollander, Thomas MacKenzie, Peter Kleinstiver,
Irina Sladecek, Gail Peterson
Decision Support Tools in Health Care

Charlyn Black
Building a National Health Information Network

Robert Butcher
Foundations for Evidence-Based Decision Making

Carol Kushner and Michael Rachlis
Consumer Involvement in Health Policy Development

Frank L. Graves and Patrick Beauchamp (EKOS Research Associates Inc.),
and David Herle (Earnscliffe Research and Communications)
Research on Canadian Values in Relation to Health and the Health Care System

Thérèse Leroux, Sonia Le Bris, Bartha Maria Knoppers, with
the collaboration of Louis-Nicolas Fortin and Julie Montreuil
*The Feasibility of a National Canadian Advisory Committee on Ethics:
Points to Consider*

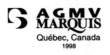

AGMV
MARQUIS
Québec, Canada
1998